HEALTH PLANNING

A Systematic Approach

SECOND EDITION

Herbert Harvey Hyman, Ph.D.

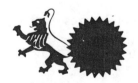

AN ASPEN PUBLICATION®
Aspen Systems Corporation
Rockville, Maryland
London
1982

Library of Congress Cataloging in Publication Data

Hyman, Herbert Harvey
Health planning.

Includes bibliographies and index.
1. Health planning.
2. Health planning— United States.
I. Title.
RA393.H95   1981   362.1'0937   81-12780
ISBN: 0-89443-379-2   AACR2

Library of Congress Catalog Card Number: 81-12780
ISBN: 0-89443-379-2

Printed in the United States of America

1 2 3 4 5

Table of Contents

Preface

I had just finished writing the 14th chapter to this second edition when I reread the "preface" to my first. That review clearly reminded me how basic concepts remain constant while the rhetoric and catch phrases of planning change substantially. An untutored reader of health planning may believe that a new planning system had been developed under the 1974 National Health Planning and Resources Development Act (PL 93-641) that had little to do with its predecessor, the Comprehensive Health Planning and Public Health Services amendments of 1966. In that first edition I wrote: "The name of the health planning agency may change, but the processes, principles and concepts involved in that planning will remain the same." And indeed that statement's truth has been borne out in my revision of this text on health planning.

A great deal has happened since the first edition was written. In fact, so much has been written in the last five years that what I initially conceived to be a tinkering with words, phrases, and an updating of statistics has resulted in the addition of over 60 percent of new material for this revision. This new material represents clarification, greater detail, and new experiences, but almost no changes in the basic concepts of health planning as originally written in the first edition.

There are many references to the National Health Planning and Resources Development Act of 1974 and its amendments in this second edition, as there should be. However, these serve mainly as illustrations of points I am trying to make. "Health planning agency" has been used throughout this edition as a generic term that applies to whatever name federal legislation or the latest buzz phrase happens to be in vogue at the time to refer to the agencies. The reader should not be deceived into thinking that the contents of this revision are dated because of their references to the 1974 health planning act. They are as valid for that act as they would be for any future legislation related to health planning.

However, the reader should also know that several important advances have taken place since the first edition. First, unlike my search for relevant literature for the first edition, I have been overwhelmed with the outpouring of materials that have been written about planning since 1975. I am fortunate to have been associated with the Bureau of Health Planning from its inception and thus made aware of the large number of contracts that were awarded to consultants, universities, and individuals to search out and update the latest knowledge and findings. Because most of the material has never found its way into print as books or scholarly journal articles, one of the benefits for the readers of this edition is to put them in touch with many of the appropriate governmental documents that only a few persons are privy to. This new body of knowledge will certainly aid students to become more sophisticated planners and to help them cope with this complex new field.

Also, a new major advance has taken place in health planning. Under the 1966 amendments, the main advance was the public's acceptance of planning as a field of endeavor. Most of the issues were centered on health planning agencies' attaining political acceptance by physicians, hospitals, other health specialties, consumers, and government. With the completion of this process, PL 93-641 was able to shift its attention to the technical process of developing health plans. That process revealed the complexities of integrating the value differences of the planning participants with the technical requirements used to identify and set goals and priorities, resources needed, and strategies for carrying them out. As a result of this process, over 200 comprehensive health plans were developed. This is indeed a major accomplishment.

In addition, the Bureau of Health Planning was given the large role of guiding, prodding, and stimulating the health planning agencies to do what the *planning law* and its regulations required of them. This was no easy task, given the antagonism that naturally exists and is directed by lower levels of government and health providers at what is perceived to be federal intrusion into their affairs. In spite of the hostility directed at perceived government interference, the Bureau did manage to provide the guidance that was so lacking under the 1966 act. Without it, it is unlikely that the health plans would have been completed in a timely manner, or that state and local planning agencies would have taken PL 93-641 as seriously as they did.

The next major step that still needs to be taken is the implementation of the goals and priorities of these health plans. Just as a major change had taken place as that first edition was being completed (e.g., the enactment of PL 93-641), so history is repeating itself with this second edition. Health systems agencies are being phased out. The new emphasis is on competition and deregulation of health facilities and services, which I examine in some detail in Chapter 14. Many conclude from this that concern for implementing the goals of the current health plans is dead.

However, I believe that they are too quick to draw this conclusion. Competition may have the positive impact of putting the brakes on cost escalation and forcing consumers to be more responsible in their use of health services. Yet, health planning will still be necessary to ensure that gaps in service are met, that little used essential services are regionalized, that inappropriately used services are eliminated, and that the location and adequacy of medical services are made available to those needing them. With our scarce resources, we cannot afford economic white elephants in the form of large amounts of unused hospital space, duplication of high cost medical technology, or the oversupply of high cost medical personnel. Planning will still be necessary to determine the proper balance between supply and need, and it will likely be under state control. The art, skills, and techniques of planning as well as the initial plans that were produced under PL 93-641 will provide the states with all the guidance they need to plan successfully for their own needs. In this planning endeavor, implementation will be the main focus.

The format of this second edition has remained essentially the same as the original text with some changes. The original chapter on implementation has been divided in two. Chapter 7 develops the concepts of regulatory or reactive implementation, and Chapter 8 details the more creative, proactive implementation process. Discussion of national health insurance has been eliminated from this text because it appears that the issue is dead and unlikely to be given serious attention for a number of years. However, in Chapter 14, I point out how the emphasis of the Reagan administration on competition and health deregulation represents an alternative form of national health insurance. This chapter thus serves both as a substitute for the chapter on national health insurance and as a prediction of what is likely to occur under the new administration.

By looking into the past, we have seen the future. It is up to us to grasp that future and make it work for the welfare and well-being of all our citizens. Deeds and acts of humanity are important, not the rhetoric and latest "buzz" words and strategies that may be in vogue. By whatever name it will be called, health planning is here to stay, and its future is as important as its beginnings have been significant and creative.

Herbert Harvey Hyman
Hunter College
New York City
September 1981

Acknowledgments

This book is dedicated to a very special person—Jerry Stolov. Few have heard of him or know of his existence. As a federal servant in the Bureau of Health Planning, he, like most of the Bureau's unsung heros, toils in the obscurity of one of its branches. The name of the branch is unimportant, but what is important is that Jerry does not let the tight limits imposed by his office hem him in. Jerry is one of those rare civil servants who truly believes that information is power and should be shared with others. His natural good humor masks his serious concerns about the health and well-being of the citizens of our nation. These concerns have been reenforced by his own family's battles with the medical establishment, many of which have been fraught with anxiety and outright hostility by the medical profession.

Through his personal efforts, I and all my readers have been truly enriched with the knowledge and information that only a rare few are aware exist in federal offices. Jerry has had the uncanny extrasensory perception of sending me reports that were relevant to the chapter I happened to be writing at the time. I never directed him to send me anything. He did this as a public and voluntary service that I or few others could personally afford had we been required to pay for them. I can truly assert that this book could not have been revised had Jerry not taken the time and interest to search out and send me reports as they became available. There is no better way I can acknowledge my true debt than by dedicating this revised edition to him.

I am also indebted to Rona Affoumado, a graduate student in my Department of Urban Affairs, who is specializing in health planning. Rona undertook the arduous and thankless but essential task of reading and analyzing a series of health plans and work programs to identify trends related to staffing, goals, functions, and financing of health planning agencies in Region II. The seeds of her excellent research efforts are sprinkled through various chapters of this book. Likewise, I want to thank Guy Alba, Director of Region II's health resources and planning division, and Frank DiGiovanni, his deputy, for the kind assistance they lent Rona and me in making themselves and their files available.

Finally, Dr. Colin C. Rorrie, Jr., Director of the Bureau of Health Planning, and his staff were kind enough to take time off from their busy schedules to discuss their activities and make reports available, as well as to help me anticipate ongoing studies and their likely dates of completion. Without this cooperation, many important details of health planning experiences would have been lost.

To all these fine governmental civil servants, both named and unnamed, I want to acknowledge my debt to you. Of course, I shoulder the responsibility for any final words that have been written in this text. I am sure that in spite of my efforts to record faithfully what I have been told and have read, I, like other authors, may have unintentionally altered their meaning to blend in with my own thought processes. Where this has unconsciously occurred, I can only offer my sincerest apologies.

In closing, I want to thank my ever-loving wife, Marilyn, and my two wonderful children, Susan and Mark, who as usual have had to do without my guidance on so many occasions.

Chapter 1

History

The elevated status that health care enjoys today—both as a major industry and as a public institution—is a phenomenon of the twentieth century and a product of technology and specialization.

During its formative years, health care was viewed as a responsibility to be assumed by individuals or by private organizations. It was not until the first decades of this century—when technological advances, special interest groups, and a growing economy signaled the beginnings of institutionalized health care programs—that health care was left to either fend for itself or become a "ward" of certain philanthropic individuals. To date, a socialized health package available to all remains a hotly debated issue in the United States, one that presupposes many questions: Are society and government mutually responsible for a country's health needs? Should individuals be left to care for themselves? This conflict involves local versus central governmental control, as well as the willingness (or lack thereof) of Americans to assume responsibility for other people. Rosen resolves this problem aptly:

> Today, the principle of state intervention and control in health matters is admitted; the only difference is in the greater or lesser efficiency of the intervention and in the greater or lesser frankness with which the role of the State is admitted.[1]

Initially, health care was viewed as necessary and of short duration. In limited form, preventive medicine, family planning, and urban health study were practiced.

During the first half of the nineteenth century, health service remained almost exclusively within the hands of private practice.

SIGNIFICANT HEALTH ISSUES: 1789–1920

The first major medical need to which the federal government responded resulted from a scourge of epidemics in the United States. The outbreak of yellow fever in Philadelphia, the first such epidemic, resulted in numerous deaths and caused major panic. Yet, the remedy, quarantine, remained under local control despite recurrences of various epidemics at 20-year intervals throughout the century. With the epidemic of 1873 (ironically, the last one) Congress instituted the national port quarantine system,[2] regulated and enforced by the Marine Hospital Service,[3] whose quarantine program was largely effective, and society quickly realized the benefits to be gained by a uniform administrative policy. Thus, out of group need, the precedent of central government intervention was established.

Health insurance to seamen, conversely, was ministered by the government from its inception in 1798. Insurance for seamen was not a new concept. Both Germany and England had established similar programs, the English program dating from 1696. Even before the 1798 congressional act, concern had been shown for the health needs of seamen in the United States. In Virginia, for example, a law, passed in 1787, called for the construction of a marine hospital at Norfolk; similarly, in neighboring North Carolina, a hospital fund was created by law in 1798, the money for which came from collections (prorated by rank) from seamen.

The government's concern, as evidenced by the congressional act of 1798 to care for the health needs of its naval defenders, is often cited as a precursor to the kind of social legislation that became the hue and cry of the labor union movement in the 1800s. It certainly kindled the debate that still rages over national health care. However, it is more likely that it was instituted not solely for humanitarian purposes, but for the practical consideration that the navy was essential to the defense of a nation that had been until only recently part of England. In addition, the cost of this piece of so-called social legislation was to be borne by the sailors themselves; it was not until later that the government was to subsidize it by levying a tax on the general population. At least one observer takes this liberalized view to task:

> As a fact accomplished, this Act of 1798 was in the nature of insurance, and it was compulsory. But in the light of the problems, thoughts, and attitudes then current, it would appear questionable to attribute to the Fifth Congress . . . an intent to institute a medical insurance scheme as such schemes are today regarded.[4]

The second major health issue resulted in the first major movement, the "sanitary reform movement." The principal issue of this movement was to clean up the filth and squalor found chiefly in cities; it was premised on the commonly accepted notion of the time that disease, illness, and death resulted from dirt. According to the specific contagion theory of epidemics, it followed, therefore, that these health blights resulted from dirt in the environment; in short, the best method to eliminate the "blight" was to remove the dirt. The movement took its impetus largely from the reports of John C. Griscom and Lemuel Shattuck, who, in their descriptive accounts of the health conditions found in their respective cities,[5] concluded that illness, premature death, and poverty were directly related. Essentially, the social temper was receptive to Griscom and Shattuck, as evidenced by the strong support for sanitary reforms. Fear of communicable diseases similarly inspired such reforms.

While people such as Griscom[6] were arguing from a totally humanitarian perspective—decrying the abuses of slumlandlords, for instance, who divided buildings into smaller apartments "in order to admit a greater number of families"—the general philosophy prevailed that the poor were somehow morally inferior. They were entitled to some basic medical care, but not in the same proportion as those who had been able to provide for their own.[7] According to Odin Anderson, the degree of charitableness toward the poor was determined by a "means" test, which was designed, states Anderson, to be "an unpleasant experience," a test designed to "discourage the seeking of relief until circumstances were very dire indeed."[8]

The reports made by Griscom and Shattuck were radical for their day. Shattuck,[9] for example, applied his study on a statistical basis, making comparisons of sanitary conditions of people relative to age, sex, race, and income levels. His interest in statistics led to his founding in 1839 of the American Statistical Society and, three years later, the passage of a law in Massachusetts that initiated a statewide program for registering vital statistics. In addition, he advocated the establishment of a state health board, charged with monitoring and regulating the health conditions within the state; a uniform nomenclature for causes of disease and death based on personal data, environmental sanitation, control of food and drugs; and vaccination against such communicable diseases as smallpox. He even discussed smoking and alcohol control, urban planning, and preventive medicine. Only the institution, in 1869, of a statewide board of health for Massachusetts (the first in the nation) became a reality. Shattuck's attempts to have some of the health board's recommendations enacted into law proved fruitless.

Although the sanitary reform movement is significant in the field of health, its prime cause was not medical improvement.

The call for sanitary reform was not based on any special medical knowledge nor aimed at any particular diseases. The data employed were social and statistical, and engineers and statisticians played a larger role than did those with medical training.[10]

The sanitary reform movement lasted until approximately 1910, when a new era in social policy and health legislation began a trend toward a more scientific approach to health. The sanitary reform movement did, however, serve to instill interest in such diseases as tuberculosis, scarlet fever, and diphtheria, as well as in infant mortality and childhood diseases. This concern helped promote the institution of preventive health measures against diseases, a concern translated into state and local boards of health. These boards would remain long after sanitary reform had become a forgotten issue.

By the 1900s the attack on overcrowded conditions (and therefore liability to disease) of the poor gained greater strength and momentum.

Disease is largely a removable evil . . . it continues to afflict humanity, not only because of incomplete knowledge of its causes and lack of individual and public hygiene, but also because it is extensively fostered by harsh economic and industrial conditions and by wretched housing in congested communities.[11]

Indeed, the cry of the time, from Europe to America, protested the social abuses wrought on those who lacked political redress. Labor laws passed from 1915 to 1920 (providing compensation for workers killed or injured on the job and protection of women and children employed in the labor market) spawned the seed of social unrest that goaded labor groups to demand a federal health insurance program. This unrest among labor was heightened by the waves of unemployment, marking the turn of the century and following World War I. The war itself played a major part in this uneasy mood in that people returned from it "shell-shocked." The great publicity given to the "war to end all wars" stressed the need on the part of government to compensate those refugees from America who had gone to Europe and fought to maintain democracy for everyone at home. The government did respond. The Public Health Service developed rapidly after 1912, and the idea that public health was a national issue assumed legitimacy. According to Rosen,[12] this trend evolved as a "natural extension of the previous view where the local community provided for such needs."

As a direct result of the sanitary reform movement, community clinics began to develop. But to bring more generalized health care to the people, it soon became apparent that some central agent of control and management was necessary. This need was met by the city and state boards of health, which expanded their role and jurisdiction into the domain of health service.

The dispensary—often an adjunct to a general hospital, existing primarily to meet the health needs of the indigent—became the model for the clinic movement. In 1900, there were only 100 reported dispensaries in the United States; by 1914, however, this number had mushroomed to around 800. Half of these specialized in tuberculosis, venereal disease, and baby and child hygiene; the others were considered "general" dispensaries. The movement toward dispensaries was adopted by industry, as a means of providing free or very low cost care for its employees. Davis and Warner offer their definition of the dispensary as "an institution which organizes the professional equipment and special skill of physicians for the diagnosis, treatment, and prevention of disease among ambulatory patients."[13] For the large public it served, the dispensary offered tests to identify communicable diseases, gave shots for their prevention, and passed out ready-made homilies of health care to be used at home for the unsophisticated patient who was generally exceedingly grateful for advice. The increased importance of dispensaries marked the advent of preventive medicine.

Although the dispensary was essentially seen as a link between the physician and the hospital, its influx into the field of medicine was short-lived. In part, the dispensary acquired a pejorative connotation within the American conceptualization of medicine; it was perceived as a "medical soup-kitchen." According to Anderson, "The dispensary concept developed only to the extent that it served to provide care at a minimum level for the poor."[14]

A major blame for the concept's failure lies in the method by which it was financed. Dispensaries subsisted on charitable donations to the hospitals with which they were affiliated or to the dispensaries themselves. Similarly, physicians often donated their services or charged minimal fees. Thus, the system existed solely to the degree to which the tenuous balance between social concerns for the poor and the economic means by which others could be charitable was maintained. Also, patient and medical professionals alike indicated dissatisfaction with this mode of operation.

Proponents of a national health insurance program felt confident, owing to the speedy enactment of workmen's compensation laws, that a similar plan could be gained for health insurance. However, they were overly optimistic. Support was not based broadly enough and, most important, much of labor, the traditional ally of liberal thinkers, did not favor national health insurance. Such a measure was seen as a "national insurance fund for the mitigation of the evil of unemployment."[15] Further, *if* such programs were to be instituted, it was believed best that they originate at the state level.

The American Association for Labor Legislation (AALL), organized in 1906 as an outgrowth of an International Association of Labor Legislation meeting in Paris in 1900, led the drive for nationalized health care; at that time, AALL members numbered a mere 165. In seven years its constituency rose to over 3,300 people interested in social reform. Essentially, this intellectual, middle-class group believed that each person is entitled to maintain self-respect by being economically self-reliant. Their definition of self-reliance, of course, hinged on the corollary that this existed only to the degree to which people were able to work when they wanted and were provided the essential needs of life (which happened to include adequate health care). From the perspective of modern theory, their philosophy was not altogether radical. Then, it was. In December, 1913, in Washington, D.C., the group introduced its proposed government-sponsored health insurance program. The plan called for disability and health insurance, emphasized preventive medicine as an adjunct to the program, stressed the program as voluntary, and established funding on a tripartite basis among employer, employee, and the public.

The plan failed. It had been met with severe opposition from organized groups, including the American Medical Association. Part of the widespread opposition to AALL's insurance package was that its realization would result in radical change: the institution of new programs. While workmen's compensation stipulated an outlay of cash funds for certain illnesses and disabilities, a national health insurance bill would require the organization and coordination of medical personnel, hospitals, drugs, and extraneous services. It represented a much greater threat to the status quo than workmen's compensation had.

The rise in number of public, private, and custodial hospitals can be traced to the same period of social development in health care as the growth in dispensaries. Essentially, hospitals are an outgrowth of pesthouses and almshouses. Indeed, the trend in the United States has been toward more custodial institutions. As recently as 1942, the number of beds in mental hospitals far exceeded the number in general hospitals. This trend once again led to more government intervention. Because society generally refused to assume the great financial and social burden of institutions for the tubercular patients, mentally ill patients, etc., the government was forced to do so.

During this same time—early twentieth century—psychiatry began moving toward the psychological treatment of mental illness.[16] The research of such psychiatrists and behaviorists as the legendary Sigmund Freud, Ivan Pavlov, and William James did much to instigate this transformation.

The development of medical technology (x-rays and clinical laboratories), as well as the discovery of anesthesia and the increasing sophistication of surgery, further encouraged the move toward broader use of hospitals. The movement occurred largely in cities where hospitals were close to professional and patient alike. Yet, for the most part, hospitals remained private or charitable institutions. ("Public" hospitals were maintained by voluntary public and private contributions, whereas private hospitals were strictly proprietary institutions.) A U.S. Bureau of the Census report for 1922 revealed that two-thirds of the operating income of hospitals within the United States was derived from patient fees. The "medical hotel," exemplified by the Mayo Clinic, Rochester, Minnesota, was a major development in hospital care. In this type of institution, rooms were given a "homelike" atmosphere in order to attract paying customers. For the most part, however, hospital expansion remained a local community responsibility.

A rise in the quality of physicians also dates from the first decades of this century and is due mainly to the Flexner report. This survey of medical schools focused on the need for well-trained general practitioners and emphasized the poor state of medical education. The report led to the closing of 29 medical schools between 1910 and 1914.[17]

Before the Flexner study, the traditional practice among state legislators was to grant training licenses to almost any physician who requested one. There was no standardization of teaching practices or means of accreditation. Essentially, training was an apprenticeship type of arrangement. The inadequacy of medical care as viewed by a professional is summed up by Dr. Alan Gregg:

> I think it was about the year 1910 or 1912 when it became possible to say of the United States that a random patient with a random disease consulting a doctor chosen at random stood better than a fifty-fifty chance of benefitting from the encounter.[18]

The evolution of health care within the United States for the most part did not take into account long-term solutions and did not, for the entire nineteenth century, verge outside the province of community responsibility. Any health-related programs generally were instituted to meet certain current needs, characterized primarily as erratic phenomena. Only the sanitary reform movement, which remained within the domain of local community government, captured the consciences of the majority of the American public. Although enlightened studies in the field of health care promoted modern concepts of preventive medicine, the institution of such programs met largely with opposition from the centers of power that would have been able to make them realities. The most progressive changes were to evolve in the early decades of the twentieth century. But again, these remained sporadic forays into the realm of modern health care and were thwarted by a public that could not be convinced to support with taxes the kinds of programs that would have been required. The trend toward government intervention in health matters was slowly, but definitely, emerging. Society's inability to control its purse strings and the creation of the federal income tax accelerated the inevitable formalized type of central help.

SIGNIFICANT HEALTH ISSUES: 1920 TO PRESENT

Prior to World War II, health care delivery and efforts to coordinate and plan health services were generally initiated by private (voluntary), non-government agencies at the state or local levels. Studies and planning efforts were usually disease oriented, categorical or fragmented in approach, directed toward specific health problems.[19] Efforts were initiated by voluntary health groups such as the National Tuberculosis Association, the American Cancer Society, and the American Public Health Association. In an attempt to coordinate the activities of these voluntary health agencies, the National Health Council was created. The experience of the depression of the 1930s, World War II, the profound rise in medical care costs resulting from the increasing imbalance between supply and demand, and the expanding role of the federal government in providing economic assistance conditioned a steady expansion of government participation in the planning, financing, and delivery of health care. This shift to increased government involvement in meeting health needs is best illustrated by examining the major health issues of the pre- and post-World War II periods and the responses of the private and public sectors to those issues.

Between 1920 and 1965 several major health issues emerged: regionalization of health facilities (provision and coordination of health facilities), alternative methods of health care delivery, financing of health care, the impact of biomedical research, and health personnel. It would appear that the most consolidated effort was initiated by the voluntary and public sectors in response to the need of regionalization of health facilities.

Regionalization of Health Facilities

Population growth, the movement from rural to urban areas, and rising medical costs were instrumental in the regionalization of health facilities as early as 1920. Regionalization was the response to such needs as adequate provision of health care facilities—expressed by many studies in numbers of hospital beds per unit of population—and facility coordination within a region.[20] Prior to 1945, the private sector played the dominant role in initiating efforts to study these needs. Each effort undertaken by a voluntary group focused on a particular locality and generally remained separate from similar efforts undertaken by other voluntary groups. As a result, criteria varied from study to study.

In 1920, the New York Academy of Medicine studied 180 private and municipal hospitals in New York City to determine if there were enough hospital beds to care for the sick. The standard measure of need used by the academy was the Public Health Service estimate that, at any given time, approximately two percent of the population would be sick. Finding that one hospital bed existed for every 200 people, the academy concluded that the health needs of the population were being met. This study marks the first formal recognition of the necessity to plan hospital needs in the United States and was followed by a number of local and regional studies.[21] These studies were obviously categorical in approach; questions of geographical distribution and availability of hospital care to all facets of the population were never studied.

A more comprehensive study of hospital needs, "The Need for More Hospitals in Rurals Areas," by A. B. and P. Mills, was published in 1935.[22] The authors studied the question of population density, the number and training of physicians, and other factors related to determining need. This was the first study concerned with health service centers, facilities of 250 or more beds designed to serve a population within a 50-mile radius of the cities where they were located.[23] Again, the emphasis was on the number of beds available to a population. The important point of this study was the Mills' concern with the question of regional health services.

Also during the 1930s, a joint committee of the American Public Health Association and the National Health Council studied the provision of full-time local health services in the United States. This study emphasized the provision of services nationwide rather than in specific localities. The Emerson Report, as it came to be called, was not released until the end of World War II.[24] The recommendations in this report concerned traditional issues of public health services: sanitation, communicable disease control, maternal and child health, vital statistics, and public health laboratory services. The report is connected to those previously discussed by its statement of minimal standards for local health services in terms of the number of health personnel and number of beds per population unit, and per capita expenditure. The study was notable for its new direction, but, by the time of its publication, public health services had so expanded that the standards recommended were inadequate.[25]

Several ambitious efforts were undertaken to coordinate health care delivery during the 1930s. In 1931, the Bingham Associates Fund, a private foundation, established a program based in Pratt Clinic and New England Hospital in Boston to encourage coordination and integration of medical services for residents in rural areas of New England. The program was conducted in conjunction with Tufts Medical School. In 1933, the Committee on the Cost of Medical Care published a report that recommended the coordination of local health services and personnel to provide maximum productivity of the scarce personnel and equipment.[26]

Thus, it can be seen that, prior to 1940, numerous studies of health care services had been undertaken by diverse participants in the private sector. These studies were conducted in response to a growing concern for adequate provision of health facilities for a growing and more transient population and health services coordination to avoid duplication of services and to combat rising medical costs.

Federal response to the issues in the 1920s and 1930s was limited. Traditionally, personal health care was provided by the private sector, primarily in a one patient-one physician situation. Further, domestic unemployment and economic instability and the ensuing World War II absorbed federal efforts and dominated federal concerns. With the conclusion of the war, however, the federal government had more time and money with which to examine those issues raised by the private sector. The passage of the Hospital Survey and Construction Act (Hill-Burton Act, PL 79-725) in 1946 was a major breakthrough in coordinating and providing health care facilities nationwide.

The Hill-Burton Act provided federal aid to states for hospital facilities. To be granted funds, however, a state had to create a hospital planning council responsible for assessing the need for new hospital construction. Because of this condition for funding, states were forced to survey existing facilities (number of beds per unit population) before they could apply for construction grants. The intent of the act was to coordinate new construction with need and with existing facilities.

In 1954, the Hill-Harris Amendments to Hill-Burton revised and expanded the program to include funding exclusively for modernization or replacement of public and nonprofit hospitals. As a result, the number of institutions applying for alterations and additions increased. Emphasis shifted from providing hospital care in rural areas to altering urban facilities. A most significant change wrought by the amendments was a shift in emphasis from construction to planning of health services. Under the Hill-Harris Amendments, state plans had to apply a new formula for assessing bed need, incorporating utilization data, projected population, and occupancy factors.

The Hill-Burton Act and amendments are often criticized as focusing too narrowly on construction, with little stress on organization and distribution of health care facilities. It should be remembered, however, that Hill-Burton not only introduced systematic statewide planning and minimum national standards for assessing hospital need, but also improved the quality of care in rural America.[27] The act and its amendments were limited because the establishment of a formal relationship among hospitals or health agencies was not made mandatory.[28]

With the passage of Hill-Burton and the expenditure of vast funds for hospital construction, the federal government firmly and irreversibly became part of the American health care system. National health planning had been introduced. This fact, coupled with the great rise in medical costs despite federal assistance, led to the formation of a joint committee of the American Hospital Association and the Public Health Service in 1958. The joint committee sponsored four regional conferences to develop guidelines for planning a coordinated community health service system. Three years following the conferences a report was issued. A rationale for areawide health planning had been provided.[29]

The joint committee recommendations were formally recognized and expanded by the public sector in 1963 when the U.S. Public Health Service issued *Procedures for Areawide Health Facility Planning*. While the joint committee studies were being conducted, the American Public Health Association and the National Health Council sponsored an ambitious project to produce a blueprint for a system of preventive and curative medical services and environmental health protection for the next ten years. Whereas the joint committee was a cooperative public and private sector venture, the National Commission on Community Health Services was largely a voluntary venture. The commission was funded by both the private and public sectors through grants from private foundations, the U.S. Public Health Service, and the Vocational Rehabilitation Administration.

The study was conducted in three parts and required four years. Part I, the National Task Forces projects, consisted of numerous autonomous studies; consequently, the recommendations of each task force were disjointed and published individually. Part II, the Community Act Studies, studied 21 individual communities throughout the United States. The findings of each of these task groups provided the basis for recommendations to be presented during the third part of the project—the Communications project. This part of the project tested public reaction to the recommendations at four different regional conferences. The commission's report, published in 1966, made the following major recommendations:

1. Community health services need greater federal participation.
2. Comprehensive health planning must be undertaken on a continuing basis.
3. Regional or areawide planning bodies must be established to correspond to problem health areas.
4. A single system must be established to provide personal health services that eventually will combine all parts of public and private health care.[30]

Concurrent with these efforts by the voluntary and public sectors to coordinate health services, the Commission on Heart Disease, Cancer, and Stroke was formed by President Johnson in 1963 to recommend steps to reduce the incidence of these illnesses through new knowledge and more complete utilization of existing medical knowledge. The recommendations of this commission were enacted into law as the Heart Disease, Cancer and Stroke Amendments of 1965 (PL 89-239). Even though the initial study was categorical in approach, the establishment of the Regional Medical Programs (RMPs) was a comprehensive response. Cooperative regional arrangements were to be organized from existing medical centers, clinical research centers, and hospitals. Fifty-six health regions were established and charged with evaluating the overall health needs within each region. Initially, the act covered only heart disease, stroke, and cancer, but the 1970 amendments expanded the program. Two important aspects of the act distinguished it from previous legislation and voluntary group emphasis on the coordination and provision of health services. First, the act provided for local participation in planning. This approach departed significantly from purely state and federal planning of facilities that were provided for in the Hill-Burton Act. Second, funding of projects was provided for both planning and operating.

Once regions were awarded planning grants, they became eligible to apply for funds to cover operating expenses of all projects in their jurisdiction. Initially, funding was devoted to continuing education and training, but this emphasis has shifted to organization and delivery of patient services, and improvement of personnel productivity and distribution.[31] Unfortunately, the RMPs were not incorporated into existing federal and state programs, causing both duplication and gaps in delivery of services, personnel training, and research.

The passage of the RMP legislation, together with the recommendations of the National Commission and the guidelines published by the joint committee, culminated in a regional comprehensive philosophy of health planning as opposed to the emphasis on facilities that had dominated voluntary concerns during the 1920s and into the 1940s. This new philosophy became law with the passage of the Partnership for Health Act of 1966.

Health Care Delivery and Financing of Health Care

The regionalization of health care is only one such issue to emerge between 1920 and 1980. The rising cost of medical services resulted in a move to coordinate and regionalize facilities in order to make more efficient use of the health care system and to avoid duplication of services. Rising costs also produced new trends in the delivery of health care and the financing of health services.

In 1933, after a three-year study of the existing system of personal health services in the United States, the Committee on the Cost of Medical Care published a report that illustrated the inability of a large portion of the population to obtain high-quality medical care, owing to rising costs. The most significant recommendation from this committee was the concept of "pre-paid medical groups." The report states that:

> medical service, both preventive and therapeutic, should be furnished largely by organized groups of physicians, dentists, nurses and pharmacists and other associated personnel. Such groups should be organized around a hospital for rendering complete home, office and hospital care. The form of organization should encourage the maintenance of high standards and the development or preservation of a personal relation between patient and physician.[32]

According to the committee, this system of health care services offered the community the maximum potential for productivity of scarce professional personnel and expensive equipment.

The concept of prepayment and group practice expressed in 1933 was incorporated into the pattern of health service delivery. In 1965, a survey conducted by the Department of Health, Education, and Welfare (HEW) of 582 group plans showed that the plans fell into five categories, depending on sponsor or consumer orientation.[33] The community-consumer plans are nonprofit plans designed to serve the general community or a particular group. These plans incorporate prepaid medical services on a private basis, not a group practice basis. The Health Insurance Program (HIP) of Greater New York and the Kaiser Plan are well-known examples of community-consumer plans. Anne Somers, a nationally respected health economist, writes that many feel the Kaiser Plan is an ideal model of a group plan. Some of its distinguishing characteristics are:

1. It is directed at a cross section of the population living in a geographic area but without rigid geographical or income limits.
2. Coordinated management and funding cover almost the whole spectrum of health care.
3. Funding is almost entirely private with respect to both capital and operating costs.
4. Paramedical personnel are used more than in conventional practice.
5. The hospital is viewed as the center of the delivery system. Insurance provides income for both the hospital and medical group.
6. Physicians are organized in a group and contract with the plan to provide services at a fixed fee per enrollee per year, regardless of the amount of service.
7. Enrollees periodically are given a choice of changing their medical plans and nonparticipants an opportunity to join the plan.[34]

Employer-employee plans took shape under the joint management of employers and unions. Workers generally contribute to a health insurance program or trust fund. One-third of these plans were found to make use of group practices that provided their own clinics or hospital facilities; the staff is paid by salary. The remaining plans made payments directly to the hospitals or physicians.

Medical society plans sponsored by various medical societies have generally been absorbed by Blue Shield. These plans emphasized the private physician-patient relationship, and the coverage was very limited.

Private group clinic plans are operated by a private group of physicians as exemplified by the Mayo Clinic, although they are not all extensive. Dental society plans are similar to Blue Shield plans: subscribers generally have a choice of member providers. These types of plans were in existence prior to the passage of the Medicare and Medicaid amendments to Social Security legislation. They are private, voluntary plans designed to provide a wide range of care, usually hospital based, at low or at least controlled costs. Also, these plans are important because they were systems of health delivery on which Congress based the Medicare legislation. They offered federal planners a variety of ways to cope with the cost of health care.

The success of the Kaiser Plan and HIP of Greater New York fostered in part the concept of the health maintenance organizations (HMOs). Section 314(e) of the Partnership for Health Act, passed in 1966, further promoted the idea of HMOs. Such organizations are distinguished from private community-consumer plans because they involve:

1. organized systems of facilities and personnel
2. a comprehensive set of maintenance and treatment activities
3. an enrolled population consisting of individuals who elect to join
4. a unique financial plan of fixed payments made in advance, regardless of the number of services received.[35]

The movement toward an alternative method of health care delivery from the single practitioner's care delivery was assured with the establishment of group plans and HMOs during the period between 1930 and 1965. This movement was supported initially by the private sector and more recently by the federal government, when it incorporated the concept of group plans into the drafting of Medicare and Medicaid bills and the Partnership for Health Act.

It is important to mention the effect that Blue Cross and Blue Shield had upon the delivery of health care and the financing of health care. There was little free cash available during the Depression and, consequently, little financial help if a medical crisis arose. Blue Cross started during the 1930s when a group of teachers made an arrangement with Baylor Hospital in Dallas, Texas, for care through a prepaid plan.[36] The idea quickly spread, and states began enacting legislation to provide this type of protection. In a period of rising medical costs and little cash, the Blue plans assured payment to hospitals for health services. Ironically, hospital costs continued to rise, especially since payment was assured. This phenomenon contributed greatly to the growing concept and need for prepaid medical plans and HMOs.

Theoretically, Blue Cross is a nonprofit, noncommercial insurance plan. Its inception and success initiated the growth of private, commercial health insurance. Blue Cross is the largest private financier of hospital care in the United States.[37] The 75 independent Blue Cross plans are linked by the National Blue Cross Association, which represents the independent plans in national affairs and provides services in marketing, education, research, and public relations. The continued growth of Blue plans was assured with the passage of the Medicare-Medicaid legislation. Blue Cross became the major intermediary between hospitals and government disbursement of Medicare payments.

Between 1920 and 1965, federal government involvement in the health care system expanded with its involvement in the funding of hospital construction and with the RMPs. It was also during this period that the question of a national health insurance program was initiated; it became a factor in the passage of the Medicare and Medicaid legislation, legislation that marked a compromise in the fight for a national health insurance policy. This legislation, unlike private insurance policies or the Blue plans, has been the strongest move yet to establish medical care on a basis of universal provision and insurance rather than on economic dependency criteria (i.e., those who have the income can purchase insurance).

The passage of the Social Security Act in 1935 signaled the acceptance of public responsibility for designated categories of the needy, deprived, and handicapped. By the end of World War II people were conditioned to disbursement of their tax monies by the government for social purposes.[38] The Social Security experience provided the philosophy and the rationale for protecting the elderly and medically indigent in a federally administered health care program.

Medicaid, Title XIX of the Social Security Amendments of 1965, extended aid to all medically indigent persons, especially children. By 1970 all states except Alaska and Arizona had Medicaid programs. The programs vary widely from state to state in size, scope of services, and age range of patients. Most programs are run by state welfare departments; little attention is paid to the quality of care or the circumstances accompanying its receipt. Because Medicaid is administered on a state-by-state basis, provision of health care for impoverished individuals has remained fragmented. A more uniform approach of government financing of health care is illustrated by Medicare, Title XVIII of the Social Security Amendments of 1965.

Medicare offers health insurance to those who are over 65 years of age and receive Social Security benefits. HEW administers the law through the Public Health Service and the Social Security Administration, and state and local agencies assist in formulating standards of participation. The law is in two parts: Part A provides hospital care insurance automatically to persons 65 and over who receive Social Security benefits. Consequently, increased hospital costs are absorbed over a large tax base. Part B of Medicare provides medical benefits such as payments for physicians and other medical bills. This part of the plan is voluntary. A key part of the legislation does require the establishment of a utilization review mechanism to determine whether the services are provided properly.[39]

One of the greatest failures of the Medicare-Medicaid legislation is that the federal government does not exert a strong enough role in providing health care to the poor and the elderly. The government provides the funding but leaves the disbursement of funds to the private sector, the traditional health provider in this country.

The Impact of Biomedical Research and Health Personnel

The health issues that were discussed previously were recognized early in the period between 1920 and 1965 and initiated responses from first the private sector and then the public sector. It was not until the 1950s that public concern increased over the lack of physicians and their unequal distribution. It is important to note, however, that efforts in health personnel planning do date back to 1910 and the study by Flexner.[40] Flexner's book exerted a major influence on established medical education standards and the improvement of physician training and education in the United States.[41] Health personnel was also an issue with the Committee on the Costs of Medical Care during the 1930s. The Lee-Jones Study, part of the committee report, was an effort to calculate personnel requirements on the basis of professional judgment or expert opinions on medical needs. These two efforts were initiated by the private sector. In spite of increased concern over the shortage of physicians, it was not until 1963 that large investments were made in training by the federal government.

Prior to the 1960s, states offered some financial assistance to medical schools within their boundaries.[42] Federal support was limited to grants for research training and biomedical research. Between 1965 and 1975 $34 billion were invested in biomedical research by both the private and public sectors. The federal government supported research through various divisions of the Public Health Service, such as the National Institutes of Health, the National Center for Health Services and Development, and the National Center for Health Statistics. Some support took the form of grants and research contracts to state and local agencies, private institutions, universities, hospitals, and individuals outside the public sector. Components of the Social Security Administration, the Children's Bureau, and HEW also administered research funds. The federal government refrained, however, from exercising any supervision or control over the manner in which medical services were provided or over the administration of the funds. The government remained reluctant to concern itself with the efficiency of the providers to whom grants were made.

The emphasis on biomedical research during the post-World War II pre-1960 decade had a profound impact on the structure and nature of medical care. The gravest impact was the deterioration of the general practitioner-patient relationship that had dominated the medical care system prior to and during World War II. The many advances made in medical technology and medical care delivery left a gap between those advances and the application to patient care. In order for the medical profession to keep pace with the advances made by medical research, the emphasis in training shifted from general practice to specialization by physicians and institutionalization of all health services within one base—usually a hospital. The institutionalization and specialization of health services brought about by biomedical and technological research greatly affected health personnel. As Kissick states, there was a divergence in the types of health personnel and a convergence of the settings in which services were delivered.[43]

The phrase *health personnel* is used to refer to all those involved in health careers from the professionally educated biomedical scientist to the practically trained nurse's aide or hospital attendant. It was estimated that in 1900 there were 200,000 health professionals who required college or professional preparation; 60 percent of these were physicians. In 1920, the number of health professionals doubled. In 1940, there were 692,000 health professionals, and in 1960 this number increased to 1,140,000, only 20 percent of whom were physicians.[44] By 1974, there were an estimated 3,885,000 health professionals, only 10% of whom were physicians.[45] The change in the percentage of physicians between 1900 and 1974 illustrates the growth in the divergence of health personnel.

During the 1950s, when shortages of physicians became a major health issue, the number of workers in health occupations increased at a rate twice that of the population growth.[46] Why, then, was there a perceived shortage of physicians? The concentration of physicians in urban areas around major hospital centers, especially in the Northeast and along the West Coast, and the fact that the most rapid growth in health occupations between 1950 and 1960 was among those who required the shortest period of training, e.g., practical nurses, x-ray technicians, and hospital attendants, generally account for the public concern over the physician shortage.[47]

Largely in response to this public concern, the Surgeon General of the United States formed a consultant group on medical education, which came to be called the Bane Committee. The objective of this group was to project the physician requirements by 1975. The Bane Report, issued in 1959, recognized that factors such as chronic illness, aging population, specialization, regional disparities, changing patterns of practice, etc., would increase the need and demand for medical services.[48] It asserted that the ratio of 141 physicians to 100,000 people was the minimum essential to protect public health. The committee recommended that the increase in physicians needed by the United States by 1975 could be met best by increasing the size of medical classes and creating new medical schools.

The Bane Report was a major effort by the federal government to plan for future medical services. It addressed, however, only the question of physician requirements, not the increased need for related health personnel. In light of this original emphasis, it is interesting that legislation, passed during the 1960s, was directed at both health professionals and allied personnel.

In 1963, under the Health Professions Educational Assistance Act, the federal government provided construction grants and student loans to assist medical, dental, and other professional schools in expanding their capacities and production of trained personnel. In 1965, the act was amended to provide formula and project grant support of basic educational costs and scholarships. The objective of these grants was to increase the supply of physicians, dentists, pharmacists, optometrists, and podiatrists. During 1964, the Nurse Training Act became law, providing grants for the expansion of teaching programs and student loans.

In 1966, a significant step was taken to cope with the divergence occurring within health occupations. The purpose of the Allied Health Professions Personnel Training Act of 1966 was to meet the growing need for supervisors of paraprofessional workers, for teachers in allied health professions, highly skilled technical specialists, and allied health professionals in new areas of medicine. This act provided for the creation of broad, multidisciplinary programs and expansion of existing programs through:

1. improvement grants to selected schools that educate professionals in three or more interrelated health fields;
2. traineeships for teachers, administrators, and specialists in various health professions; and
3. project grants for developing, demonstrating, and evaluating new curricula to train new types of health technologists.

Together, these acts provide for most aspects of health personnel training. Individually, however, they represent a fragmented approach in planning of health personnel. The Health Manpower Act of 1968 (PL 90-490) is a more comprehensive approach to such planning. This act was passed in response to a report published by President Johnson's National Advisory Commission on Health Manpower in 1967. Title I of the act covers Health Professions Training; Title II covers Nurses' Training; Title III covers the Allied Health Professional Program; and Title IV covers Health Research Facilities. Under each title, funds were dispersed through construction grants, grants given directly to health training institutions, special project grants, student loans, and scholarships. Though planning for health personnel training has advanced since the Flexner report in 1910, the issue of distribution of medical services and personnel still must be dealt with by both the public and private sectors.

The impetus given in the 1960s to increasing health personnel was so successful that Congress became concerned about a potentially severe glut of health professionals, particularly physicians, in the 1980s. The number of active physicians had increased from 261,000 in 1963 to 340,000 in 1975, and a projection of 440,000 during the 1980s and almost 600,000 by 1990 could be made. This translates into an increase from the 1980 rate of 198 physicians per 100,000 population to a projected rate of 244 by 1990, or 70 percent more physicians than called for in the Bane Report.[49] In response to this dramatic change, Congress passed the Health Professions Educational Assistance Act (PL 94-484) in 1976 to maintain an appropriate balance between the population's need and the supply of health professionals available. The act contains several strategies for achieving this goal. It restricts the number of foreign medical graduates practicing in the United States by requiring them to take a more difficult medical examination and to pass a more difficult English test than had been required in the past. Furthermore, by limiting the number of graduate medical education positions to 16,000, the number of foreign students able to compete with Americans for these openings will decrease. It is expected that the number of foreign medical graduates practicing in the United States will decrease by 50 percent in 1990 from 44,000 to 22,000.[50]

The act also addresses the problem of physician maldistribution. There is a scarcity of physicians in rural areas and urban inner cities, compared to suburban and other urban areas. As of September 1977, 2,200 physician shortage areas, i.e., areas having less than one primary care physician for every 4,000 persons, had been documented. It has been estimated that approximately 18,000 physicians would be needed to meet the needs of these shortage areas,[51] and a National Health Services Corps program was established in early 1970 to meet these needs. In return for a certain number of years of practice in underserved areas, the government will pay for a physician's education. From the initial assignment of 13 newly graduated physicians in 1971, the Corps has grown so that 9,000 scholarships were awarded in 1979 to increase substantially the number of physicians practicing in these underserved areas.[52] Because almost half remain in these areas after their tour of duty has been completed, this is a hopeful sign that the needs of designated underserved areas may be met in the foreseeable future.[53]

PL 94-484 also addresses the imbalance between the number of primary care physicians and the number of specialists. The number of active primary care physicians increased from 125,000 in 1963 to 152,000 in 1975, but their percentage among all practicing physicians decreased from 48 to 44 percent.[54] Through various incentive programs, the act is intended to increase the number of incoming graduate medical students in general or family practice to 50 percent.

Through these various strategies, PL 94-484 seeks to reduce the imbalance of health professions maldistribution and increase the number of family practitioners in order to raise the quality, access, and availability of medical services.

CONCLUSIONS

The responses to some of the key health care issues reveal certain patterns with respect to the two main criteria from which the issues were examined: (1) who identified the health issue and responded to it (the private sector, the governmental sector, or a combination?), and (2) what was the nature of the response from a planning point of view (fragmented and narrow in scope, or broader and more comprehensive with a view to the future?).

With regard to the first criterion, the primary response to health issues no longer comes from the private sector, as it did before 1920, but instead comes from the government. Prior to the 1920s, the local and state governments were the most likely governmental levels to become involved in health issues and their resolution. From the 1920s to the mid-1960s, the federal government played an increasingly important role in solving health problems. The nature of this involvement has, however, not been a solo act on the part of the various levels of government. The usual pattern of response has been the formation of a blue ribbon commission headed by a prestigious physician or health leader from the private sector. Increasingly, the commissions have been federally funded, and usually a majority of their members have been from the private sector with only a minority representing government or the consumer and the public interest. The commission's recommendations have generally been the basis for legislative action by the federal government and often have called for the use of public funds to implement them. Thus, the role of the private sector has continued to be influential, but the government's influence, as holder of the purse strings, has assumed greater importance as national decisions were required for solving health problems. It can be concluded that a partnership has been developing between the private and governmental sectors in the solving of health issues. This partnership can be evidenced by the important role the private sector has been given in implementing federally sponsored programs, whether ambulatory outpatient clinics, the recent development of HMOs, or the training of physicians and allied health personnel.

With respect to the second criterion, almost all the health planning from the act of 1798 that provided assistance to maritime personnel to the present has been primarily of the reactive type. Only after a health problem had been identified and assumed to be of major significance for a large segment of the population have there been attempts to solve it. Except in a few instances, such as Shattuck's report and the Hill-Burton legislation, most of the responses have been concerned with solving the immediate problem within a narrow scope. The plans have been related to a narrow field, such as professional personnel or hospital facilities, but seldom has more than one of the health fields been brought into the planning focus at one time. In the mid-1960s, the emphasis began to shift to analyzing an entire field of professional and allied health personnel needs. This new direction has been especially evident with respect to the RMP, which originally combined research, planning, and dissemination of information on three health disease entities (heart disease, cancer, and stroke) and later widened the scope to include other diseases. In short, there has been a greater receptivity and need to look at the health field in a much more comprehensive manner than had been true prior to the 1960s.

The third conclusion to be made is that, beginning in the 1960s, decision making has involved more consumers from all economic levels in the planning and analysis of health needs. While prestigious health leaders and government officials have been the main participants in the past, the recent emphasis on consumer involvement in RMPs signals a shift to widen the base and, thus, include more voices representative of the diverse public interests.

NOTES

1. George Rosen, *A History of Public Health* (New York: MD Publications, 1958), p. 465.

2. The change from local control of quarantines to federal control came at the influence of similar legislative enactments on a national level in Europe. England, for example, established such national quarantine measures following the cholera epidemic there in 1848, which also led to the creation of England's General Board of Health.

3. The Marine Hospital Service had been set up to regulate naval hospitals run by the government for American seamen; the first hospital was founded in Massachusetts. The Marine Hospital Service is also the forerunner of the present U.S. Public Health Service.

4. Harry S. Mustard, "The Development of the Health Services, 1875–1915," in *The Uneasy Equilibrium, Private and Public Financing of Health Service in the United States, 1875–1965*, ed. Odin W. Anderson (New Haven: College and University Press, 1968), p. 22.

5. Griscom was describing the conditions of the poor as well as the sanitary conditions in New York City, while Shattuck studied health conditions in Boston.

6. John C. Griscom, *The Sanitary Condition of the Laboring Population of New York with Suggestions for Improvements* (New York: Harper, 1845). The problem of housing in New

York City was considered acute, exacerbated by the steady stream of immigrants pouring daily into the city. Overcrowding and dilapidated houses were common. It was not until 1850 that the city sought to remedy the problem by building tenements, designed to be economical housing for the poor, and a new concept in urban architecture.

7. The concept of providing for oneself, as it was defined in the nineteenth century, consisted of having saved sufficient funds to take care of the eventual medical costs. However, these costs were low since hospitals were not common and most treatment was done in the home.

8. Anderson, *Uneasy Equilibrium*, p. 52.

9. Lemuel Shattuck, *Report of a General Plan for the Promotion of Public and Personal Health Relating to a Sanitary Survey of the State* (Boston, 1850, reprint ed., Cambridge: Harvard University Press, 1948).

10. Anderson, *Uneasy Equilibrium*, p. 23.

11. Rosen, *Public Health*, p. 464.

12. *Ibid.*, p. 468.

13. Michael M. Davis and Andrew R. Warner, "The Hospitals and Physicians," in Anderson, *Uneasy Equilibrium*, p. 33.

14. *Ibid.*, p. 35.

15. A member of the U.S. House of Representatives introduced a bill in 1917 to establish a commission to prepare a plan for a national insurance fund against unemployment. It called for the inclusion of sickness and disability insurance programs. The bill was favorably recommended by the Committee on Labor to the Congress for a vote. In Congress, however, it failed, the vote taken 40 minutes before Congress was to adjourn for the session. Samuel Gompers' opposition to the bill was that he believed such a commission would be biased and recommend compulsory health insurance. Gompers felt it should be voluntary and urged instead a study of such methods.

16. The move in the field of psychiatric research away from the organic theory of mental disorder—in which body and mind were polarized dualities—propelled psychiatry out of the laboratory and into the public sector, where answers to psychiatric disorders were sought in behavior. Also, it established the psychological tone that later led to the advent of the social worker concept and, much later, therapy.

17. Abraham Flexner, *Medical Education in the United States and Canada* (New York: The Carnegie Foundation for the Advancement of Teaching, 1910). Dr. Flexner personally visited medical schools in order to make his survey.

18. Anderson, *Uneasy Equilibrium*, p. 32.

19. Ernest L. Stebbins and Kathleen N. Williams, "History and Background of Health Planning in the United States," in *Health Planning: Quantitative Aspects and Quantitative Techniques,* ed. W. A. Reinke (Baltimore: Waverly Press, 1972), p. 3.

20. Joel J. May, *Health Planning: Its Past and Potential* (Chicago: University of Chicago, Center for Health Administration Studies, Health Administration Perspectives Number A5, 1967), p. 13.

21. *Ibid.*, p. 14.

22. A.B. Mills and P. Mills, "The Need for More Hospitals in Rural Areas," *The Modern Hospital* 44 (1935):50–54.

23. May, *Health Planning,* p. 15.

24. Haven Emerson, *Local Health Units for the Nation.* A report for the American Public Health Association, Committee on Administration (New York: The Commonwealth Fund, 1945).

25. Stebbins and Williams, "History of Health Planning," p. 8.

26. I.S. Falk, C.R. Rorem, and M.D. Ring, *The Costs of Medical Care* (Committee on the Cost of Medical Care) (Chicago: University of Chicago Press, 1933).

27. Stebbins and Williams, "History of Health Planning," p. 8.

28. May, *Health Planning*, p. 30.

29. *Ibid.*, p. 39.

30. National Commission on Community Health Services. *Health Is a Community Affair* (Cambridge: Harvard University Press, 1966).

31. Stebbins and Williams, "History of Health Planning," p. 9.

32. Falk, Rorem, and Ring, *Costs of Medical Care*, p. 109.

33. L.S. Reed, A.H. Anderson, and R.S. Hanft, *Independent Health Insurance Plans in the United States, 1965 Survey* (Washington, D.C.: U.S. Government Printing Office, 1966).

34. Anne Somers, *Health Care in Transition: Directions for the Future* (Chicago: Hospital Research and Educational Trust, 1971), p. 114.

35. Stebbins and Williams, "History of Health Planning," p. 13.

36. O.W. Anderson and M. Lerner, *Health Progress in the United States 1900–1960* (Chicago: University of Chicago Press, 1963), p. 303.

37. Health Policy Advisory Center, *The American Health Empire* (New York: 1970), p. 148.

38. Erwin Witkin, *The Impact of Medicare* (Springfield, Ill.: Charles C Thomas, 1971), p. 7.

39. *Ibid.*, p. 31.

40. Flexner, *Medical Education*.

41. Stebbins and Williams, "History of Health Planning," p. 3.

42. William L. Kissick, "Health Manpower in Transition," in *Economic Aspects of Health Care*, ed. John McKinlay (New York: Milbank Memorial Fund, 1973), pp. 257–294.

43. *Ibid.*, p. 264.

44. *Ibid.*, p. 260.

45. Bureau of Health Manpower, *Health Manpower Projections* (Washington, D.C.: Health Resources Administration, DHEW, undated, about 1977).

46. Kissick, "Health Manpower."

47. *Ibid.*, p. 262.

48. G. Bane, *Physicians for a Growing America*. Report of the Surgeon General's Consultant Group on Medical Education, U.S. Public Health Service No. 709 (Washington, D.C.: U.S. Government Printing Office, 1959).

49. Bureau of Health Manpower, *On the Status of Health Professions Personnel*. A report to the President and Congress, DHEW Publication No. 78-93 (Washington, D.C.: Health Resources Administration, 1978), Table II-8, p. II-30.

50. *Ibid.*, p. IV-7-9.

51. *Ibid.*, p. II-26.

52. Health Resources Administration, *Health Resources News* 6, no. 8 (September 1979): 1.

53. U.S. Dept. of Health and Human Services, *Health: United States—1980* (Washington, D.C.: Public Health Service, 1980), p. 80.

54. Bureau of Health Manpower, *Status of Health Professions Personnel*, p. IV-45.

Chapter 2

Issues in Medical Technology

The proliferation and control of life-dealing medical technologies raise serious ethical questions to which little thought has been given in health legislative and planning circles. Important inventions and applications of technology to alleviate illness or specific medical conditions raise questions of priority when these developments are taken as a whole. Where should the limited staff, facilities, and financial resources be allocated? To cancer research or treatment? To automobile accident prevention or standard housing for the poor? No easy answers can be given to the numerous questions raised, because they involve different values, priorities, and groups of persons with an interest in these issues. They are both planning and political questions and, as such, require the involvement of many persons and groups concerned with the public interest.

The allocation of health care resources, the organization of the health care system, and the cost and financing of health care involve many of the same issues. Where do physicians practice? What kind of training do they receive? Who serves the poor of the urban and rural areas? Why is there controversy over whether there are enough physicians? What impact does the organization of medical services have on the consumer? Why have the costs of health care been increasing at a more rapid rate than other services; yet, there appear to be disproportionate benefits in return for these higher costs?

The need for rationalizing the health care system and the federal initiative resulted in the first comprehensive health planning effort, the Partnership for Health Act. As the predecessor to the National Health Planning and Resources Development Act of 1974, it was the first planning strategy to involve community leaders in attempts to resolve these issues.

As the field of technological invention continues to expand and devices for saving, sustaining, and controlling life are being developed at an enormous pace, there is strong indication that the decisions being made in these crucial areas must be examined from many sides—not only who makes the decisions, but also their larger implications. Ethics, values, and moral judgments all have an important part to play in decision making; even more important is the need to reconsider who the decision makers should be. As a guide to this sort of thinking, a leading physician has said "... medicine is not now and never has been our private preserve but is something in which all people have a vital stake."[1] It is worthwhile remembering that "vital" has the meaning of "pertaining to life" as consideration is given these serious questions.

Technology has been defined as the knowledgeable combination of information and skill, of know-what (science) and know-how (technique).[2] According to Webster, technology is the "totality of the means employed to provide objects necessary for human sustenance and comfort." Several questions arise from this definition: What are the "objects necessary for human sustenance and comfort"? What is an acceptable level of "human sustenance and comfort"? For whom? And most crucial, Who is to define these qualities? These are the first of many issues that must be examined in any evaluation of the new medical technology and what it portends for both consumers and providers, now and in the future.

Glancing at the recent past reveals that the last decades have seen a veritable explosion in all the technologies, with the area of medical innovation second in popular novelty only to the conquest of space programs. The 1970s began to display the harvest of the early discoveries, which are increasingly becoming part of standard medical practice.

In *Future Shock,* Alvin Toffler has aptly named the present condition, "the accelerative thrust."[3] One may wonder if all this speed and proliferation is a blessing, or even if it is necessary. Ninety percent of all scientists who ever lived are alive today, and one can assume that, as a group, they are exceedingly prolific and continuously at work. But when it is further recognized that a time lag of some 10 to 15 years occurs between the discovery of a new technique and its application,[4] it is clear that the explosion is only beginning; society is on the threshold of a technological boom in the medical arts that will grow ever more complex in the next decades.

Medicine, traditionally the domain of physiologists, with increasing emphasis on biochemistry, microbiology, pharmacology, and genetics, has made new alliances, which seem incongruous; yet outstanding discoveries have resulted. The newest partnerships of medical practitioners are with engineers (mechanical, chemical, and electrical), physicists, mathematicians, and an array of highly skilled technicians.[5] This begins to raise questions concerning the appropriateness and validity of current medical education. As a "medical engineer," should the new physician's training be further grounded in the "hard sciences," or is the existing pattern of a mutual alliance between two independent sciences valid?

Serious questions are raised with respect to yet another area: the computer in medicine. Should the physician's training include computer applications, or should the coalitional arrangement be continued? One physician has commented that ". . . it would appear that all the functions of a doctor are being taken over either by other people or by machines,"[6] consequently leaving only two avenues open to the physician of the future, either as full-time researcher or a quasi-social worker, "helping people adjust to their diseases."[7] The entire meaning and direction of medical education would be radically altered if such a prediction came to pass, and it is necessary to focus now on the trends and indications that, should there be no intervention, may some day defy solutions.

SAVING LIVES

So far the approach has been circuitous. The issues confronting health planners are complex, involving changing rules and roles. Changing technologies have an impact on the health care and delivery system, as well as on the moral and ethical questions that are now being confronted with respect to efficacy and safety.

In a section of the *American Journal of Public Health,* in February 1974, it was reported that "presently", more than 1,500 manufacturers produce 12,000 kinds of medical devices, most of which lack adequate control." Because of this, the *Journal* called for legislation to control the "testing, sale, and utilization of all medical devices." In its concern for patients' safety, Congress passed the Medical Device Amendments of 1976, which give the Food and Drug Administration (FDA) a vastly expanded responsibility to oversee the marketing of some 8,000 medical devices. The term *medical devices* includes techniques, drugs, mechanical devices, and procedures. These devices are also divided into three main medical categories: preventive, diagnostic, and treatment. Preventive devices, such as immunizations, protect persons from disease. Diagnostic devices, such as computerized axial tomography (CAT) scanners, are used to identify disease. Treatment devices, such as open heart surgery or hemodialysis, either relieve or limit the spread of disease.[8]

To begin to carry out this responsibility, FDA developed 19 panels of experts to recommend how 3,500 devices should be classified into basic categories. The 1976 amendments described three of these categories. Class 1 category devices are subject only to general controls, which include premarket notification, adherence to good manufacturing practices, and record keeping requirements. Class II medical devices must meet FDA's performance standards, which relate to their construction, components, ingredients, and properties. A manufacturer must seek premarket approval of a medical device both when general controls would not ensure its safety and efficacy and when there is insufficient information available to develop performance standards. Premarket approval is the overriding regulatory requirement for Class III devices, which include life sustaining, life supporting, or implanted devices.[9]

It is not the intent here to make an exhaustive study of these devices, but rather to emphasize the enormity of the field. In fact, a quarterly journal called *Biomaterials, Medical Devices and Artificial Organs* was added to the ranks of established medical publications in 1973, in an obvious response to an expressed demand. The editor of the publication has a Ph.D. in medical and chemical engineering.

The first area requiring examination, not only for its growing appeal to the medical profession, but also for its equally strong appeal to the public, is that of prosthetics. The use of a prosthesis, the addition of an artificial part to correct a defect of the body, has been possible for some years, but today the art is moving beyond the mere attachment of limbs to devising a system whereby the limbs may be controlled by the wearer by electronic impulses to create more lifelike effects with increased mobility and utility.

Surgeons, cooperating with engineers, have devised electrically controlled stimulating mechanisms that act on existing organs. The most famous of these is the pacemaker, which by tiny electrical shocks keeps the heart beating regularly. Pacemaker implantations are now almost commonplace, although their history began with much doubt and many problems in technical proficiency. As the state of the art has progressed to even more miniature and complex materials and functions, it is worth the pause to question whether enough control of the "testing, sale, and utilization" is actually all that is required. It may also be useful to consider, for instance, the vast expense of continually improving what may have reached its limit of efficiency.

The past decades have undoubtedly produced tremendous advances in saving lives; the preponderance of research (and its funding) and applications have been directed toward the four leading causes of death in the United States and major industrialized nations, which are heart disease, cancer, stroke, and accidents (although advances reducing the number of deaths from the latter cause have been more educational than technological). What is most disconcerting is that, while the efforts have been mobilized against these major killers and cripplers, the number of deaths attributable to these causes has not changed proportionately. For example, while there has been a 10 percent reduction in death rates due to heart disease from 1950 to 1976, there has been an increase in the death rate due to malignant neoplasms (cancer) of about 12.5 percent during this same period.[10] On the positive side, nephritis, pneumonia, tuberculosis, and premature births, leading causes of death in 1940, are no longer on the list of the top ten causes of death as of 1970.[11] Environmental factors and inoculation procedures, as well as the chemical therapies and antibiotics that were developed during those 30 years, are generally considered responsible for the marked changes.

Some of the applications of the new medical technology, which by their nature are more costly, require more diverse technical input and generally must be used in large medical facilities and centers, raising questions as to their best use and continued development.

The heart-lung machine, from its earliest use in 1952, has been crucial in the evolution of open heart surgery and paved the way for numerous technological developments.[12] Hyperbaric oxygen therapy (HOT) units, also with their beginning in the mid-1950s, have greatly increased the success rate of heart surgery with difficult cases, and today there are entire HOT units attached to large hospitals. The high pressure oxygen environment has proved helpful to patients suffering from multiple attacks.

The defibrillator, long a standby for emergency reviving of heart attack victims, has recently undergone streamlining, and has emerged as a portable unit, greatly reducing cost and immensely aiding utility.[13] Paralleling this advance has been the development of such self-contained systems as the "MAX," which may be moved to the patient; provides a total support unit for heart attack victims, as well as intravenous apparatus; and may double as a stretcher or even an operating table should such need arise.[14] Powered by batteries, it can work without electrical outlets. Many other less spectacular but more convenient devices are available for rescue type operations and may be used by only semiskilled or nonprofessionals with a clear understanding of how the apparatus works. This makes it possible for more people to carry out rescue work without waiting for full professionals and can often mean saving a life.[15] The Emergency Medical Services Systems Act of 1973 (PL 93-154) provided funding to states and their subdivisions to develop coordinated emergency medical services (EMS) systems. The availability of specially trained EMS technicians and specially equipped ambulances has reduced mortality and enhanced treatment for persons who have emergencies such as burns, cardiac conditions, poisoning, trauma, accidents, or neonatal and behavioral conditions. The complete EMS system is based on detecting and reporting the emergency, dispatching an EMS team and ambulance, providing treatment at the scene or transport to an emergency facility, treatment at the emergency facility, and transfer, if required, to another facility for care.

The ventricular bypass, transplanted hearts, and the gradually emerging artificial heart all became possible because of greatly increased knowledge of immunosuppressive system drug therapies, new materials, and the lifesaving properties of the heart-lung machine. Not only does the machine function effectively during operations, but it also sustains patients with failing transplants.[16] Under these circumstances, whether the cause be in the immunosuppressive system or in the availability of suitable donor organs, many patients are submitted to "incredible measures" to be kept alive until the physicians can find means to reverse conditions.[17]

An ironic twist has now placed the heart-lung machine, once considered the *summum bonum* that enables many lives to be saved, at the center of a controversy over the valid definition of death. Conventional medical and legal texts define death as the failure of the heart and lungs; with the aid of the heart-lung machine the patient may be minimally maintained for some extended period. Recently, a group of physicians suggested different criteria for the establishment of death, criteria that relate to the functions of the nervous system and brain and have precedence in setting time of death in potential donor patients.[18]

The serious question of fixing the time of death has many moral as well as legal ramifications. Cases of extraordinary recovery have been found after readings of flat-line (death) recordings on an electroencephalogram (EEG) and complete arrest of the circulatory system. Physicians face these uncertainties continuously, and they may "be subject to serious legal risk if the presence of death is not clear" when they act in cases of transplant donors, since "to hasten the death of anyone, even a person whose death is imminent, is still a homicide."[19]

Not only has it been said that "death is too important a matter to be left to physicians,"[20] but the definition of death has not been resolved to everyone's satisfaction. Yet, "dying is continuous with living,"[21] and consideration of another type of intervention of medical technology also lends itself to profound questioning.

Hemodialysis began as an early invention by a Dutch physician, Willem Kolff, in the 1940s, to purify the blood outside the body in stimulated solutions acting as the kidneys would, if functioning normally.[22] Renal failure and its treatment, hemodialysis, still have many problems, although the technical equipment is more sophisticated. Transplants have been tried but with little permanent success. It is estimated that the survival period of a kidney transplant patient is five years. Since the passage of Section 2991 of the Social Security Act in 1972, the federal government has paid most of the expenses of dialysis or transplantation. There has been an increase in the number of transplants from 1,460 in 1970 to 3,504 in 1976;[23] at the same time, the number of patients treated for chronic renal disease has increased from 2,456 in 1970 to 17,229 in 1976. Costs have also greatly increased—from $286 million in 1974 to an estimated $1.7 billion in 1980.[24]

Concerned, Congress is trying to contain the rapidly rising cost of the program. The cost of home dialysis ($12,480 in 1977) is significantly less than that for outpatient center treatment ($23,400 in 1977); yet, in spite of substantially similar survival rates, the percentage of persons treated in the home has decreased from 39 percent in 1971 to 13 percent in 1976.[25] Physician bias is said to be the major reason for this increasing emphasis on outpatient treatment. In contrast, Great Britain has 66 percent of these patients on home treatment.[26] With the number of persons living with this condition expected to rise to 55,000 in 1984, compared with 15,000 in 1974, it can be readily predicted that the estimated cost of $3 billion for the program will find Congress raising serious questions about the use of the various treatments and may well result in rationing care for those with the poorest prognosis for survival.[27] More important, the National Institutes of Health (NIH) spent only $13.3 million of its total 1977 budget in research on the causes of chronic renal failure and development of more efficient hemodialyzers. This research budget is less than two percent of the cost of treating those with the condition.

Like the determination of the exact moment of death or the length of time a patient should be continued on the heart-lung machine with no improving signs, dialysis, or as it has been called "life on the machine," presents an enigma. If a patient who ceased treatment was not declared a suicide by his or her life insurance carrier, then one may ponder the thought that life on the machine is not life in the sense that we usually understand it.[28]

Having grappled with the already monumental questions of what is death, perhaps it is time to confront the question of what is life? It is useful to examine the balance sheet of costs and benefits as decisions are being made to spend ever increasing amounts on research, development of new equipment, applications, and the entire battery of technological devices, and to place greater emphasis on the human qualities of life, aside from medical intervention, such as living conditions and the environment. Also worthy of consideration is the moral obligation to keep every patient alive. Should all this effort be continued and to what point?

The Office of Technology Assessment (OTA) was established by Congress in 1975. Its main purpose is "to examine current Federal policies and current medical practices to determine whether a reasonable amount of justification should be provided before costly new medical technologies and procedures are put into general use."[29] In one of its first publications, *Assessing the Efficacy and Safety of Medical Technologies,* OTA examined 17 recently developed and widely used medical devices with respect to the costs and benefits of these various technologies.[30] Of the 17, only 5 received high marks for both safety and efficacy: (1) treatment of Hodgkin's disease, (2) cast application for forearm fracture, (3) drug treatment for otitis media in children, (4) drug treatment for hypertension, and (5) amniocentesis. For the other 12, the report raised many questions. For example, it was suggested that hysterectomy may be overused, that physicians may fail to use procedures less risky than appendectomy, that a procedure such as tonsillectomy may be overused, and that the use of procedures such as coronary artery bypass surgery or mammography should be reduced for certain types of persons. The study clearly demonstrated that only with careful assessment is it possible to determine the efficacy and safety of a medical device. Unfortunately, too often in the past, medical devices were not adequately assessed before they were widely used and accepted as efficacious solely because of their widespread usage. Creation of OTA and passage of the 1976 amendments to the Food and Drug Act aim to correct this deficiency.

There is a great deal of confusion regarding the cost effectiveness of medical technology. There are those who contend that medical technologies, while high in costs, actually save lives and reduce the costs of medical care. In a study of 16 surgical contributions, Orloff found that the $21 million awarded for research by NIH in 1970 "involved a saving of $2.83 billion in 1970, a benefit-cost ratio of 134."[31] He goes on to show very favorable benefit-cost ratios for the use of medical technology on a number of specific diseases, such as acute nephritis, heart block, body surface burns, and duodenal ulcer. In reviewing changes in the cost of medical care from 1930–1975, Mushkin, Paringer, and Chen conclude that "expenditures were reduced some 17% rather than increased by the advances in medicine."[32] They recognize that their study shows a different conclusion than the studies of Fuchs, Feldstein, or Gaus.[33] However, none of the studies used comparable methodologies. The only conclusion that can be drawn at this time is that no one really knows the cost-benefit impact of medical technology or its relationship to the rapidly increasing medical costs.

IMPROVING PATIENT CARE

Essential to the improvement of patient care at any stage along the health continuum is the ability to screen and diagnose the patient's condition accurately. Many tools are at the physician's disposal: the electrocardiogram (EKG), phonocardiograph, image analysis linked with a computer, and radiology, to list a few in the area of heart ailment detection. Scanners, employing radioisotopes, are useful in identifying brain tumors and even larger areas of malignant cells. Ultrasonics, especially in predicting the condition of the fetus, have greatly enhanced obstetrical practice without any harmful side-effects to either mother or fetus.[34] Ultrasonic devices have also proved valuable in detection of and surgery for eye disease, principally because of the accuracy obtained in soft tissue and in such small areas as the eye.[35]

Thermography, the science of heat mapping, has won favor in the medical community since it was learned in the early 1960s that malignant growths could be detected as "hotter" spots and even distinguished from benign growths.[36] A useful preventive measure based on thermography has been the development of mammography, the examination of the female breast. Another predictive aspect of thermography is in determining potential stroke victims, and readings of thermograms are expected to become as routine as temperature measures on the hospital charts of patients.[37]

Monitoring patients in the hospital has become an extremely well-developed procedure, from the intensive care and coronary care units (ICUs and CCUs) with their amazing array of machinery, wires, and screens to portable bedside units that record heart, blood pressure, and brain impulses. From the sophisticated to the simple, the tools have been designed to assist the professional staff, and even patients in maintaining continuous and immediate feedback on all vital signs. In this respect, the hospitals are the legatees of the space development program, which pioneered long-range monitoring that could be adapted to nursing stations to render it effective for patient care.[38]

Surgical monitoring, using consoles that may be placed outside the operating room to reduce crowding, has produced greater efficiency while maintaining the functional aspect.[39] Numerous other mechanical/electrical/electronic devices have been engineered and are being continually revised and improved to perform ever more startling feats. But the most significant of all the devices, and the nexus of the entire technological revolution in medicine, has been the application of the computer to medical practice. One of the most intriguing is the Multiphasic Screening Laboratory (MSL), a self-contained unit that moves the patient through a variety of tests, both for checkup purposes and for hospital admissions. Here is the most striking of partnerships made eminently clear: the patient becomes an active party in the diagnosis. Guided by a technician, without any other professionals present, the patient responds to a number of tests in sequence by entering modules and communicating with the computer. Even the patient's medical history can be obtained in this manner, including a wide assortment of secondary questions that arise as a result of previous answers.[40]

As if this is not enough, a procedure known as "telediagnosis"[41] has been devised; the patient is interviewed over a television screen by a physician who may be miles away, and the teletype console carries the important information to the physician's terminal station as a "printout." The implications for this type of procedure are almost limitless, for the advantages of long-distance teleprocessing can even employ telephone lines to link a patient in a remote or underserved area with a highly sophisticated medical center many miles away. This, of course, could hold down the cost of building these extremely expensive technologically advanced centers in areas where the population does not call for them, yet avoid leaving large segments of the population completely unserved or underserved. In this way, telediagnosis could help offset the problems of medical delivery imbalance and ensure quality care for all, while staying within reasonable financial and personnel bounds. The implications for the use of the computer have been extended as far as a national health network that could provide the latest medical information, instantly, to any physician anywhere.[42] The technology now permits the transmittal of x-rays through the closed circuit telediagnosis unit, and conceivably could provide the physician with sufficient information so that "treatment" might end without the patient ever being in the presence of the physician. Here again, certain unpleasant side-effects may result from the advances of technology. In the case just described, what psychological effects would this impersonalization (or depersonalization) leave on the patient and the physician? Is the patient merely symptoms? Is the physician merely a computer with a face and voice? What of the human values of the physician-patient relationship? As patients become more sophisticated about the machinery, do they also become more engrossed in their own state of health and the maintenance thereof? Do the number and type of mechanical devices directly relate to improved well-being, or are there other mitigating factors that must be taken into account? All these questions raise issues with the decision-making process: Who is doing it, for whose interest, and with what result?

In addition to advances in technological diagnosis, there has also been progress in the field of automated therapy. Arising from the successes of the intensive care monitoring devices, burn treatment centers have been established in which the practices of physicians are programmed into a computer that analyzes the data and recommends treatment. From this trend, it has been estimated that much of a physician's routine work could be eliminated by the diagnostic-treatment aspects of computerization.[43] If such tasks are more readily transferred to associate personnel, technicians, and the computer, what will be the role of physicians in the future? Their function as it is known today may become obsolete, and patients will be left with the medical researcher or the medical caseworker, with all other functions conducted by the auxiliary sources. Is this the direction in which medicine should go? The consequences of these current issues must be carefully weighed, since their future implications have a profound impact on what may be considered desirable medical care.

SHAPING FUTURE LIVES

Up to this point, consideration has been given to the many issues involved in therapeutic and remedial intervention as well as diagnostic and preventive measures implemented by the new technology. However, population control is another area influenced by new technology. It is important to recognize that fertility control measures and abortion methods act as a population curb through individuals rather than as a planned societal effort, although the effects are felt by the entire society. As consumers become more actively involved in the total health care delivery system, it becomes increasingly urgent that they know the choices open to them in order to make decisions in their best interests.

Chemical contraception has progressed far, but there are those in the drug industry who feel that, in order to gain greater advances, new contraceptive drugs should be given "conditional approval" while still in the experimental testing stages.[44] Harmful side-effects of these drugs are not always controlled, even though efforts are made to do so; therefore, the serious question of whose interests are most at stake, consumers or drug manufacturers, must be raised.

There is considerable speculation about a new procedure of implanting a capsule of progesterone as a birth control device, effective until removed or cancelled by injection, and affording a safe, long-lasting birth control method for the user. By eliminating chances for error, increasing safety from harmful side-effects, and lessening physician visits due to contraception failure, the method would seem to be most attractive. Is this the best direction health care delivery can take in the area of managed births? Are there other possible avenues? The subject of abortion must be dealt with as well. The great question of "when does life begin?" is asked. A storm of controversy greets the subject from moral, religious, political, and even business interests. Who speaks for the public? Is there a way of protecting and preserving the public's interests among the many divergent views?

There is speculation about an effective patient-administered after-pill that can terminate a known pregnancy. The chemical prostaglandins are being investigated as potential total fertility control drugs, and some have said that, when birth control is perfected, the entire procedure will be as "silent as taking aspirin,"[45] and quite as unobtrusive and private. Is this the course to be pursued? Is the public interest best served by the independent actions of individuals, just as conception is a matter of personal choice? What will the impact be on future generations? It would seem reasonable that certain societal policies could be fashioned concerning these matters, which so profoundly affect society as a whole.

Another interesting aspect of chemical technology is the development of intravenous feeding. This provides complete nutrition to the critically ill patient and permits other procedures to be performed; however, under normal conditions, it has been found that tampering with nutritional habits has certain inherent dangers.[46] Vitamin therapies, frequently seen as fads among certain groups, are also found to be quite helpful in the management of particular medical problems, yet they are being examined by regulatory agencies in order to establish limits and controls to prevent negative effects. Is intervention by controlling agencies the most desirable end? Who is to benefit from these interventions? To what extent shall there be free choice of diet and nourishment without the constraint of regulation, or is this measure necessary to safeguard health?

Obviously, for every decision made, many alternatives are not selected; therefore, outcomes are not known for each of the alternatives. While it is generally believed by medical practitioners that the body chemistry usually does not require chemical intervention, an ever growing plethora of pills and potions are offered, although in fact the concept of "less is better" might be more appropriate. It is further understood that no drug, however beneficial, is totally without risk to the person taking it. What may save one life may cause complications in another. Tolerances vary among individuals, and it must be recognized there are no foolproof safeguards.[47] The stamp of approval by the FDA, supposed to indicate safety, is, in fact, no more than a general approval, without regard for individual difference. Penicillin and the host of antibiotics that have been developed since the 1940s to combat bacteria have proved immensely successful in controlling and managing infections.[48] However, care must be taken in prescribing and administering these potent drugs, or harmful consequences may ensue. Self-prescription and drug abuse continue to be an enigma of our times, particularly in pain relievers and mood-altering drugs, which can produce changes in the perception, sleep patterns, and even personality of the person taking them. Dealing with these problems poses questions concerning control of sales and distribution outlets.

The moral, ethical, and practical implications of imposing stricter drug controls must be weighed against their potential effect on medical progress.[49] Desirable control of resource allocation and undesirable restriction of potential benefits should be of foremost concern when all suggestions of regulating medical practices are made. Should free rein be given technological explorations? Should there be a concentration on further refinements of those already developed? Are there other areas where research time and money may be more profitably and rationally spent? Apart from determining which programs shall be encouraged, the numerous issues raised in this chapter must be confronted. What is the optimal level of health? Maximal? Minimal? Who shall decide? Who is to live? When is death? Are more facilities required? Special units? Long- or short-term care? Are certain illnesses inherently more critical than others? Do these form a *prima facie* priority? Should there be more or less control and by whom? Where shall the technological wealth be housed—within hospitals? Universities? In centralized outpatient centers? Who will determine the channels of accessibility to needed resources? Financial interests? What is to be done, given the limited funds for an untold number of demands? Are inequities in care and treatment to be tolerated in a society with so much know-how?

These questions, and others that arise not so much from a moral and ethical base, but are directly related to past patterns of health system delivery and financing, also point up the need for careful evaluation of goals and objectives in order to cope conscientiously with the fragmented cross-purpose conditions currently prevailing in the U.S. health care system.

For many years, there has been serious concern about health service and its delivery in the United States. The availability of care, its costs and quality, the way in which services are provided and administered, and the opportunity for users of health services to be appropriately involved are some of the primary targets of this concern. As far back as the 1920s, when the Committee on the Cost of Medical Care published its landmark study, most of today's critical and still unmet health problems were foreseen and predicted. Since then, emphasis and focus on U.S. health needs have blown hot and cold. The prominence given to health at the federal level of government has depended almost entirely on the special health administrations. In any case, there has been little consideration given to the broad underlying unresolved issues and to the many interrelated complex factors of health care and its delivery. In addition, many are reluctant to subscribe to any fundamental change in the traditional health care pattern; this, in conjunction with the persuasive powers of provider agents and agencies, has worked to prevent development of any effective national policy to combat the flaws in the present health care system. One conclusion is little disputed, however. In the United States, there is a crisis in health care.

Overview

The health crisis in America today afflicts all people both financially and in terms of the quality of health care they receive. The problems of the health care system were summed up in a recent editorial in *Fortune:*

> Whether poor or not, most Americans are badly served by the obsolete, overstrained medical system that has grown up around them helter-skelter, without accommodating very well to changing technology, expanding population, rising costs, or rising expectations.[50]

As already indicated, the twentieth century has brought with it dramatic advances in medical technology that have drastically altered the patterns of disease. However, the patterns of the delivery of medical care have remained static. Immunizations and antibiotics, applied within a system devoted to care of acutely ill patients and public health intervention, have all but eliminated infectious diseases as a major cause of death. Meanwhile, the rates of disability and death due to chronic diseases, the most outstanding of which are heart disease and cancer, have greatly increased. Medical science has not yet discovered specific weapons against chronic diseases, but it has made giant strides in developing knowledge about prevention, early diagnosis, and long-term management of these diseases. Yet, the health delivery system has not been adequately modified to encourage the application of this knowledge; the system is still designed to provide care for infectious diseases. The following appeared in one issue of *Scientific American:*

> In sum, the technology and medical procedures available for coping with the diseases that afflict the population have been expanded and improved, but the structure of the system that deploys the technology and resources has tended to remain fixed in a mold determined by medical and social circumstances that are quite different from those that exist today. The result is a mismatch between the technology of medicine and the apparatus that delivers care.[51]

The health service industry is now the third largest enterprise in America, employing 5.1 million persons in over 700 job titles as of 1976.[52] Expenditures for health services during 1978 amounted to $192.4 billion, or $863 per person. This represented 9.1 percent of the gross national product, up from 4.5 percent in 1950, 5.3 percent in 1960, and 7.5 percent in 1970. Of the increase in health expenditures between 1969 and 1978, 63 percent could be attributed to inflation, 7 percent to population increase, and 30 percent to intensity of use, e.g., greater number of inpatient days, greater use of high-cost medical technology, and increased number of medical staff per inpatient. The federal government spent $43.3 billion on Medicare and Medicaid benefits in 1978.[53] Despite the huge amounts of money currently being poured into the health system and the stunning technological developments that the health industry has provided, the fact remains that a great number of people in the United States, particularly the poor, minority groups, and the elderly, fail to receive adequate health services. The following examples can be cited:

- In 1971, the Census Bureau reported that the life expectancy for black males decreased between 1960 and 1968, while for white males, life expectancy increased. The infant mortality rate and the maternal death rate among blacks continues to be three times as great as it is for whites. For all Americans, there are 13 countries in the world with lower infant mortality rates.[54]
- On the average, the elderly must live on less than one-half the income available to young couples or a single person, yet their medical expenditures are six times that of a youth, and two and one-half times that of a person between the ages of 19 and 64.[55]
- A poor child in the United States is three times more likely to be mentally retarded, fifteen times more likely to be defective at birth, and three times more likely to be prematurely born than children of higher income families.[56]

The unmet health care needs in the United States are not limited solely to these groups. Soaring costs have forced many middle-class Americans into the ranks of the medically indigent. Even many of those who are fortunate enough to have adequate health insurance are unable to gain access to needed care because of the uneven distribution of health personnel and facilities. (For example, in some neighborhoods in New York City, there is less than one physician in private practice to serve each 12,000 residents.) Absence of early preventive care, unnecessary surgery, and poor quality medicine, as evidenced from comparisons of U.S. health indexes with those of other industrialized (and some less industrialized) countries, occurs among all income groups.

The cause of these myriad interconnected problems can be traced to three forces that have changed the nature of the delivery of health services in the United States: (1) the technology of medicine, (2) the character of the population, and (3) the nature of U.S. disease problems. It can be shown that, to a large degree, the conflict among these forces of change, and the present organization of health resources has accounted for the problems that affect the delivery of service, the quality of care, the high cost of medical care, and other manifestations of the "health crisis." In effect, the cause of the problem is that ". . . we persist in our old ways, fail to restructure our health services to meet the new situation, and try to solve the health problems of the latter half of the 20th century with the social machinery inherited from the 19th century."[57]

Although the effects of medical technology are profound in terms of the current state of medicine and what it is capable of doing, equally important are its effects on the health industry by, for example, increasing specialization and the division of labor. In addition, the advances in medical science have caused changes in the character of the population: the long-term decline in the birth rate, the lowering of mortality in the early years of life, and the lengthening of the life span due to medical advances all have shifted the age composition of the American population to one with a greater proportion of older people. The combination of an older, possibly more illness-prone population and a general population that is more highly educated to the availability and use of health services results in a population increasingly demanding a greater quantity of health services.

Health Care Resources

The changes in medical technology, the population characteristics, and the nature of disease have been thrust on a system that operates in response to market forces of supply and demand. In this respect, single practicing physicians may be seen as medical entrepreneurs who sell their services on the open market as any other small businesspeople. Likewise, the voluntary hospital limits its services to those who are able to pay either through private or public sources. This market-oriented system of services is derived from an earlier time when the health enterprise was simpler and smaller. When more resources, hospitals, and facilities were needed, the delivery of health services grew, largely by accretion, without a necessary restructuring of organization. Thus, this piecemeal approach of growth, based on unstructured market responses to medical needs and coupled with the increases in demand for medical services due to the new medical technology, has led to serious maldistribution of health care resources (both personnel and facilities) in terms of need.

Physicians, selling their medical services on the open market, tend to practice in those communities that can best afford their services, resulting in large disparities in the geographical location of resources, both on a national level and within individual communities. In a study conducted by the American Medical Association (AMA),[58] figures showed that the distribution of medical services in various sections of the United States was closely linked to the affluence and appeal the population segments had to physicians. By comparing data for six states with high per capita and household incomes with data for an equal number of states with low incomes, it was found that the more affluent states averaged 160 practicing physicians per 100,000 population, or almost double the 87 physicians per 100,000 population in the less affluent states, not including physicians employed by the federal government. In addition, large metropolitan areas average far better than nonmetropolitan or rural areas in attracting physicians; however, poverty-stricken areas of the cities are unable to attract the services of private physicians. Where physicians do practice in ghetto areas, they tend to be older and more poorly trained than those practicing in more affluent areas.

Distributional problems in the type of medical practice (specialists versus general practitioners) are also inherent in the market-oriented medical system. The boom in medical technology has brought a concomitant increase in the number of physicians who specialize. The consequence of medical specialization is that, whereas there has been little change in the physicians per population rates, there has been a decline in the number of physicians in general practice. For example, in 1963, there were 34.4 general practitioners per 100,000 population, declining to 25.1 in 1975, although there was a 16 percent increase in the number of active physicians during this period.[59] On the other hand, there is a general surplus of medical specialists. During this 1963 to 1975 period, there has been an increase in specialists in internal medicine (60 percent), pediatrics (51 percent), obstetrics/gynecology (26 percent), and surgical specialties (26 percent.[60] Although there is an acknowledged shortage of primary care physicians, the increase in the number of internists and pediatricians has compensated somewhat for the reduction in the number of family physicians.

It is this decline in the number of primary care physicians that has left millions of people in urban areas without a family physician and, thus, dependent on hospital emergency rooms and clinics for their care. Physicians who provide primary care are in short supply because specialties frequently offer greater rewards in terms of prestige, self-esteem, and money. The imbalance between the number of primary physicians and specialists may also have other complicating effects: there is some evidence to show that an excess of some specialists, e.g., surgeons, may lead to excessive use of some treatments, e.g., unnecessary surgery.

The improper management and utilization of health care resources, in particular of personnel resources, is another contributor to the health care crisis. Health care represents one of the nation's most rapidly growing fields of employment, totaling 1.7 million in 1970 and rising to 5.1 million in 1976.[61] Despite this increase, poor distribution, coupled with inadequate utilization, training, and organization, aggravates the shortages of personnel in one area, while causing surpluses in others.

There is growing recognition that the shortage of active physicians may be coming to an end. It is estimated that the number of active practitioners will rise from approximately 444,000 in 1980 to approximately 594,000 in 1990,[62] which will be more than enough physicians to meet the basic needs of the U.S. population. While there may be enough physicians to meet overall need, two issues remain to be solved. The first is the poor geographical distribution of physicians. As of 1977, 2,187 shortage areas had been identified in the United States. These areas required an estimated 18,000 physicians to meet their basic needs.[63] While part of this shortage has been made up in the past by the utilization of foreign medical graduates, the passage of the Health Professionals Educational Assistance Act of 1976 has reduced the number of foreign medical graduates permitted to practice in the United States. It is anticipated that, when the act is fully implemented, less than 50 percent of the present number of foreign medical graduates will be eligible to become a part of the U.S. active practitioner supply. While the increased number of American medical graduates may partially compensate for this reduction, certain states, such as New Jersey and New York, that have depended to a great degree on foreign medical graduates and certain types of institutions, such as mental hospitals and public-supported hospitals, may find it difficult to replace this source of medical practitioners.[64] However, federal policy is to increase the number of slots in the National Health Service Corps and promote the utilization of physician's assistants to meet medical needs in shortage areas.

A second issue that the increase in the number of active medical practitioners may not solve is the imbalance between general, or family, physicians and specialists. As noted earlier, the percentage of general practitioners among active physicians has declined. The Health Professionals Educational Assistance Act of 1976 has as one of its major goals to increase the percentage of medical graduate students in primary care, especially family medicine, to 50 percent in 1980. Medical schools dependent on federal funding have reluctantly accepted the federal goal. However, a study of first year residents showed that 9 percent of the students in first year residencies in internal medicine were not in the program in the second year. Further, a large percentage of these students were specializing in various areas of internal medicine. A similar phenomenon was observed among pediatrics residents. Thus, while on the surface medical schools appear to be meeting their federal obligations, in the long run there may be no real change in the emphasis on medical specialties.[65]

The discussion of the problems in health care resources would be incomplete without mentioning the serious problem of misuse of existing health care facilities. In recent years, the number of general hospital beds in the nation has increased at a greater rate than the population itself. Between 1960 and 1976, the ratio of beds per 1,000 population rose from 3.6 to 4.6, an increase of 28 percent in the face of increasing doubt regarding the justification for hospital expansion.[66] A national standard of 4 beds per 1,000 population in 1978 has now brought a halt to bed expansion in most regions of the United States.

In every study of facilities utilization, varying percentages of patients who should be using more appropriate facilities are found. Patients who could be treated in physicians' offices or are able to receive x-ray or other laboratory services from ambulatory care facilities are found occupying hospital beds instead. Not only does this practice of unnecessary hospitalization translate into high medical costs, but also it results in a tremendous waste of facilities that could be used to better advantage. In addition to indicating that too many patients are hospitalized unnecessarily, studies also show that those patients who are hospitalized tend to stay longer than the time needed for complete recuperation from their illnesses. It has been found that hospitalization is far less frequently used in better organized systems. Health maintenance organizations (HMOs) in particular have been found to be more efficient users of health resources. Abernethy and Pearson noted that "after adjusting for age, sex and other factors, HMOs use 30 to 50 percent fewer hospital days, fewer physicians, and provide health care at a cost of 10 to 30 percent less than the traditional fee-for-service system."[67] This has been accomplished with no measurable difference in health outcome between the two systems.

The prevalence of overhospitalization in the United States can be traced to the method by which medical care is currently financed. The extensive use of third party mechanisms, such as Blue Cross, Blue Shield, Medicare, Medicaid, and private insurance programs, has resulted in a decreased amount of out-of-pocket payment for the patient. After a designated deductible is paid by the patient, the third party mechanism will continue to pay the bill until such time as treatment is ended. Therefore, there is no real incentive to cut costs by remaining in the hospital for a shorter period of time. Both the patient and the physician, who usually determines the patient's length of stay in the hospital, realize this. In addition, there is no incentive to use outpatient care services or services provided in the physician's office, services usually less expensive than hospitalization, simply because, in most cases, insurance does not cover them. Insurance does

.cover inhospital treatment and services rendered in the hospital. Thus, when routine diagnostic testing is needed, more likely than not it will be performed in the hospital. Consequently, a major thrust to the overutilization and misappropriation of hospital facilities stems directly from the financial payment mechanism for medical care. In many cases, patients could be equally well cared for in extended care facilities, such as nursing homes, following hospitalization, in lieu of continued hospitalization. There are also patients in nursing homes who could be in residential facilities or boarding homes or who would benefit both physically and mentally from services delivered to them in their own homes. Many times, the care rendered would be equal to the care given in hospitals or more appropriate for the patient's condition. Viable alternatives and, in many cases, less expensive alternatives would be a better use of health care resources than costly hospitalization. With PL 92-603, Congress established the Professional Standards Review Organization (PSRO) to ensure that federally funded programs such as Medicare and Medicaid were used in an efficient and effective manner. PSROs were mandated to reduce lengths of stay in hospitals, to disapprove payment for unnecessary hospitalization, and to ensure a minimum quality of medical care. Although PSROs are still rather young organizations, the Health Care Financing Administration recently evaluated 108 active PSROs and their 1977 activities. Comparing these PSROs with 81 inactive PSROs, it found no statistical difference in inpatient hospital utilization. However, it did find significant reductions in hospitalization in the Northeast and North Central regions of the United States, an actual increase in the South, and a slight decrease in the West. Overall, it was estimated that the reductions saved about 940,000 days of Medicare-sponsored hospital days.[68] Thus, while the program cannot be considered a major success in cost containment at this point, it has the potential for inducing major reductions in unnecessary hospitalization in the future. Furthermore, it can be seen that health care resources are poorly utilized from a survey of hospitals that maintain expensive facilities so rarely used they fail to warrant the initial expense or continued funding for their upkeep. In 1967, 31 percent of the hospitals that had open heart surgery facilities had not used them for a year.[69] In addition to the cost of maintaining such facilities and the staff needed for their operation, there is a risk to the patient that these underutilized facilities will have deteriorated in quality by the time they are used. Recognizing this as a major quality and cost problem for hospitals, the Department of Health, Education, and Welfare (HEW) approved a set of national guidelines for health planning in 1978 that set standards for costly, infrequently used hospital services as a way of rationing their future use. Standards were set for obstetrical, neonatal, and pediatric inpatient services; open heart surgery units; cardiac catheterization units; radiation therapy treatment; CAT scanners; end-stage renal disease units; and the supply of hospital beds.[70]

Organization of Services

The mismanagement of resources is partly a function of the fragmented manner in which resources are organized for the delivery of health services. Many believe that there is a severe need for reorganization and rationalization of the delivery system because the present one is a throwback to another generation when the concept and treatment of medical disorders was different. In order to ensure comprehensive care to the entire population at the point of actual delivery of service and reduce the chances of wrongly allocating and utilizing resources, there must be a change in the organizational structure of the system to ensure that the capability, responsibility, and authority exist to accomplish these goals.

The system of health care has been described by some as a "no system system,"[71] or as a "cottage industry of small entrepreneurs [physicians]."[72] Characterizing the system of health care as a cottage industry should not be taken to imply

> that the industry has spurned the development and use of sophisticated technology and scientific knowledge or that it relies solely on the uneven skills of individual craftsmen who learn their "trade" through trial and error. What is meant is that unlike other industries that have undergone organizational, as well as technological revolution, the organizational structure of the health industry in essence retains its preindustrial format, relying to a large extent, on small, independent firms."[73]

In economic terms, the health care delivery system has been characterized as "the epitome of the *laissez-faire* era and the greatest of oligopolies."[74]

Most medical care is performed today by the solo practitioner, or the physician who is in practice alone. The solo practitioner, although backed by consultation with other physicians, by laboratories, and often by a hospital, operates so small an enterprise that its very size may ultimately mitigate against efficiency. It has been found that, until a certain scale of operation is reached, it is difficult to utilize scarce medical and technological skills to their best advantage. Thus, the solo practitioner ends up wasting a great deal of skill on tasks that do not require his or her expertise. This decrease in efficiency can severely reduce the physician's ability to provide quality care to suit the varied needs of the patient population. More important, however, one report has concluded that

> the linkages among physicians are loosely structured, inconvenient to many patients, susceptible to episodic rather than continuous care, very often inefficient and expensive, and relatively difficult to maintain. Moreover, the burdens upon the average physician are often so great that they limit his time and narrow his perspective in keeping abreast of both medical advances and social change.[75]

Solo practice medicine has had its very distinct merits in providing personal care to those in need. However, this form of medical practice developed at a time when illness was episodic and could be managed by the single family physician. Solo practice is no longer feasible, either economically or as a source for effective comprehensive medical care, because of the growing incidence of chronic disease, the overwhelming movement toward specialization, the greater need to manage medical practice, and the need and desire for a health care system that goes beyond mere medical attendance. By requiring the patient to go to different physicians and hospital facilities, sometimes for each disease or episode (leading to great variations in the quality and level of care rendered), the "nonsystem" of medical care delivery promulgates a pattern of health care that can be characterized as fragmented and lacking integration and coordination, failing to deliver the comprehensive and preventive care now needed.

Rapid medical technological growth has placed the hospital in a strategic position in health care delivery, causing a serious imbalance in the traditional organization of health services. A technological gap has developed and is widening between the care provided in physicians' offices and the care performed in hospitals by highly specialized medical personnel using complex technical equipment. This disparity is fostered further by the lack of adequate and overall linkages between medical groups and solo physicians with general hospitals to create a single, integrated health facility system. The present organization of the delivery system is also fragmented by the growing disparity between smaller hospitals unable to afford highly specialized personnel and equipment and lacking access to the new medical knowledge and techniques, and the larger and, in most cases, university-based teaching hospitals financially able to provide advanced equipment and specialized staff. Planning and coordination of services have been hampered by this "nonsystem" of autonomous and competitive medical facilities, resulting primarily in the wasteful duplication of services with its negative effects of increased costs and lower quality of care. The fragmented system of care is also compounded by the existence of two distinct hospital systems in most parts of the United States, private hospitals and "charity" hospitals, inevitably resulting in a dual quality system of care.

Financing System

When the pattern of financing mechanisms for health care is examined, the most striking observation is that the present form of financing was instituted at a time when the financing problems were different from those in today's health care economy. The serious nature of the problem is evident when one considers the role the financing mechanism plays in the overall organization of services and on the ability of consumers to receive and pay for needed medical care. Deficiencies in the financing mechanism have been influential in denying access to much needed care for many Americans and for reinforcing the existing highly inefficient system of delivering medical services. An overview of the financial flow through the system and how care is presently financed serve to point to the serious flaws of the mechanism.

In fiscal year 1977, aggregate national health expenditures, which include government expenditures both for construction or improvement of physical facilities and for medical research, were $169.9 billion. Of that amount, $149 billion was spent for personal health care (health services for the direct benefit of the individual, i.e., hospital care, physicians' services), or 87 percent of all health expenditures in 1977. Medical care is financed both publicly and privately, but the private share has been the larger by far. Even with the advent of more publicly financed medical care programs, such as Medicare and Medicaid, private sources still accounted for 59 percent of the total health expenditures in fiscal year 1977 and 60 percent of the personal health expenditures.[76]

Two sources provide the income flow for the health system. Individuals and families who pay directly for service also pay indirectly through taxes to federal, state, and local governments, health insurance, and, to a lesser extent, by contributions to charities. The other income source is the employer, who pays the employees' share of payroll taxes, makes contributions for health insurance premiums, and pays corporate income taxes. The income sources are funneled to government and private financial intermediaries who are private insurers, government, and other third parties who receive the funds from these two income sources and purchase, or reimburse individuals who purchase, health services. Private and public insurance has become the major form of financing medical care, accounting for $98.5 billion of the $149 billion spent for personal health care.[77]

It certainly can be stated that insurance coverage has, at the public and private levels, helped to provide for the consumers' need for protection. Statistics show that about 78 percent of the population under the age of 65 have some form of private insurance protection, mainly for hospital and surgical coverage; 77 percent of those working (ages 19 to 64) are protected through insurance plans; 96 percent of those over 65 have publicly supported insurance coverage.[78]

Actually, the health care finance system has not functioned well in distributing the burden of expenditures among individuals. Where most people do have some form of health insurance, there are serious gaps in the health insurance system that leave many with no protection at all or with inadequate protection against certain expenses. The following indicates the nature of the problem in 1977:

- The uninsured were concentrated among the poor. Twenty-two percent of people with family incomes of less than $3,000 and 21 percent in families with incomes of $3,000 to $5,000 were uninsured.
- Sixteen percent of nonwhites were uninsured, compared with ten percent of all whites.[79]
- Among the categories of people less often insured were the unmarried (24 percent were not insured), the widowed (29 percent), the divorced (30 percent), and the separated (49 percent).
- People with various kinds of disabilities were also often uninsured. Among those limited in some degree by disability in pursuit of their major activity, 30 percent of those under 65 were not insured. Among those unable to carry on their major activity, as many as 51 percent were uninsured.
- The uninsured were also often to be found among the unemployed. In many instances, even brief periods of unemployment resulted in a loss of protection, despite many efforts to extend coverage during interruptions of work and sustained unemployment.
- Occupations in which coverage is relatively limited include service workers (26 percent) and farm workers (52 percent).[80]

In addition, as a result of this method of payment, there have been serious dislocative effects on the actual services that are rendered, as well as on the organization of medical services. Health insurance provides relatively good coverage for inpatient care and for surgery, yet it excludes equally important out-of-hospital services and limits access to them.

Public and private financing of health care has also reinforced the existing system of delivery, including its defects. Medicaid and Medicare, both public insurance programs, were designed by Congress to be built into the existing delivery system. The result, as time has shown, was disastrous, since the cost to those people the program was to have benefited was increased. One reason for this was that the usual mode of service delivery helped to produce a financing response that totally lacked cost control measures and failed to restrain the use of high-cost facilities and procedures. It was economically favorable for both patient and physician to utilize hospital services, since those services were covered; thus, less expensive alternatives, which were not insured benefits, went underutilized.

The financial mechanism has also effectively modified the behavior of the patient and the provider in the health care market. Insurance does not always completely cover bills for medical service; however, it does reduce the price the consumer must pay. This, in effect, tends to increase demand for services, particularly those covered by the insurance program. (This percentage reimbursement for the cost of care is the largest for hospital and surgical services, and the least or nonexistent for preventive or ambulatory services.) Increased demand, in many cases, is the result of the provider's decision that medical care is needed for the consumer and is not initiated by the consumer personally. In an economic sense, increased demand results in increased prices, and increased demand for certain types of medical service has been spurred by insurance coverage that has added to health care costs rather than offset them. An indication of how health coverage has increased utilization of services and costs is seen from the following findings of the Governor's Steering Committee on Social Problems on Health and Hospital Services and Costs:

> Most so-called health insurance is, in effect, "sickness" insurance, providing coverages mainly for in-patient hospital care, the costliest ingredient in the system, when, in fact, much care could be given equally well on a fairly less expensive ambulatory basis. The Health Insurance industry itself estimates that almost 20% of all surgery performed in a hospital could be performed equally well in a doctor's office or an out-patient clinic—and probably would be if it were covered by insurance. It has been estimated that about 25% of all hospital admissions are essentially for "insurance" purposes.[81]

Between fiscal years 1965 and 1977, private insurance benefits increased from $8.7 to $40.4 billion, and public expenditures on personal health care rose from $9 to $58 billion. On the other hand, direct individual payments also rose from $14.9 to $46.6 billion. Of this total increase between the years 1965 and 1977, 7 percent is attributed to population growth and 30 percent to increased per capita utilization of care, combined with the rising level and scope of provided services as a result of technological and medical advances. The remaining 63 percent resulted from price increases.[82]

Cost of Medical Services

One of the more deleterious aspects of the crisis of medical care is its high cost, making it inaccessible to the near poor and a growing number of middle income families. Inflationary medical costs account for more than 75 percent of the increase in hospital care expenditures and nearly 70 percent of the increase for physicians' services.[83] While it is true that, since World War II, both the Consumer Price Index and its medical care component have been steadily rising, indicating a general trend toward overall inflation, medical care prices have risen far more rapidly than the Consumer Price Index, which reflects all consumer items. In the 1960s, hospital charges rose four times as fast as other items in the Consumer Price Index, and physicians' fees rose two times the rate. During the years 1966 to 1970, when all consumer items rose 19.7 percent, costs of overall medical care, particularly hospital charges and physicians' charges, rose 29.1 percent, 71.3 percent, and 30 percent, respectively. Hospital care and physicians' services are, therefore, primary contributors to the inflation of medical costs. This tendency continued during most of the 1970s.

Rapidly accelerating medical care prices affect every American who at some time may have to pay for medical services. While it is true that Americans with moderate to low incomes and those who require medical attention because of advanced age and severe disabilities are more drastically affected by excessive increases in medical prices, such increases are not uniquely problems of the poor, aged, or chronically ill. Ultimately, they affect all those who must decide either to delay, curb, or forego completely, needed medical attention because of its prohibitive cost.

There are several reasons for the rising costs of medical care: the impact of new demands for the services of a limited number of practitioners; the failure to develop and emphasize less costly but equally effective services and facilities as alternatives to the use of expensive hospital facilities; the failure to plan and coordinate services, resulting in unnecessary duplication of services and underutilization of more complex services; and most important, the inefficient use of high-cost hospital services. These problems may be eliminated, although not easily, through a comprehensive national policy.

Other, more complex causes of the inflationary cycle of medical costs are not easily correctable, since they are both inevitable and necessary to the provision of more effective services. Costs are a function of technology. Thus, the use of more complex medical technological equipment and the concomitant need for more highly trained and specialized personnel will continue to increase the costs of care. An increasing proportion of the aged in the population and the greater incidences of long-term and, therefore, expensive chronic illnesses will also serve to increase the costs of providing medical care. Also, medical costs will continue to rise because of nonmedical phenomena. Some alternative forms that may tend to lower health care costs are prohibited by law. For instance, in some states, it is illegal to form a group practice, although this is changing, and often physicians and dentists are prohibited from using trained aides and assistants to their highest capabilities. The nature of the medical "market" also tends to discourage cost containment, since the health care market is not the same as a market for commercial products. In the medical market, which is not a purely competitive market system, a great deal of information is hidden from consumers because not only are they unable to pass judgment on the quality or kind of care they receive but also they are not in the position, especially at times of emergency, to shop around for the best physician and quality of service at the best price—all of which translates into higher and higher costs. Finally, it is now widely recognized that the prevailing methods of reimbursing providers under health insurance reduces the incentives to contain costs, because, increasingly, one party sets prices for services, a second receives them, and a third pays for them. The result is that no one really is concerned about rising prices when everyone knows that the bill will inevitably be paid. While medical prices are becoming more and more prohibitive, effectively eliminating increasing numbers of people from receipt of care, little has been done to deal adequately with this complex problem.

Medical (and Dental) Education

Another manifestation of the medical care crisis is that the majority of medical and dental schools are verging on financial insolvency. While most institutions of higher learning have been hard hit as a result of the steadily rising costs of education, the financial woes of the schools committed to providing highly technical medical and dental educations have been still greater. Two major reasons for this are (1) the greater dependence on expensive techniques, supplies, and machinery for teaching purposes; and (2) the larger disparity between the actual costs of education per student and the amount charged for tuition (the gap between costs and tuition are, in some cases, as high as $20,000 per student per year, for which the school must absorb the difference). These reasons, among others, make medical and dental education an increasingly expensive proposition for schools. Compounding this already grave situation, the government presently is seeking to decrease substantially the amount of assistance to medical and dental schools, an action that will force the schools either to diminish the size of classes or to increase the tuition to even greater heights, a move that will effectively limit the number of students able to afford medical and dental educations.

The problems discovered in analyzing the U.S. medical and dental education systems are not simply that available personnel cannot meet the demand for services and that prospects for increasing these numbers are dimming; nor do they only concern the financial problems of the schools, although these are certainly important problems. There are gaps in the emphasis of medical and dental school educations that make it difficult to separate the reasons for the crisis in health care from what is being taught and emphasized in the curricula. "The medical and health care professional education system has not been adequately responsive to the needs of our society, although there are new concrete and specific signs of awareness that major change is necessary."[84]

It has been seen that some of the major unmet needs in the health care system revolve around the skewed distribution of medical professionals and resources in favor of research and specialization of service. While there is an ever expanding need for primary care physicians to service a growing population, the trend has been for greater numbers of physicians to turn to noncommunity-related medical practice. Most personnel studies report that the United States is short of physicians, principally primary care or general practitioners, and medical schools have made some effort to produce a different mix of students. "Between 1965 and 1970, medical school enrollment per class increased from 9,200 students to slightly over 10,000, an increment of 900 in six years. [But], of 8,367 medical school graduates last year (1970), only about 2 percent (187 students) became general practitioners. The rest took specialty training or entered research or other areas."[85] From 1968 to 1974, there was a definite growth in the number of medical graduates choosing residencies in one of the primary care areas (general practice, family practice, internal medicine, or pediatrics). The percentage of graduates choosing primary care residencies increased from 29.5 to 31 percent during this period, with the major increase coming in general or family practice, growing from 2 to 7.2 percent. On the other hand, medical graduates choosing surgical specialties fell from 37 to 31.1 percent between 1968 and 1974. With the passage of the Health Professions Educational Assistance Act of 1976, this trend is guaranteed to be emphasized and continued.[86]

However, as noted previously in this chapter, it is not clear whether these changes presage real or surface improvements in the proportion of primary to specialty care physicians. Many argue that medical schools have been the cause of this trend toward specialization and that they have resisted changing their current research-oriented curriculum and training emphasis to one of community services. In addition, health professionals have defined health and medical care in highly restrictive terms. Curricula tend to emhasize the treatment of the more obscure (but probably more interesting) and specialized medical disorders at the expense of needed emphasis on preventive medicine and more community-related diseases. Some disorders, such as mental health, drug abuse, and alcoholism, although accounting for very significant problems, have received very little attention in medical school curricula. Ultimately, the extent to which the nation's health care problems will be met and solved will depend on the willingness and ability of medical schools to train their students adequately and to offer them the curricula necessary to take on their new roles in providing quality health care services for all.

Consumer Responsibility and Public Participation

There is a growing national concern for consumer participation in matters relating to the provision of health, education, and welfare services, and in community development. With the greater emphasis on decentralization of service delivery, the concept that consumer representatives should share in local decision making is becoming accepted by many people—particularly those in the public sector. However, one of the problems with this concept is the need to define a middle ground position of community responsibility that merges private initiative with public accessibility.

The reason that consumer participation is necessary at all touches on several important dysfunctional areas of development within the health care industry.

> The health field, as presently constituted, lacks the economic incentives or accountability of the market place and its discipline of consumer choice. Health care exists in a "no-man's-land" where the ultimate buyer, the patient, does not make the decisions as to whether or not to purchase services, nor does he have the opportunity to influence the purchasing power of his health care dollar by having available alternatives. The patient is therefore seeking avenues of influence over the organization and function of the health care system."[87]

The rationale for consumer involvement in decisions concerning the receipt of health care is, therefore, a strong one. Not only is consumer participation an opportunity for patients to retrieve the bargaining power dissipated through third party payment mechanisms, but also to ensure that the services and care provided will be of high quality, at a reasonable cost, and relevant and responsive to the needs of those for whom they are intended. Community participation in health services also serves to raise the consciousness of people regarding the definition of good health care and how to get it.

More Rational Health Care Services

In recent years, health care has been moving in many directions at once, prompted by the development of new medical inventions and techniques; the advent of federal programs involved with special problems, such as heart, cancer, child health, and migrant workers; and the creation of new funding sources through Titles XVIII and XIX of the Social Security Act. Also contributing to the confusion are the increased benefits won in union contracts and the willingness on the part of the general public to experiment with new forms of health delivery through group practices, prepaid group health insurance, ambulatory care clinics for the urban poor, and mobile medical vans that bring services to the client. The first half of the 1960s saw the beginning of this thrust. Policy planners laboring to improve health delivery and fiscal systems became overwhelmed. The many changes fomented many old questions and raised some new questions. The confusion created an awareness for a much needed rational approach to health care.

Originally, it was thought that the Regional Medical Program (RMP) could serve such a planning purpose. However, the resultant legislation weakened the intent to provide for comprehensive regional planning that could deal with the new medical knowledge and also develop a new health planning and delivery system. Something more was required, something that could provide a link between the political structures of the established health components from which the RMP had been divorced.[88]

As counterpoint to RMP, the Comprehensive Health Service Amendments Act of 1966 (PL 89-749), along with its Partnership for Health Amendments of 1967 (PL 90-174) represented a more orthodox but powerful approach in coordinating the many existing health services and institutions into an integrated system "to assure comprehensive health services of high quality for every person."[89]

The objectives were clear-cut:

1. "to encourage the states to develop and carry out comprehensive health planning both for the state as a whole and within the regional and local areas."[90]
2. to contain or reduce the rapidly escalating costs that have not returned benefits proportional to their increased expenditures.

Improved efficiency would be sought through comprehensive health planning, while improved services would be provided to people at the same or lower cost. Both efficiency and effectiveness of programs were emphasized.

How was this to be done? First, a serious constraint was placed upon the agencies that were to be established to meet these goals. They were not to interfere "with existing patterns of private professional practice of medicine, dentistry, and related healing arts."[91] Since the act mandated a partnership of the producers, whose practice was not to be interfered with, and a majority of consumers of those services, it was felt that a radical approach to health care was not as important as integrating and coordinating the existing service institutions. However, the concept of involving a majority of consumers was considered a major departure from tradition. This was due to two factors. The first was the increasing militancy and aggressive behavior of the black and Spanish-speaking leaders who demanded and were granted active policy-making roles in community mental health, as well as antipoverty and model cities programs. Involving them in comprehensive health planning (CHP) was merely an extension of this accepted policy on the part of the Kennedy and Johnson administrations. The second factor was the strong endorsement by the National Commission on Community Health Services for community participation.[92] When it became evident that the majority of new health planning agencies would be private, nonprofit organizations, the 1967 amendment was passed, calling for the inclusion of local government representatives on the health planning boards. Thus, the first step was to ensure the participation of these three constituencies.

The second step was to designate a statewide body as the health planning agency. Because this was Section 314(a) of the legislation, the statewide agencies became known as "A" agencies. The state agencies were given the responsibility for formulating a state plan for current and future health needs of their populations. These plans had to be submitted to and approved by the secretary of HEW before they could be implemented and funds could be authorized.

Since the mandate called for planning programs with consumers and providers who were closest to the people who use health services, it seemed logical that the states be divided into regions or areawide jurisdictions, each with its own health planning body. These agencies, known as the "B" agencies after their authorization in Section 314(b), were to have boundaries drawn with final approval by the state "A" agency and to receive up to 75 percent federal funds for developing, coordinating, and evaluating areawide plans. The agencies could be nonprofit, private, or public. About 75 percent eventually developed as nonprofit, private agencies, patterned after existing health and hospital areawide health facilities agencies, many of which became the "B" agencies for their areas.

While the "B" agencies in a sense were formed and approved by the state "A" agencies, there were no clear-cut relationships stated in the law to determine what the responsibilities and authority of the "B" agency were. This was a recognition on the part of congressional lawmakers that the relationship was political and, consequently, would vary for each state, based on past relationships between the local communities and the state. However, it was clear that the "A" agency had to approve the areawide plans before they could be submitted to Washington for federal assistance.

A further recognition of the political characteristic of planning was shown by the passage of a law authorizing two types of grants for areawide "B" agencies. The first was a grant to assist local health leaders in identifying and designating the appropriate agency to assume and develop the CHP role. The federal government recognized that competing groups existed within an area and that time was required to work out delicate relationships before real planning would be possible. In view of the fact that "B" agencies were to have very little authority to take action and impose sanctions on resistant health providers and other potentially recalcitrant people, maximum emphasis was to be placed on earning goodwill and encouraging the cooperation of all key personnel and their constituents concerned with health services. The second type of grant was to be awarded to "B" agencies created with minimal or no problems. These were to be given grants to begin planning the services and facilities needed and to consider alternate ways of integrating health delivery components into a coordinated system.

The third step in developing competent planning agencies was the authorization by the act of grants to public or nonprofit private institutions or universities for the training of health planning professionals and citizen board members in the knowledge and functions of a comprehensive health planning agency (CHPA). This was necessary because there were few professionally trained health planners who had a broad and comprehensive view of planning health services. The health and hospital planning facility agencies were quite competent in planning for the "bricks and mortar," and many of the public health trained professionals were equally adept at planning health services. But there were few who understood the tools and methodologies for planning both the facilities and the program services or who could take into account the environmental, economic, social, and demographic factors related to the communities. Likewise, the board members of the "B" agencies had a wide variety of backgrounds and knowledge. Training them to understand their responsibilities and to develop a common conceptual base for comprehensive planning was important for a meeting of the minds between staff and board. Funds were authorized under Section 314(c) for these training purposes.

Section 314(d) was a forerunner or demonstration of the current emphasis on revenue sharing. Block grants were given to state health and state mental health agencies for planning, training, and implementation costs in developing limited health programs. These were authorized, based on the acceptance of a state health plan, by the secretary of HEW.

Finally, Section 314(e) authorized federal grants for training, broadening, and initiating new services to public or nonprofit private agencies. While the sums of money were limited, they were made available as incentives to local agencies to try new directions in the provision of health services or different delivery systems. Also, it was hoped that this would give some added power to the "B" agencies in securing the cooperation of the numerous autonomous health service agencies.

The Partnership for Health Act began as a new attempt at bringing together the many strands of categorically funded programs and research that the federal government had financed over the years in order to raise the quality of health care. In the process of sitting together, the consumers, providers, and government officials would be in a position to confront the many nagging problems noted earlier in this chapter and to make a concerted attempt at finding solutions. A later document prepared by the CHPA outlined the process by which this planning meeting of the minds could take place. It recommended analyzing the health resources, needs, and problems of the regions; selecting goals and priorities for solving these problems; developing both current and long-range policy and action recommendations; and, finally, developing criteria for evaluating the results.[93]

The Partnership for Health Act was a major breakthrough in congressional efforts to foster truly comprehensive health planning. The vagueness in the act concerning what could be expected by the partners and their planners, their limited authority to carry out their major responsibilities, the wariness of providers toward their new consumer partners, uncertain funding, and the inability to overcome the initial political problems caused by the union of three formerly antagonistic forces were instrumental in

58   HEALTH PLANNING

preventing most of the CHP regional and state agencies from carrying out their mission. After eight years, Congress reviewed what had happened and decided to modernize the CHP planning model. The National Health Planning and Resources Development Act of 1974 (PL 93-641) was the product. This far-reaching health planning law will be discussed in detail in the following chapter. In one way or another, Congress hoped that its new creation would be able to deal more effectively with the problems of health care.

NOTES

1. Louis Lasagna, *Life, Death and the Doctor* (New York: Alfred A. Knopf, 1968), p. 3.

2. Kenneth Vaux, ed., *Who Shall Live?* (Philadelphia: Fortress Press, 1970), p. 107.

3. Alvin Toffler, *Future Shock* (New York: Bantam Books, 1971).

4. Gerald Leach, *The Biocrats* (Harmondsworth, England: Penguin Books, 1972), p. 16.

5. Norman V. Carlisle and Jon Carlisle, *Marvels of Medical Engineering* (New York: Sterling Publishing Co., 1967), p. 11.

6. Michael Crichton, *Five Patients* (New York: Alfred A. Knopf, 1970), p. 135.

7. *Ibid.*

8. Shelly B. Frost, Zita Fearon, and Herbert H. Hyman, *A Consumers Guide to Evaluating Medical Technology* (New York: Consumer Commission for the Accreditation of Health Services, 1979), p. 10.

9. Office of Technology Assessment, *Assessing the Efficacy and Safety of Medical Technologies* (Washington, D.C.: U.S. Government Printing Office, 1978), pp. 69–70.

10. Office of the Assistant Secretary for Health, *Health: United States—1978*, U.S. Public Health Service No. 78-1232 (Hyattsville, Md.: DHEW, 1978), Tables 28 (p. 180) and 31 (p. 192).

11. John H. Dingle, "The Ills of Man," *Scientific American*, September 1973, p. 82.

12. Carlisle and Carlisle, *Medical Engineering*, p. 16.

13. *Ibid.*, p. 86.

14. *Ibid.*, p. 87.

15. *Ibid.*, p. 85.

16. Jurgen Thorwald, *The Patients* (New York: Harcourt Brace Jovanovich, Inc., 1972), p. 281.

17. *Ibid.*

18. Robert S. Morrison, "Dying," *Scientific American*, September 1973, p. 59.

19. Lasagna, *Life, Death and the Doctor*, p. 226.

20. Morrison, "Dying," p. 87.

21. Carlisle and Carlisle, *Medical Engineering*, p. 87.

22. *Ibid.*, p. 112.

23. Eli A. Friedman, Barbara G. Delano, and Khalid M.M. Butt, "Pragmatic Realities in Uremia Therapy," *The New England Journal of Medicine* 298, no. 7 (February 16, 1978): 369.

24. Actuary Office, "Annual Projected Costs of Medical Services: Medicare Dialysis and Transplant Patients: 1974–1984," mimeographed (Washington, D.C.: Social Security Administration, 1977), unpaged.

25. Friedman et al., "Uremia Therapy," p. 369.

26. *Ibid.*, p. 370.

27. Actuary Office, "Projected Costs," unpaged.

28. Leach, *The Biocrats*, p. 252.

29. Office of Technology Assessment, *Assessing Efficacy and Safety*, Foreword.

30. *Ibid.*, pp. 23–55.

31. Marshall J. Orloff, "Contributions of Research in Surgical Technology to Health Care," in *Technology and the Quality of Health Care*, Richard H. Egdahl and Paul M. Gertman, eds. (Germantown, Md.: Aspen Systems Corporation, 1978), p. 96.

32. Selma Mushkin, Lynn C. Paringer, and Milton M. Chen, "Return to Biomedical Research, 1900–1915," in *Technology and Quality*, Richard H. Egdahl and Paul M. Gertman, eds. (Germantown, Md.: Aspen Systems Corporation, 1978), pp. 105–120.

33. Victor Fuchs, *Essays in the Economics of Health and Medical Care*, (New York: National Bureau of Economic Research, Columbia University Press, 1972); Martin Feldstein, *The Rising Cost of Hospital Care* (Washington, D.C.: Information Resources Press, 1971); Clifton R. Gaus, *Biomedical Research and Health Care Costs*, Testimony before the President's Biomedical Research Panel, September 29, 1975.

34. Carlisle and Carlisle, *Medical Engineering*, p. 72.

35. *Ibid.*, p. 74.

36. *Ibid.*, pp. 79–82.

37. *Ibid.*

38. National Aeronautics & Space Administration, Technology Utilization Division, *Medical Benefits from Space Research* (Washington, D.C.: U.S. Government Printing Office, 1970).

39. Carlisle and Carlisle, *Medical Engineering*, p. 97.

40. John H. Knowles, "The Hospital," *Scientific American*, September 1974, pp. 132–134.

41. Crichton, *Five Patients*, p. 108.

42. Carlisle and Carlisle, *Medical Engineering*, p. 93.

43. Crichton, *Five Patients*, p. 128.

44. Leach, *The Biocrats*, p. 32.

45. *Ibid.*, p. 50.

46. Sherman M. Mellinkoff, "Chemical Intervention," *Scientific American*, September 1973, p. 104.

47. *Ibid.*, p. 112.

48. *Ibid.*, p. 106.

49. Joseph Fletcher, in Vaux, *Who Shall Live?*, p. 130. Dr. Fletcher has criticized the positions of both the FDA and NIH for employing "over simple" ethics and paying lip service to the credo that the "patient comes first, in his individual capacity" while overlooking the very real fact that any chance distribution of "medicated" and "control" groups runs the risks and potentials inherent in any experiment.

50. *Fortune*, Editorial, August 1970.

51. *Scientific American*, April 1973, p. 15.

52. National Center for Health Statistics, *Health Resources Statistics: 1976–1977* (Washington, D.C.: U.S. Government Printing Office, 1979), p. 5.

53. Office of the Administrator, *Health Care Financing Review* (Washington, D.C.: Health Care Financing Administration, 1979), pp. 1–4.

54. Bureau of the Census, *Pocket Data Book, U.S.A., 1971* (Washington, D.C.: U.S. Government Printing Office, 1971), p. 64.

55. Social Security Administration, Office of Research and Statistics, "The Size and Shape of the Medical Care Dollar" (Washington, D.C.: U.S. Government Printing Office, 1970), p. 30.

56. National Center for Health Statistics, "Vital and Health Statistics Data from the National Health Survey" (Washington, D.C.: U.S. Government Printing Office, 1970).

57. Milton Terris, "The Need for a National Health Program," in *Toward a National Health Program,* the 1971 Health Conference (New York: New York Academy of Medicine), pp. 24–31.

58. American Medical Association, *Distribution of Physicians in the United States, 1970* (Chicago: 1971). A more recent study, *Supply and Distribution of Physicians and Physician Extenders* (Health Resources Administration, GMENAC Staff Paper no. 2, 1978), shows that there continues to be an increasing disparity between physicians practicing in metropolitan and nonmetropolitan areas between 1970 and 1976. (Table 11, p. 42 of the report.)

59. Bureau of Health Manpower, *On the Status of Health Professions Personnel: A Report to the President and Congress,* Health Resources Administration No. 78-93 (Washington, D.C.: Health Resources Administration, 1978), p. IV-46.

60. *Ibid.,* p. IV-46.

61. Office of the Administrator, *Health Care Financing Review,* p. 5.

62. Bureau of Health Manpower, *Status of Health Professions Personnel,* p. II-30.

63. *Ibid.,* p. II-26.

64. *Ibid.,* pp. II-9, 10.

65. *Ibid.,* pp. IV-23-26.

66. Office of the Assistant Secretary for Health, *Health: United States—1978,* p. 356.

67. David S. Abernethy and David A. Pearson, *Regulating Hospital Costs,* (Ann Arbor, Mich.: AUPHA Press, 1979), p. 50.

68. Health Care Financing Administration, *Professional Standards Review Organization: 1979 Program Evaluation,* Health Care Financing Administration No. 03041 (Washington, D.C.: Office of Research, Demonstration, and Statistics, 1980), pp. xi and xii of Executive Summary.

69. U.S. DHEW, *Towards a Comprehensive Health Policy for the 1970's: A White Paper* (Washington, D.C.: U.S. Government Printing Office, 1971), p. 11.

70. U.S. DHEW, "National Guidelines for Health Planning," *Federal Register* March 28, 1978, 43 FR 13041 *et seq.*

71. William L. Kissick and Samuel P. Martin, "Issues of the Future in Health," in *The Nation's Health: Some Issues,* Sylvester E. Berki and Alan W. Heston, eds., *The Annals of the American Academy of Political and Social Sciences,* 1972, pp. 151–154.

72. *Ibid.*

73. Paul M. Ellwood, Jr., "Models for Organizing Health Services and Implications of Legislative Proposals," *Medical Cure and Medical Care* 50 (1972): 75.

74. Kissick and Martin, "Issues in Health," p. 153.

75. Committee for Economic Development, *Building a Health Care System*, p. 35.

76. Office of the Administrator, *Health Care Financing Review*, Table 3, p. 24.

77. *Ibid.*, Table 5, p. 27.

78. Office of the Assistant Secretary for Health, *Health: United States—1978*, Table 166, p. 406.

79. *Ibid.*

80. Committee for Economic Development, *Building a Health Care System*, pp. 63–64.

81. Governor's Steering Committee on Social Problems, *Report*, p. 23.

82. U.S. Social Security Administration, *Social Security Bulletin* 35 (1972): 63–64.

83. U.S. DHEW, *A White Paper*, p. 19.

84. Governor's Steering Committee on Social Problems, *Report*, p. 21.

85. Office of the Administrator, *Health Care Financing Review*, Table 7, p. 32.

86. Bureau of Health Manpower, *Status of Health Professions Personnel*, Table IV-9, pp. IV-22-26 and IV-53.

87. Kissick and Martin, "Issues in Health," p. 152.

88. Roger M. Battistella, "Comprehensive Health Care Planning: New Effort or Redirected Energy," *New York State Journal of Medicine* 4 (1969): 2350–2370.

89. Preface to PL 89-749, U.S. Congress, November 3, 1966.

90. Battistella, "Redirected Energy," p. 2364.

91. Preface to PL 89-749.

92. National Commission on Community Health Services, *Health Is a Community Affair* (Cambridge: Harvard University Press, 1966), pp. 154–182.

93. U.S. DHEW, Public Health Service, Office of CHP, *Information and Policies on Grants to States for CHP*, August 1967.

Chapter 3

National Health Planning and Resource Development Act of 1974: A Systems Approach to Planning

On January 4, 1975, PL 93-641, National Health Planning and Resources Development Act of 1974 became law, replacing PL 89-749, the Partnership for Health Act. This new law is comprehensive in scope, specific in its language, powerful in its authority, and clear in its intent. The act essentially abolishes the Comprehensive Health Planning (CHP) Agencies, Hill-Burton, and Regional Medical Programs as individual programs and consolidates them into a single new program. The congressional committees studied the records of each of the three health programs, noting their strengths and weaknesses. The resulting act aims at maintaining their strengths while overcoming their weaknesses.

The Senate committee's report found that

> . . . the CHP program is one which began with great enthusiasm in 1967 and 1968, flagged without substantial financing or federal support until approximately 1971 and is now again receiving substantial support and initiative from the Department. It is a program which in many communities has been very effective but in others has either never existed or has lacked adequate funding, staffing and authority with which to make substantial changes in the health system.[1]

The act is patterned primarily after the Partnership for Health Act with its emphasis on a consumer-provider partnership, comprehensive planning, regulation, and evaluation, and a close relationship among regional, state, and federal governments. The act is divided into two major titles. Title XV concerns the development and functions of the areawide and state planning agencies. Title XVI focuses on health facilities planning and is essentially a substitute for the Hill-Burton Act.

Seven principles guided Congress in developing PL 93-641.[2]

1. widespread citizen involvement with a consumer majority
2. adequate funding
3. emphasis on implementation of a plan's goals and objectives
4. linkage of new resources to a health plan's goals
5. competent, technically sound health planning
6. federal government leadership role in the planning process
7. comprehensive planning, including a community's environment, life style of its people, and genetic factors

FINDINGS AND PURPOSE (SEC. 2)

The act identifies many national problems requiring attention. Among these are the need to provide "equal access to quality health care at a reasonable cost," inflationary increases brought about by the infusion of large federal sums, the "lack of uniformly effective methods of delivering health care," the poor distribution of services, the greater emphasis on the more costly services of hospital care rather than utilization of less expensive and more appropriate alternative medical services, the failure to involve the provider of health services in the planning and improvement of health services, and finally inadequate efforts made to educate the public in proper personal health care and the availability of services.

Certain deficiencies have long been known to exist in the medical service system: the imbalances in the distribution of services, the need to contain the rapid spiraling costs, and the negative contribution the federal government has made to the inflationary forces through passage of Medicaid, Medicare, and other expensive medical programs without attendant efforts to forecast and restrain these inflationary forces. The findings imply the acceptance of the medical system as it exists, with its emphasis on disease and treatment rather than on prevention and diagnosis of the causes. The act implies that cost containment can come about by use of alternative treatment services, such as health maintenance organizations (HMOs), by reducing duplicated and little used expensive service modalities, or by providing outpatient rather than inpatient services.

TITLE XV—NATIONAL HEALTH PLANNING AND DEVELOPMENT

National Health Priorities (Sec. 1502)

The act for the first time sets forth national health priorities requiring areawide and state health plans. Of the ten priorities, seven are related to improvement in the efficiency and effectiveness of the health care system. These priorities embody health problems discussed quite extensively in the last decade and focus on such concepts as coordination, integration, comprehensiveness, continuity, uniform cost accounting, quality of care, and use of less expensive care. The other three priorities call for providing medical services to "underserved" populations, educating the public to the effective use of available services, and promoting prevention of disease through study and implementation of recommendations related to nutrition and environmental factors affecting health. The 1979 amendments added additional priorities, e.g., providing appropriate mental health services, fostering competition in the health care sector, containing the cost of medical care through greater efficiency and appropriate use of health services, and eliminating duplicate or unneeded services.

These priorities are consistent with the health problems identified in the findings. The importance of the priorities is that they chart a major course of deliberation and action for the planning agencies to follow and at the same time serve as a general set of criteria by which the secretary of Health and Human Services (HHS) can evaluate the work of the health planning agencies. The references to health education and prevention appear to be priorities for emphasis in the future rather than at the present time. The first priorities are concerned with setting the existing health delivery system in order. The priorities are action-oriented because Congress expects efforts in their implementation to take place as soon as feasible.

The act also calls for the establishment of a national council to advise the secretary on changing health priorities. In addition, the secretary is expected to receive guidance from the areawide and state health planning agencies and other medical and health associations. However, it is the secretary who determines the priorities.

The council, originally composed of 15 members, was increased to 20 members by the amendments. Of these, 16 are voting members, and 4 are ex officio government officials. Of the voting members, 50 percent must represent consumers, and two of these must be representatives of rural and urban medical underserved populations.

Health Systems Agencies (Sec. 1511–1516)

The basic unit upon which the whole system rests, according to the act, is the health systems agency (HSA).

Boundaries (Sec. 1511)

Several criteria for establishing boundaries are prescribed by the act. Among these are population size, the presence of a medical center with "highly specialized health services," and a size large enough to ensure the availability of the full range of health services for the area's population. The act gives the governor of each state the responsibility for designating boundaries. It is expected that the governor would give first priority to the health planning area boundaries that exist. The population size is expected to be within the range of 500,000 to 3,000,000 persons, but the act allows for exceptions for those areas where the population is highly concentrated, as in Chicago, Los Angeles, and New York City, or quite sparse or spread out as in the Midwest, Southwest, and Far West. Also, the boundaries are expected to be consistent with the Standard Metropolitan Statistical Areas (SMSAs), but again exceptions can be made with the approval of the secretary. The intent of Congress is to have a smaller number of large planning regions rather than many small regions.[3] Of the 205 health service areas designated, 15 cut across the boundaries of two or more states.

One implication in the wording of the act with respect to boundaries is its emphasis on action. The secretary and Congress are aware that sound health planning and the promulgation of plans must precede the ultimate passage of national health insurance. Consequently, Congress foresaw a general acceptance of the existing health regions rather than another prolonged conflict in the creation of new boundaries. In spite of congressional emphasis on coordination between HSAs and other organizations, particularly the Professional Standards Review Organizations (PSROs), only 45 health service areas are coterminous with PSRO areas.[4]

Legal Structure of HSAs

The HSA for the region can be (1) a nonprofit private corporation or public benefit corporation; (2) a public regional planning body, if it had been in existence at the time the act was passed; or (3) a single unit of general local government, provided its jurisdiction is similar to that of the health service area. The major debate in Congress was over permitting local jurisdictions to choose the legal structure for its HSA. Since 75 percent of the "B" agencies have been organized as nonprofit private corporations, there was a strong move to accept this as the standard for all HSAs. However, the political conflicts that would ensue in the other 25 percent of the regions to convert their legal structures into nonprofit private bodies and the concern of Congress to implement the act as rapidly as possible led to the compromise of giving the regions the three options of organization previously noted. As of November 1979, 202 HSAs had been designated. Of these, 177 are private, nonprofit corporations; 25, government-sponsored. In addition, among the 57 State Health Planning and Development Agencies (SHPDAs), eight are covered by Section 1536 requirements that give these states and trust territories the responsibility for both HSA and SHPDA functions.[5]

Staff of HSAs

The act specifies the minimum size of staff at five to include expertise in at least the following areas: (1) administration, (2) the gathering and analysis of data, (3) health planning, and (4) development and use of health resources. However, for larger populations, one additional staff member for every 100,000 population in the region could be authorized. Consultants could be hired as needed for special assignments, but not to engage in routine agency activities. The implication of this type and size of staff is that the HSA is expected to perform technical planning and have an adequate staff to carry out this function. The 1979 amendments require the HSA staff to have three additional areas of expertise: an understanding of mental health; an ability to perform financial and economic analysis; and a knowledge of public health matters, such as prevention of disease. Through specifying these areas of expertise, Congress aimed to overcome the deficiencies of the predecessor CHP "B" agencies by ensuring a minimum size professional staff with basic areas of knowledge and competence.

Governing Body of HSAs

The governing body is to consist of 10 to 30 members, although a larger body would be acceptable if it authorizes an executive committee of 10 to 30 members "to take such action (other than the establishment and revision of the plans . . .) as the governing body is authorized to take" (Sec. 1512(b)(3)(A)). The intent of Congress is action, which in its deliberations it concluded would be inhibited by a large, unwieldy governing body.

The governing body is to be made up of a majority (up to 60 percent) of consumers who are residents of the region, the balance being health providers who must also reside in the area. Government officials are also to be included as either consumers or providers. The consumers are to be "broadly representative of the social, economic, linguistic and racial populations, geographic areas of the health service area, . . ." (Sec. 1512(b)(3)(C)(i)). In addition, officials of Veterans Administration hospitals or HMOs located in the region are required to be appointed as ex officio members.

The 1979 amendments added greater specificity to the original act by requiring the HSA governing body to include consumers who represent the handicapped and major purchasers of health care, such as labor unions and business corporations. On the provider side, the amendments increased the percentage of direct providers, e.g., physicians, dentists, nurses, optometrists, podiatrists, physician's assistants, and other health professionals, including administrators of health facilities, on the governing body and executive committee from one-third to one-half. Finally, they require that persons with expertise in mental health, either consumers or providers, be included on an HSA governing body.

The selection process has also been altered so that the governing bodies do not become self-perpetuating. The 1979 amendments now require that each HSA develop a process by which one-half of the members are selected by a means other than nomination by the current members of the HSA governing body. To ensure the competence of the governing body members, particularly the consumer members, both the HSA and the health planning centers must provide education, information, and technical assistance on an ongoing basis. These amendments were added to overcome the tendency of HSAs' professional staff to cater to the more knowledgeable provider members, as well as to make it easier for both consumer and provider members to carry out their responsibilities.

PL 93-641 differs from its predecessor in its conflict of interest section (Sec. 1512). One clause of this section states that a member of the HSA governing body may not vote on any issue in which he or she has an interest. While this is generally understood and accepted practice, the fact that it is stated explicitly underscores its importance and gives greater credibility to the decisions made by HSA decision-making units.

The HSA can form subarea councils with an advisory capacity, provided their composition is similar to that of the governing body. Again, the act, by this option, gives the HSA maximum flexibility in forming smaller councils, which may be necessary in either highly concentrated or very sparse geographical areas within its boundaries. At the same time, it permits the HSA to have a more diversified body that is closer to the needs and priorities of the varied constituencies residing in the region. However, authority for final decision making is to be maintained in the governing body of the HSA.

The act spells out the major responsibilities of the governing body. It is responsible for the day-to-day operation of the HSA with respect to staffing, budgeting, and setting of agency standards of operation. It is responsible for developing a long-range plan called the health systems plan (HSP) and a short-range plan called an annual implementation plan (AIP). In addition, it has the responsibility for approving contracts, issuing annual reports, meeting six times a year with at least one meeting each quarter, and conducting its business in well-advertised, open public meetings with adequate notice. A quorum consists of at least one-half its membership, and a majority vote of the members present and voting is required to validate an HSA action. According to this formula, as few as three members in a ten-member governing body or eight in a thirty-member body can set policy for the HSA. Since the act does not specify that a minimum number of consumers or providers must be present as part of the simple majority required to hold a legal meeting, it is possible that many decisions made by the HSA may reflect the positions held by its most active members, be they providers or consumers.

While this threat to the democratic process is possible according to the act, the openness of the meetings, the requirement for broad representativeness of the consumer members, and the inclusion of a wide variety of provider and governmental constituencies are safeguards that Congress sought to build into the governing mechanism to balance the danger of control by a small clique of the HSA's governing body.

Functions of HSAs (Sec. 1513)

The HSA is required to perform certain functions in order to ensure that the act's national priorities are adhered to and quality health services are available to residents within its region. The HSA is required to make a diagnosis of the problems and needs of the population as well as the deficiencies in resources through the collecting and analysis of data that are available from its own efforts and those of other agencies. Based on this diagnosis, the HSA must develop a long-range plan (HSP), consisting of goals and priorities and subject to revisions based on open public hearings. The HSP in turn serves as the basis for the HSA's development of an AIP, in which specific objectives and priorities among the projects are identified and programs are designed to achieve the objectives. The HSA is expected to involve regional health providers in the implementation of its AIP. The HSA is required to provide them with technical assistance and to make grants available for carrying out certain parts of the plan. The act provides from its Area Health Services Development Fund grants to the HSA to implement such programs. The fund authorized $25, $75, and $120 million for fiscal years ending on June 30 of 1975, 1976, and 1977, respectively, but these were never appropriated. Under the 1979 amendments, the authorization has been drastically reduced to $20 and $30 million for the fiscal years ending September 30, 1980 and 1981, respectively. Part of the reason for the earlier failure to appropriate these funds and subsequent reduction is that Congress has not given specific guidance for their use. Since they were originally conceived as demonstration funds to replace those in the defunct Regional Medical Program (RMP), the use of these funds is severely restricted to planning and developing projects; they cannot be used to pay the costs of delivering health care services.

The ambiguity surrounding the use of the funds, plus the availability of many other federal, state, and private grants, raises the question of how significant this small sum of money can be to stimulate implementation of HSP/AIP goals and objectives.

The HSA is also responsible for other functions. Among these are coordination of its activities with those of other agencies involved in health planning or services, review and approval of specified federally funded programs designated for the region, recommendations to the state agency with respect to the need for new health facilities in accordance with its HSP and AIP, and for modernization, construction, or conversion of facilities to different medical uses.

The HSA is obligated to review all health facilities in its region within three years of its establishment and every five years thereafter. However, Congress made it clear that the HSA's "recommendations carry no sanctions; they are intended to serve as a basis for regulatory decisions to be made by the state health planning and development agency."[6] Finally, the intent of the act is to encourage the use of quantitative analysis and the systems approach to plan development. In this way, Congress believes that the broad goals of improving the health of the region's population; increasing accessibility, acceptability, and continuity of care; restraining cost rises; fostering competition; and reducing the potential for duplication of services will be achieved. Furthermore, the 1979 amendments make more explicit the fact that HSPs should add to their emphasis on inpatient and long-term care services those services that relate to prevention, ambulatory and home health care, and alcohol and drug abuse. Prior to the passage of the amendments, HSPs may or may not have included such goal-oriented health service components. Further, the amendments recognize the importance of implementing HSP high-priority goals and objectives. Consequently, HSPs now need to be updated only every three years instead of annually, although AIPs still must be updated each year as a means of demonstrating progress toward their short-range objectives and of showing the HSA's public accountability.

State Health Planning and Development Agencies (Sec. 1521-1526)

Designation of SHPDA (Sec. 1521)

Governors designate and the secretary of HHS approves the naming of SHPDAs, which have the "authority and resources to administer the state administrative program" (Sec. 1521(b)(1)(B)) and are capable of carrying out the functions assigned to them. The SHPDA may delegate some of its responsibilities to other agencies with the consent of the governor and approval of the secretary. In addition, the Statewide Health Coordinating

Council must be established by the governor before SHPDA is approved. The state agency has up to two years to demonstrate its capacity to carry out its responsibilities and functions. If, after four years, the secretary has not given full approval to a SHPDA, all federal funds designated for "the development, expansion, or support of health resources in such state [will be cut off]until such time as such an agreement is in effect" (Sec. 1521(d)). Either the governor or secretary has the right to terminate the agreement upon 90 days' notice. However, the secretary must consult with the National Council on Health Planning and Development and provide the state with a hearing before termination.

Responsibilities of SHPDA (Sec. 1522)

The act identified a number of responsibilities the SHPDA must perform, most of which are administrative in nature. One of these is the development of an administrative mechanism with proper authority to carry out the agency's functions. It must set forth personnel standards, hire professionally trained staff, provide consultation to the Statewide Health Coordinating Council (SHCC), ensure that its deliberations are held in public meetings, and coordinate its activities with those of other health agencies operating on a statewide basis. In addition, it must make provisions for its own annual evaluation, make periodic reports to the secretary on its activities and fiscal health, and review and modify at least every three years the state plan.

State Functions (Sec. 1523)

The SHPDA, or another agency within the state, may be delegated certain functions to perform as part of its agreement with the secretary. Among these functions are the following: (1) the completion of a state plan through the coordination and integration of the individual HSA plans, (2) the implementation of those parts of the plan that fall within the jurisdiction of the state government, (3) assistance and consultation to the SHCC in its review of the state's medical facilities plan, and (4) serving as the "1122" designated planning agency of the state for review and determination of need for medical facilities and programs. In addition, the SHPDA must review and report on the status of all institutional health services in the state periodically and at least once every five years. Although findings of these reviews carry no sanctions against the institutions, it is hoped they will serve as a means of improving services while reducing duplication of programs and facilities. The SHPDA is required to review and render its recommendations on all health facilities proposals within a period of one year after an HSA has made its recommendations to the state. If the SHPDA makes a decision inconsistent with that of the HSA, it is required to submit a report to the HSA on the reasons for its contrary decision.

Essentially, the SHPDA plays the role of coordinator, integrator, and final decision maker within the state on all health matters. However, while the agency is the key decision maker, the act intends that it take its primary guidance from the recommendations of the HSAs in their plans and review of health facilities and services. From this perspective, the SHPDA becomes more a reactive and review agency than a creative developer of its own plans.

Statewide Health Coordinating Council (Sec. 1524)

The SHCC is an advisory body to the SHPDA. It has at least 16 members, a majority of whom must be consumers, and consumer members from rural and urban medically underserved areas must be included. The governor appoints the chairperson, although the SHCC members may appoint the chairperson if the governor fails to do so. While the governor appoints all members to the SHCC, each HSA must have at least two members—one consumer and one provider—appointed to the SHCC from a list of two or more nominees for each seat to which the HSA is entitled. However, in states with more than ten HSAs a minimum of one representative per HSA may be appointed, provided the consumers comprise the majority of the SHCC. Each HSA within the state has the same number of representatives on the SHCC. In addition to the HSA representatives, the governor can appoint up to 40 percent of other representatives, including officials from government, except that the majority of those so appointed must be consumers of health care. Finally, one-half of the providers on the SHCC must be direct providers of health care, and if one or more Veterans Administration hospitals are located in the state, then one of their chief medical officers must be made an ex officio member. Its meetings are open to the public and held at least quarterly. A number of functions are assigned to the SHCC:

1. It annually reviews the HSPs and AIPs prior to their submission to the secretary.
2. It reviews and revises the individual HSPs that serve as the basis of the state plan; it revises the HSPs to ensure appropriate coordination and to "deal more effectively with statewide health needs."
3. It holds meetings open to the public on the state plan with at least 30 days' notice.
4. It reviews the budgets of the HSAs and advises the secretary about these.

5. It reviews and makes its own recommendations on HSA planning grants to the secretary.
6. It advises the SHPDA on the performance of its functions.
7. It must approve or disapprove state-formulated plans, such as a state alcoholism plan. The secretary will withhold funding for such SHCC-disapproved applications until reviewing the SHCC's decision. If the secretary overrides the SHCC's recommendation, the reasons for the decision must be given in writing.

Rate Regulation

Although the act initially authorized the secretary to make grants to six states for the purposes of documenting and developing standards relating to the effectiveness of regulating the rates of various components of health delivery, the 1979 amendments offer grants to any state that intends to regulate such rates.

General Provisions (Sec. 1531-1536)

The act includes provisions and criteria for review changes in the health system and requires the secretary to provide technical assistance to HSAs and SHPDAs. It authorizes the secretary to establish a national health planning information center and five regional centers for the study and development of health planning and makes the secretary responsible for reviewing in detail the operation of the HSAs and state agencies at least once every three years to ensure the competency of their operations. The secretary is also asked to develop standards and guidelines with respect to the operation of the regional and state planning agencies and their outcomes as measured by the effect of health services on the well-being of people.

TITLE XVI—HEALTH RESOURCES DEVELOPMENT

The goals, financing, and regulation of health facilities and plans related to them are dealt with in Title XVI. It is the replacement of Hill-Burton and mandates a relationship between the development of health systems and state health plans on one hand and the facilities that these plans call for on the other. In the past, the relationship between health planning and health facilities planning has been haphazard at best.

Financial assistance is made available primarily for the following four priorities: (1) modernization of health facilities, (2) development of new outpatient medical facilities, (3) new inpatient medical facilities in areas of very rapid growth, and (4) conversion of existing facilities to new health uses. The act calls for the secretary to prescribe general regulations for the operation of state agencies and HSAs.

General Regulations (Sec. 1602)

The secretary is required to promulgate regulations that (1) identify the priorities under the title that the states must meet with respect to populations served, location of such facilities, the feasibility of a health system area financing such facilities, comprehensiveness of services, and, finally, the compliance of existing facilities with local fire, building, or life safety codes and regulations; (2) prescribe specific projects according to these priorities; (3) require the state facilities plan to guarantee access and availability of service to all residents and particularly for those residents unable to pay for such services; and (4) provide guarantees to the secretary that any health agency or institution receiving funds under this title is, in fact, complying with the regulations and is carrying out the projects as stated. Those agencies must make periodic reports to the secretary.

State Medical Facilities Plan (Sec. 1603)

Before any project grants can be awarded, a State Medical Facilities Plan must be developed and approved by both the SHCC and the secretary. The plan is to be based on a survey that identifies the available and needed health facilities, inpatient and outpatient, and those requiring modernization. It is to identify the state's priorities and the specific projects that are required to implement those priorities. Section 1604 outlines the process for the approval of projects consistent with the Medical Facilities Plan.

Allocation of Facilities Finances (Parts B, C, & D)

Three types of funding are made available for the implementation of the Medical Facilities Plan: allotments, loans and loan guarantees, and project grants.

Allotments

The secretary allocates funds to each state based on its population, financial need, and need for medical facilities projects; no state receives less than $1 million. A maximum of 20 percent of the allotment can be used for construction of new inpatient facilities, but not less than 25 percent is to be used for outpatient facilities for medically underserved populations, with one-half going to the rural underserved. If a state fails to use the funds allotted to it within two fiscal years of the year for which it was allotted, these funds may be reassigned by the secretary to other states. However, allotment funds were never appropriated as authorized by Congress.

Loans and Loan Guarantees

A fund is to be established in the Treasury Department from which the secretary of HHS may draw to loan to nonprofit private entities for medical facilities. These loans will be provided at an interest rate three percent lower than the existing market rate. The amount of loans available to each state is based on its population, financial needs, and the need for medical facilities according to its state plan. As with allotments, unused allocation of loan funds may be redistributed to other states.

Project Grants

Of the allotments assigned to each state, 22 percent are allocated for project grants. These grants are to be used for construction or modernization projects "designed to (1) eliminate or prevent imminent safety hazards as defined by federal, state, or local fire, building, or life safety codes or regulations, or (2) avoid noncompliance with state or voluntary licensure or accreditation standards" (Sec. 1625(a)). The grants are available to public or quasi-public agencies and will pay for up to 75 percent of the cost of the projects, although they will pay 100 percent for projects located in urban or rural poverty areas. The secretary requires a guarantee that the projects funded under these grants can be completed by the funds requested.

Area Health Services Development Fund (Part F)

The act creates an Area Health Services Development Fund for each HSA from which grants may be drawn for implementing projects that are of high priority and an integral component of the HSP and AIP. No funds will be allocated by the secretary until the region's HSP and AIP have been developed and approved by both the SHCC and the secretary. A development grant may not be greater than $1 per person in the health service area. These funds have not been appropriated as of 1980.

Additional Grants under the 1979 Amendments

A new section was added by the 1979 amendments in order to provide grants and technical assistance to hospitals and state agencies to discontinue unneeded hospital services and/or convert them to other health services recommended in the HSP and AIP. The secretary approves all such requests and determines the size of the grant. The grant may be used to liquidate outstanding debts related to the institution; to plan, develop, or purchase equipment; to deliver alternative health services; or to provide termination pay for personnel losing their positions as a result of discontinuance. The amendments authorized $30, $50, and $75 million, respectively, for fiscal years ending September 30, 1980, 1981, and 1982.

WHAT THE ACT DOES

The National Health Planning and Resources Development Act of 1974, including its 1979 amendments, is a major step forward in a congressional effort to bring a more integrated approach to health planning and implementation. Integration is effected on two levels. On one level, federally funded health planning and implementation programs, CHP, RMP, and Hill-Burton, are united in one program. This greatly simplifies the administration of the program. On the second level, the act provides greater power and authority than had existed under the previous legislation to gain compliance of private and public health providers with the goals, objectives, and priorities of plans formulated by HSAs and SHPDAs.

The carrot and stick approaches are used to gain compliance. In the carrot approach, medical institutions are given incentives, technical assistance, and financial inducements in the form of outright project grants, loans, or demonstration funds if they comply with the HSP and AIP priorities. On the other hand, the stick approach can lead to rejection of institutional projects or possible loss of other funds, such as Medicaid depreciation dollars, if institutions fail to comply with the planning goals and priorities. The fact that the authority for gaining approval or disapproval resides in one health planning system rather than three independent agencies concentrates the authority of the HSAs and state agencies and means they will have to be taken more seriously than in the past.

The act also creates an integrated decision-making mechanism for health planning. The key to this mechanism is the SHCC, which must approve the state plan. Since 60 percent of SHCC's members are from the HSAs, plans developed in the regions are guaranteed acceptance, in most cases, at the state level. The act also requires an integration of the HSA plans so that they can be collectively oriented toward the achievement of statewide priorities. In addition, the State Medical Facilities Plan requires review by the HSAs with respect to the needs for health facilities in their regions, and consistency with their long- and short-range plans. Consequently, the state plan becomes an integrated document of the goals and priorities for the entire state of which the Medical Facilities Plan is an important component. This is in contrast to the past, where the Hill-Burton agency, CHP planning, and RMP often worked at cross purposes with each other.

The act sets forth some national priorities; Congress expects the new health planning system to be guided by them. In the past, each planning agency defined its own priorities. Through these priorities, which will be changed as circumstances require, a concentrated effort can be made to resolve some of the major medical problems that beset the nation's population. While these priorities initially focused on the efficiency of the health system itself, the emphasis in the 1979 amendments is on the effectiveness of the system, as shown by its efforts in disease prevention, ambulatory care, home health services, and mental health deinstitutionalization. The importance of maintaining a healthful environment and of stimulating competition in the health system, primarily by means of HMOs, has also been recognized. This shift shows congressional intent to contain cost while improving the quality of care. Progress must be made toward these goals before Congress can be expected to pass some form of national health insurance. To avoid an inflationary impact such as that previously engendered by the sudden influx of Medicaid and Medicare funds, the medical system must be put on the most efficient base possible.

Consistent with the setting of national priorities, the act proposes a systems-oriented planning process to ensure that these priorities, as well as other health problems, are surveyed, analyzed, and reviewed for inclusion in a final HSP and an AIP. Previously, the CHP agencies were left to their own devices on how they should plan, who should be involved in that planning, and the nature of the staff they should hire to do the planning. This is no longer left to chance; the act spells out all of this. In addition, technical assistance is to be provided in the form of one national and five regional centers for the hiring of consultants as the individual needs of the HSAs and SHPDAs require.

The systems approach is oriented primarily to the use of quantitatively stated goals, objectives, and output measures that can be evaluated for achievement and comparison among the HSAs and SHPDAs. Fuzzy, broadly conceived goals are no longer acceptable. Precise objectives and specific programs, stated in quantitative terms, are required. The first set of national guidelines for health planning, which was concerned with standards for hospital beds and use of high-cost specialized medical technology such as computerized axial tomography (CAT) scanners and cardiac catheterizations, were intended to provide federal guidance. Future federal funding of HSAs and SHPDAs, and even the health institutions that are expected to implement the region's planned goals and objectives, may well be dependent on their capacity and desire to implement national standards at the state and local levels. In a period when the national budget for the purchase of medical services is reaching its limit, it is important for Congress to know what it is buying with its federally funded medical programs.

The act places great emphasis on the democratic decision-making process. It does this in several ways. It opens to public scrutiny, to a far greater degree than in the past, the deliberations of the planning agencies. This is done by a minimum number of open public meetings per year, the availability of documents and reports that pertain to each agency's business, and a final review by the public of any HSP, AIP, State Health Plan (SHP), or Medical Facilities Plan proposed by the various elements of the health planning system. Through these means, through the definition of the composition of the governing bodies, and through the emphasis on consumer majorities, the act creates a mechanism of checks and balances to ensure that the interests and needs of all are heard. The 1979 amendments carry this process one step further by ensuring that medically underserved populations are included on the governing bodies and that the process for appointing HSA governing body members is open.

The act is also concerned with the health planning system's responsiveness to the real needs of the region's population, as shown by its encouragement of subarea councils. While these councils are advisory in nature, Congress intended that they serve in a more than advisory capacity. The grass roots voice and needs of the population of all the sections of the regions are expected to be heard through these subarea councils, and their goals and priorities are to be incorporated into the region's HSP and AIP in the same way that these regional plans are integrated into the state plans. Thus, through a "bottom up" planning, starting with grass roots communities in each HSA, and open public meetings, a more democratic process for planning becomes possible. Special interests will have a more difficult time securing passage of pet projects and will find it necessary to compete with the needs of people and institutions in other communities and the articulated goals and priorities contained in the health plans themselves. To ensure the solvency of the democratic process, the act provides sufficient funds to staff the health planning agencies so that they are not reliant upon the benevolence of the medical institutions that in the past have had the funds to contribute to the CHP agencies and thereby influenced the decisions of the governing boards. By law, these institutions are not permitted to make contributions to the HSAs or SHPDAs. The 1979 amendments specifically require both staff and health planning center expertise to provide education, technical assistance, and information to board members, especially to consumer members.

The act recognizes the fact that certain populations and certain communities in the HSA regions have been more disadvantaged than others in obtaining quality medical care. It specifically identifies the urban and rural medically poor, the people unable to pay for medical care regardless of where they live, the underserved populations residing especially in rapidly growing suburban communities where medical services have not kept pace with the population growth, and the old and inadequate public and private medical facilities that no longer serve their populations well. These geographical areas and categories of population are given high priority in the planning and expenditure of funds for medical services.

Finally, the act is more concerned with providing quality health services than with construction of new medical facilities. One of the key influences in the congressional consensus behind this act was the expectation that it would result in far better medical services at a lower cost. Ninety percent of the $750 million 1973 budget was appropriated for Hill-Burton and RMP, compared to 10 percent for planning. In PL 93-641 the percentages are substantially altered. Forty percent of the $245 million 1975 budget are appropriated for planning. This is an initial increase of $30 million over the 1973 budget for planning and rises to a total of $170 million for fiscal year 1977, more than double the amount devoted to planning for 1973.

WHAT THE ACT DOES NOT DO

It is acknowledged in the act that the present medical system can work if it can be made to operate in a smoother fashion. Its emphasis is on efficiency, continuity, availability, accessibility, comprehensiveness, and integration of medical services. While the act suggests innovations, these innovations are designed mainly to implement ideas that have already been tested and accepted, such as HMOs and various forms of group practice and outpatient services. The act recognizes the deficiencies of the present system: fragmentation and poor allocation of services to disadvantaged groups, lack of continuity of services, duplication of costly services, and lack of standards to evaluate quality of care.

By its emphasis on these values and on the implication that each health systems region must contain one major medical facility center, the act in effect accepts the regionalization concept of quality medical care. In this concept, several levels of medical care are envisioned with the most routine and general care rendered by physician's assistants in the neighborhood, supported by outpatient ambulatory clinics staffed by general practitioners. These in turn would be supported by community-based hospitals with some specialized services. The community hospitals would be backed by larger teaching hospitals, and at the core would be the medical schools and hospitals with their super-specialty services and research into the causes of disease. Administrative and decision-making linkages would be required in such a regional medical system. This system would ideally guarantee quality care at the lowest cost for the medical services required to meet the health needs of the population.

The problem with such a medical system is that it assumes a disease orientation to health rather than the causes of health problems in the socioeconomic, physical environment of the region.

Although the 1979 amendments indicate that emphasis is beginning to shift to the positive aspects of health and well-being, it is not yet clear whether this new emphasis will be of sufficient magnitude to overcome the medical disease orientation of the health care field. If it fails to achieve this change in emphasis, the act will reenforce a system that is more efficient in treating the sick than in correcting the environmental conditions that produce the sickness.

A corollary of this point is that the indicators the act specifies for use in evaluating health outcomes are primarily disease-oriented, e.g., mortality rates, morbidity rates, and staff or hospital bed-to-population ratios. This may make it virtually impossible at a later date to change the nature of the indicators to positive ones such as nutrition levels or robustness of health. Those indicators would require another data base entirely instead of the management information system being developed nationally in support of the act's HSAs. The cost and burden to change the data/monitoring system may be far too great to obtain support from Congress and the medical practitioners whose training, competency, and orientation are embedded in the current disease-oriented health indicators. Thus, the use of such indicators reenforces the orientation of the system toward medical care rather than the very different goal of good health.

Not surprisingly, the act barely mentions environmental health planning and does not mention socioeconomic factors related to health conditions. Yet, studies have been made that show the real effect of noise, air, and water pollution on the physical and emotional well-being of people. Even though the 1979 amendments give greater priority to the environment and wellness, it is unlikely that the disease indicators will show much improvement in the near future, even with the world's best medical system.

The act is concerned with moving quickly to resolve some of the more evident problems identified in its introduction. Consistent with its action emphasis, it specifies a maximum-sized governing body for the HSAs of 30 persons, unless an executive committee of 10 to 30 members is established. While no one would argue that "action now" is needed, the question is whether the equal emphasis on the democracy of the structure and the involvement of diverse public interests will actually result in action. The democratic process has always been a slow, cumbersome one in which decisions on basic issues are generally not made until a consensus has been formed in their support. The actual composition of the HSAs and the SHCCs lends itself to representation from a wide scope of health and medical constituencies, each of which has its own interests and orientations for solving problems. Without any bloc large enough to force its collective will on the governing bodies, either the consensus desired for identifying and accepting goals, objectives, and priorities will be very slow in developing, or the boards will have to find a way of subverting the interests of the many to the needs of a few in order to develop their plans. Since there will in most instances be three levels of planning and decision making (the subarea, the regional, and the state), the "action" the act was designed to encourage turned out to be slower than anticipated. This is evidenced by the slowness of the Bureau of Health Planning in completing and releasing a full set of regulations, by the 36-month period required to develop the first set of national guidelines instead of the 18 months called for in the act, and by the fact that not all SHPDAs are fully designated as of 1980.

The act also demands knowledgeable board members. For the most part, even the college-educated with their capacity for abstract and conceptual thinking find the systems approach to planning difficult to comprehend, but necessary if they are to render judgment on the work of the technically trained professional planners. Forecasts, simulation techniques, operations research methods, and program evaluation and review techniques (PERT) and critical path charts used by technical planners to justify their recommendations may disenchant and, in many cases, completely mystify the grass roots consumers as well as many of the medical practitioners who do not customarily think in these terms. Several consequences flow from this type of planning. First, many board members may lose interest, leaving a small group of board members representing a narrow constituency to make the major decisions on goals and priorities. Second, it greatly enhances the influence of the technical planners in the development of the HSPs and AIPs. Third, since technical planners do not like to make forecasts without a heavy investment in research and the collection and analysis of data, a further delay may be entailed before they even develop their recommendations for board consideration. Thus, to the democratic decision-making delays noted earlier are added the technical delays of the study-research process. But the graver consequence is the potential exclusion of the broad base of provider and consumer involvement in the decision-making process due to the heavy emphasis on the technical, systems approach to planning.

In a recent assessment of one HSA, it was noted that many of the project review committee meetings failed to have a majority of consumers as required by the bylaws. Since this is one of the committees that reviews highly technical medical issues, without proper education consumer members can easily become confused and simply stop attending meetings.

No act that has all benefits and no costs can be created. The purpose of pinpointing what the Act does (its benefits) and what it does not do or does in a negative way (its costs) is to alert the health planner and the public to what has to be guarded against if some costs are to be averted. Regardless of its potential dangers, the National Health Planning and Resources Development Act of 1974 represents a major advance over previous congressional efforts to build some rationality into the health planning process that will bring benefits to people. As with all other improvements, many more steps and shifts in direction will occur in the future as experience and greater knowledge open up new avenues for progress in bringing about better plans and planning for the well-being of people.

Financing the HSAs

The passage of PL 93-641 and its 1979 amendments was intended to overcome past financing problems of the HSAs. The act forbids the HSA to accept funds or contributions of services or facilities "from any individual or private entity which has a financial, fiduciary, or other direct interest in the development, expansion, or support of health resources" (Sec. 1512(b)(5)). This section was included in order to avoid conflicts of interest that were evident in the funding of the predecessor health planning agencies.[7] Private funds can be contributed provided the contributors have either no or only a general interest in the health care field. Local or state tax levy funds can be contributed in support of the HSA's activities.

With respect to federal distribution of funds, the dollars actually spent under PL 89-741 (Partnership for Health Act) were almost 40 percent of the amount authorized by Congress. It should be noted that it is not unusual for Congress to appropriate less than the authorized limit. Thus, during the life of the program, Congress actually appropriated only $92 million of $152 million authorized and spent only $60 million, or about 25 cents per capita. In only one of the seven years in which the program operated did the federal agency actually spend all of the appropriated dollars. PL 89-741 was never the favorite of any president, and there were repeated attempts to kill the program during the term of one. This accounts for the low percentage of funds actually spent once they were appropriated by Congress.

In contrast, PL 93-641 authorizes 50 cents per capita or twice the amount of the previous law. Further, these funds do not have to be matched by the HSAs. If the HSAs can raise supplementary funds, these are matched dollar for dollar up to a maximum of $200,000. The records show that only a very small proportion of HSA funds, an average of 3.4 cents per capita, come from supplementary matching grants. HSAs tend to live within the means of their yearly federal funding grants.

By initially setting the minimum funding level at $175,000 for a fully designated HSA, Congress took into account the costs of hiring a basic five-person professional staff to carry out the mandated functions of the HSA. With the additional requirement that the staff members have expertise in economic analysis, mental health, disease prevention, and public health services, the 1979 amendments are incrementally increasing the minimum funding level to $260,000 by 1982. HSAs with small populations have generally been funded at a higher than minimum level because of the demands placed on them to meet all their responsibilities.

This method of funding has tended to overcome problems that affected the CHP agencies. First, HSAs are no longer influenced by organizations and agencies that gave matching funds to their predecessors for the purpose of obtaining special favors. In fact, PL 93-641 specifically states that "non-Federal funds . . . shall be funds which . . . are otherwise contributed to the agency *without conditions* as to their use . . ." (Sec. 1516 (c)(ii); emphasis added). This does not prevent health providers or consumers with substantial influence from exerting it in other ways, however.

Second, the mission of HSAs is no longer confused. Unlike their predecessors, HSAs are required to develop comprehensive health plans within a specified period of time. Failure to meet this deadline means that HSAs cannot achieve a fully designated status. This status carries with it both higher levels of funding and additional responsibilities that are predicated on the completion of approved HSPs and AIPs, including review of new institutional services, approval or disapproval of federally funded programs, and evaluation of existing health care services. Thus, planning has become more important than project review. HSAs are now perceived as planning and implementation agencies. Their regulatory function of project review is now appropriately viewed as a significant component of implementation and is no longer confused with the planning function.

Third, HSA staff, particularly its administrators, no longer must divert their energies to fund-raising. Finally, by allocating a minimal level of support, Congress ensured that all HSAs, regardless of the size of their populations, would be able to carry out their basic functions required by the law. Of these, training and education of board members, collecting and analyzing data, and planning were initially given greatest emphasis. With the passage of the 1979 amendments, the emphasis has shifted to imple-

mentation (including project review), community involvement, and advocacy of public issues.

As mentioned earlier, funding under PL 93-641 has been at a higher level
than under its predecessor. However, this applies only to those HSAs that
have been fully designated. It has taken about two years for most HSAs
to attain full designation. During this time, most of the HSAs received
from 30 to 40 cents per capita, depending on the availability of funds. At
the end of 1979 there were still three HSAs that had not received fully
designated status, five years after the law was implemented.[8] Table 3-1
illustrates variations in the funding formula of some fully designated agencies from 1976 to 1979.[9] These figures indicate that Congress has appropriated sufficient funds for fully designated HSAs to meet their responsibilities. The major variation is shown for the two HSAs receiving the
minimal funding grant of $175,000, Southeast Alaska and Nevada, with
per capita grants of $3.49 and 66 cents, respectively. All the other randomly
selected HSAs have per capitas within 6 cents of the 50 cents called for in
the initial legislation. Due to inflation and additional responsibilities

Table 3-1 Sample Funding Formulas for HSAs

HSA	Population	Federal Share* 1979	Per Capita for† 1979	1978	1977	1976
Southeast Alaska	50,198	$ 175,000	$3.49	$3.50	$3.50	$2.90
C. Arkansas	459,506	223,859	.48	.48	.44	.35
South Florida	1,491,743	840,057	.56	.55	.58	.34
Maine	1,072,588	563,641	.53	.54	.47	.29
Health Planning Council—Boston	2,198,510	1,097,653	.50	.50	.45	.29
Nevada	266,954	175,000	.66	.66	.66	.54
Eastern Ohio	758,975	417,494	.55	.55	.50	.32
Utah	1,226,142	597,342	.49	.48	.43	.27

*The federal share includes both the basic grant and the supplementary federal
matching funds. Matching funds average 3.4 cents per HSA nationwide in 1979. The
per capita amounts are higher for those HSAs with matching funds because their share
of the matching is not included in any of the per capita figures noted. For example, if
these matching funds were added, Southeast Alaska would have per capita of $5.89
and South Florida, 64 cents for 1979.

†Additional data taken from Bureau of Health Planning Memo, dated February 1,
1980, to Regional Health Administrators regarding "FY 1979 Funding Information-
HSAs and SHPDAs."

assigned HSAs in the 1979 amendments, this level has been increased to 60 cents.

As noted previously, there is a difference between funds authorized and those appropriated by Congress. Table 3-2 shows, for example, that the initial amount authorized for HSAs in 1975 was $60 million, but no funds were appropriated because funds left over from the three predecessor programs (CHP, RMP, and Hill-Burton) were used to get the HSAs and SHPDAs started. In 1976, $90 million was authorized, but only $64.09 million (70 percent) was appropriated and almost all of it was obligated. By 1978, $125 million was authorized, but only $109.5 million (88 percent) was appropriated. For 1981, $165 million has been authorized with $87 million (53 percent) appropriated. These data show the variability with which Congress maintains its funding of the health planning programs. The low 53 percent appropriation for 1981 reflects a major decision by the President and Congress to balance the federal budget and thus decrease the initial funding of most federal programs across the board. However, it should be pointed out that this decrease from 50 cents to about 33 cents per capita represents a more severe cut than the 9 percent reduction for funding the SHPDAs.[10] It reflects a shift in federal and congressional emphasis from planning for quality, accessibility, and availability of health care to regulation and cost containment, functions lodged primarily with the state agencies.

Table 3-2 Authorizations, Appropriations, and Obligations under PL 93-641 for Health Systems Agencies and State Agencies, 1975–1982 (Dollars in Thousands)

Agency	1975	1976	1977	1978	1979*	1980	1981	1982
Health Systems Agencies:								
Authorized	60,000	90,000	125,000	125,000	125,000	150,000	165,000	185,000
Appropriated	-0-	64,090	101,498	109,494	110,142	124,717	87,000	
Obligated	-0-	63,353	96,170	103,560	105,973			
State Agencies:								
Authorized	25,000	30,000	35,000	35,000	35,000	35,000	40,000	45,000
Appropriated	-0-	19,000	25,859	31,835	33,235	32,000	32,000	
Obligated	-0-	18,317	24,139	28,889	29,205			

*PL 93-641 was extended for one year.
Source: Bureau of Health Planning Memo, February 1, 1980, to Regional Health Administrators, "FY 1979 Funding Information-HSAs and SHPDAs," Report 42 (HSAs) and Report 40 (SHPDAs).

While the prohibition against accepting contributions from those with a direct interest in their decisions frees HSAs from obligations to such contributors and thereby enables them to make more objective planning and regulatory decisions, it also has a negative impact. With the substantial reduction announced in the 1981 budget, HSAs either must drastically cut back on the functions they perform, or must engage once again in fund-raising activities to offset the loss of federal dollars. Yet, the pool of potential sources is severely reduced by the law's restrictions on who may contribute. To be sure, there are general purpose sources of funding, such as banks, corporations, and foundations, but the competition for these resources is intense and most likely will limit how much HSAs will be able to obtain from them. Thus, while the HSAs have been able to carry out their responsibilities with the funding levels called for in the 1979 amendments, they are more handicapped than their predecessors when funding levels are suddenly reduced. They have both a more limited pool of resources from which to draw nonfederal funds and less experience in how to compete for them.

The 1979 amendments do provide limited assistance for those agencies that must cope with unusual situations, e.g., heavy travel expenses because of a large geographical territory as in some of the Rocky Mountain states or greater staffing requirements because of an extremely large, dense population as in New York City or Chicago. Five percent of the HSAs' national funding level is set aside to assist such HSAs in meeting these unusual expenses. The $1.7 million appropriated for this purpose in the 1980 budget is simply too small to offset the almost $40 million reduction proposed for the 1981 budget, however. Until the Congress can ensure funding stability, HSAs will continue to plan under conditions of uncertainty and potential crisis situations.

NOTES

1. Committee on Labor and Public Welfare, *Report on the National Health Planning and Development and Facilities Assistance Act of 1974,* U.S. Senate, 93rd Congress, November 12, 1974, p. 13.

2. Paul G. Rogers and Lee S. Hyde, "Planning for Quality Health Care," in Health Resources Administration, *Health in America: 1776–1976.* Public Health Service, No. 76-616, pp. 117–126.

3. Committee on Labor and Public Welfare, *Report on Health Planning Act,* p. 44.

4. Comptroller General of the United States, *Status of the Implementation of the National Health Planning and Resources Development Act of 1974,* No. HRD 77-157 (Washington, D.C., November 2, 1978), p. 9.

5. U.S. DHEW, *Directory: Health Systems Agencies, State Health Planning and Development Agencies and State Health Coordinating Councils* (Hyattsville, Md.: Health Resources Administration, November 1, 1979), inside cover page.

6. Committee on Labor and Public Welfare, *Report on Health Planning Act,* p. 51.

7. *Ibid.,* p. 47.

8. *Health Resources News* 7, no. 2 (April 1980): 1.

9. U.S.DHEW, *Directory.* The difference between the 48 and 56 for South Florida, for example, represents matching supplementary funds.

10. These figures are taken from the Report of the comptroller general (see note 4), the 1979 amendments (PL 96-79), Sec. 1516, and information supplied by the Bureau of Planning, Hyattsville, Maryland.

Chapter 4

Planning for Health

The previous chapters have explained the historic evolution of planning and have shown how crises generate planning efforts. Again, American society finds itself in another crisis. Today's crisis is one of choice from among the numerous problems, potential solutions, and new, technical innovations. In the absence of any clear-cut policy for selecting among priorities, the marketplace model of permitting each group, agency, or organization to proceed independently, regardless of other participants and varying needs, has culminated in a chaotic situation in which the various health thrusts seem to point in different directions at the same time.

PL 93-641 was passed in the hope that through planning some form of rational system could be developed that would help organize the health industry into a more coherent state. The great concern in our new age of resource limitations, made more acute and etched more sharply on our psyches by the oil crisis, is how to utilize available resources to meet the health needs of our society most effectively. Therefore, we are concerned with the concept of planning as it applies to the present health situation. Can planning resolve such questions as: (1) Should more money be put into renal dialysis treatment or into cancer research? (2) Should citizens have a real voice in determining the health priorities of their communities? (3) Should the consumer be required to pay the direct costs of some health care, even if a national health insurance plan is enacted? (4) Should there be one coordinated system of health care or many, independent systems? Such questions gain significance, not only because the health industry has become "big business," but also because it has become well over a $200 billion industry and is continuing to grow rapidly. Critics have begun to question whether the U.S. economy can afford such large expenditures when there are so many other needs that must be met from the same funds.

PLANNING THEORY

In almost all planning schools, whether devoted to urban planning, regional planning, or health planning, there is usually a course devoted to planning theory. Kaplan defines theory as "the device for interpreting, criticizing and unifying established laws, modifying them to fit data unanticipated in their formation, and guiding the enterprise of discovering new and more powerful generalizations."[1] The important fact for Kaplan is that theory inevitably depends on fact and testable hypotheses to confirm its validity. In the process, a theory can be broadened so that generalizations and predictions can be drawn from them. A theory is true "if the predictions made on the basis of [it] are in fact fulfilled."[2]

In spite of the numerous books being written on planning and the publication of the *Journal of the American Planning Association,* there is very little that has been written or tested about planning theory. In an undated chapter of a proposed book on planning theory, Dyckman explored the historical antecedents to the modern style of planning.[3] He noted at the outset of his extensive exploration that there was a "failure of American planning to produce any influential statement of its 'theory,' despite a growing amount of serious intellectual work."[4] He attributes this to a number of factors. Among these are the planner's confusion between science and theory because of an emphasis on pragmatism and the uncertainty about "identification of planning as a distinctive process or activity."[5] Later, when the city planning profession began to flourish, planners became interested in applying science to human affairs. In this application, however, they tended to be more concerned with the efficiency or means of making cities better places to live without asking to what ends. This was accepted because planners were generally sympathetic to the city reform movement with its emphasis on individualism, its antiurban bias, and the myth of the agrarian American. Their rationalistic approach to the decision-making process provided a pseudoscientific support for the beliefs of the reformers.

After World War II, the planners were strongly influenced by the national economic planners, exposure to other professions, and particularly the latest social science techniques. This exposure reinforced the planners' concern with rationality, techniques, and procedures. These procedures in turn gave the planners an aura of prestige and acceptance as they applied scientific pragmatism to the problems of the cities. The marriage of public administration tools and economic methods, used by the planners to find the most efficient way to improve cities, was largely accepted by the reformers and city officials who found that "social planning might not be inconsistent with democratic control."[6] In spite of all the changes that have taken place over the years, Dyckman found that the emphasis continued on the means of planning rather than the end. As he states in his conclusion: "The state of planning theory at this point of great growth [1960s], in the United States planning profession remains partial and planning is increasingly great, . . ."[7] Fifteen years later, there was even greater emphasis on sophisticated procedures. Health planners have also been captivated and enamored of the latest procedures and methods as they apply to health planning.

Dyckman is not the only one to find a lack of planning theory. Faludi, in his compilation of writings on planning theory, came to the same conclusion that "there has been surprisingly little written on what planning theory is or ought to be."[8] He has discovered that there are a number of normative prescriptions of what planning ought to be, but they are not based on any empirical studies, with the exception of vague references to bits of experiences.[9] More recently, there have been schematic frameworks for research, especially by Friedmann and Bolan.[10] Both cite a number of variables and hypothesize how they appear to be related to each other, but thus far little has been done to test these relationships. For example, in his behavioristic framework, Bolan hypothesizes that there is a relationship between achievement of planning goals and the following characteristics: (1) limited scope, (2) easily predictable consequences, and (3) easily communicable issue.[11] Friedmann identifies hypotheses for testing, such as "innovative planning is typically uncoordinated and competitive."[12] In addition, both ask numerous questions requiring further study.

Planning educators are becoming more concerned with the development of planning theory. This theory is necessary if planners are to have their own scientific base and body of knowledge to explain the hows and whys of planning. Planners, now, are like gamblers who have before them a number of shining balloons, each claiming to bear within it a secret message of what planning is all about. There are only two darts to throw and no real clues. Since a start must be made, it is hoped that even if the planners miss the target, a little more knowledge will be gathered and the possibilities narrowed through logic, creative thinking, and the empirical testing of ideas. Until there is a theory that provides some explanation, planners must, as Dyckman notes, content themselves with a pragmatic approach with its emphasis on techniques and procedures. These continue to supply the planner with the necessary status to be sought in order to support the policies of the decision makers. This is a serious time for the United States. Goals are not clear, and conflict between traditional and emerging goals is characterized by a search for new directions of unknown consequences. The opportunity exists for planners and participants from other disciplines to give thought to the results of planning rather than only to the best means to achieve results. While a lack of planning theory may exist, much is available on the planning process, planning models, and definitions.

DEFINITIONS OF PLANNING

Lack of agreement on how planning should be defined is one of the first problems. The lack of theory is a contributing factor because it permits each planner to conceptualize a personal definition. As a result, there are definitions that focus on comprehensive planning and those that aim at a specific function (social, economic, physical) of planning, as well as subfunctional categories such as personnel, health, and welfare planning. In addition, there are definitions that include the systematic aspect of planning, concerned with logic and rationality. Further, there are definitions that emphasize auspice or responsibility for planning, such as regional or city planning where the focus is on both the geographical boundaries and the governmental unit responsible for implementation. Finally, there are definitions that concentrate on the essence of the planning function itself where the emphasis is on either the process and procedure of planning or the substance of planning. This approach considers the basic problem Dyckman noted in the planner's preoccupation with means rather than ends. The importance of further analysis of health planning rests on the fact that PL 93-641 specifically emphasizes the comprehensive aspect of health planning. Unless this term can be carefully defined, particularly in the absence of any theoretical formulations, debate over the meaning of comprehensive health planning will continue, and the absence of clarity will encourage each health planner to define the term on an individual basis.

Comprehensive planning has been officially defined by the Executive Office of the President as (1) preparation, as a guide for long-range development, of general physical plans with respect to the patterns and intensity of land use and the provision of public facilities, including transportation facilities; (2) programming of capital improvements based on a determination of relative urgency; (3) long-range fiscal plans for implementing such plans and programs; and (4) proposed regulatory and administrative measures which aid in achieving coordination of all related plans of the departments or subdivisions of the governments concerned and intergovernmental coordination of related planned activities among the State and local governmental agencies concerned.[13]

The main thrust of this definition is on the physical aspect of planning. Holeb indicates that the scope of activities of comprehensive planning at the local level is determined by the relationship of the agency to the municipal decision makers.[14] Thus, some planning agencies are involved in housing only, some in housing, zoning, transportation, etc. However, until recently, comprehensive planning has not included social aspects of planning, although many have been concerned with economic planning. Thus, the comprehensive aspect of planning is an ambiguous term that is used as a catch-all phrase to mean whatever the planner, agency, or theoretician wants it to mean along the dimensions of what is planned, the geographical size of the area being planned, the time orientation, and the level of power or authority required to assist in the implementation of the plan.

On the other hand, the term *comprehensiveness* is used by Friedmann as a qualifying characteristic for defining what he means by allocative planning.[15] In his definition, comprehensiveness refers to the interdependence of three characteristics: (1) explicitly stated objectives, (2) major alternative uses of available resources, and (3) external conditions that may affect the implementation of these objectives. These characteristics refer to the rationality and logic of the planning process rather than the setting of boundaries dealing with function, scope, and power, the definition used by the federal government. It can be seen from Friedmann's usage that there is no consensus of opinion on what is meant by comprehensiveness in planning.

More agreement is afforded the definition of functional planning which generally refers to a limited specialized area of study such as physical planning, social planning, economic planning, or sectors within these categories such as housing, land use, or transportation planning. Whereas the term *comprehensive* is subject to wide interpretation, functional planning, because of its specificity, is regarded as more intensive.

The two become linked as Altschuler notes: "City planning's most important functions are (1) to create a master plan to guide the deliberations of specialist planners, (2) to evaluate the proposals of specialist planners in the light of the master plan. . . ."[16]

The same characteristics of comprehensive planning also apply to functional planning, except they are limited to the specialty under consideration. The planning activities and the power to implement the scope of the function being planned are all characteristics that have to be specified when discussing a functional planning effort. Comprehensive and functional definitions are concerned with both means and ends, but, as will be seen in the discussion of allocative planning, the ends are fairly well given while the means are open to change.

Planning as rational, future-oriented action is one of the more common definitions accepted by planners and scholars. Banfield defines planning as

> the process by which he (planner) selects a course of action (a set of means) for the attainment of his ends. It is 'good' planning if these means are likely to attain the ends or maximize the chances of their attainment. It is the process of rational choice that the best adaptation of means to ends is likely to be achieved.[17]

This definition infers a dependence on rationality in order to select the best means to achieve a desired end. As a political scientist, Banfield assumes that the ends are usually dictated by elitist decision makers, among whom planners are seldom included. The ends are usually given to the planner, who must devise rational means, a course of action, to achieve them. As a general definition, geographical boundaries, comprehensiveness, and time horizons are rarely considered basic characteristics of this definition. The emphasis is on process, rationality, and the power or authority required to carry out the plan.

Other planning theorists concur with Banfield's definition, but with some variation. Davidoff and Reiner define planning as "a process for determining appropriate future action through a sequence of choices."[18] Faludi defines it as "the application of scientific methods to policy-making,"[19] while Friedmann refers to it as "the application of scientific and technical intelligence to organized actions,"[20] and, finally Dror defines it as "the process of preparing a set of decisions for action in the future, directed at achieving goals by preferable means."[21]

All of these definitions have a number of characteristics in common. They all stress a planning process. The process permits a series of alternative choices (means) to achieve some action or objective (end). The study and investigation required to define these means and ascertain alternatives have usually been the main emphasis of planners. This is accomplished by the planner's use of design methodologies that have become increasingly sophisticated in an attempt to link data with needs, criteria, economic and political feasibility, and the efficient use of resources. They all stress the future and, as such, are predictions of what will happen in some time period if the alternatives are carried out. All imply value judgments, generally consistent with those of the local governing elite. Finally, all imply that planning is continuous and, therefore, dynamic.

Whether planning takes place within the framework of an approved master plan or is concentrated on some functional sector, these definitions indicate that through monitoring and evaluating, the objectives and/or more usually the means are adjusted in order to attain goals. For example, in the last decade we have witnessed a succession of alternatives to improve the lot of the urban poor. Voluntary social services supplemented by public welfare was succeeded as the dominant alternative by the anti-poverty and model cities programs, and these in turn are being succeeded by special revenue sharing and economic development programs. Fried-mann hits hard at the type of planning implied by these definitions.

> Planning practice is chiefly concerned with incremental deci-sions, and planners generally avoid taking the long view. . . . Planning is conservative, and planners are ordinary bureaucrats who crave the security of a career, the promise of regular advancement and the prospect of eventual pension.[22]

Such planning practices tend to emphasize maintenance of the status quo.

The final group of definitions are those that stress planning for funda-mental change in societal structure. Friedmann defines innovative plan-ning as one of the "basic forms of planning concerned with actions that produce structural changes in the *guidance system* of society."[23] Mayer, relying on Parsonian social system theory, states that the only way to solve human problems is to change the structure of the social system. He states that the "underlying assumption is that the source of social problems lies somewhere in the social order, the organized set of relationships which exist among individuals engaged in a system of interaction."[24]

The essence of these last definitions is that basic problems in society are not often solved by incremental or adaptive modifications of social systems that are responsible for the problem in the first place. What is required instead is new direction and possibly destruction of the existing social system and the establishment of a new social structure if real change is to take place. Consequently, these definitions advocate radical changes, possibly irrational strategies and a conscious breaking up of the equilibrium in the social system in question. As Mayer so well states: "It is more basic in the sense that it gets at more fundamental roots of social problems. It is not reductionist; it does not reduce social problems to characteristics of individuals. It is more realistic in the sense that it affects everyone involved and not just those who take advantage of individualized resources."[25]

Reviewing these definitions reveals the complex issues involved in plan-ning and the reason that more has not been accomplished in planning theory development. The nature of the variables requiring evaluation are basic to the manner in which society functions and are thus more likely to meet with resistance from decision makers. If Friedmann's characterization of the typical planner as conservative and unwilling to rock the boat is correct, it is unlikely that such a planner would undertake the type of studies required in developing planning theory. It would mean studying such variables as the roles of the planners and the people with whom they normally work, the planning strategies used, the actions taken, the formal and informal decision-making structure, the sources of power, their own ideological leanings and those of the decision makers, the types of objectives promoted, and the resources recommended for implementation. When one seeks studies that have been completed on some of these variables, it is not surprising that they have been made by theorists from the social sciences, especially political science, such as Banfield, Altschuler, Dahl, Meyerson, Gross, Gans, and Munger, to name a few. Not being directly involved on a daily basis with the participants or the social, economic, and political systems being studied, they can more easily analyze and offer insights into the planning-power relationships. Unfortunately, many of the variables requiring study are not touched upon by the social scientists. The scientists have little interest in planning methodologies, time horizons, scope of planning, or geographical boundaries within which planning is done. Yet, studying these variables is important for a deeper understanding of how planning functions. Until such studies are accumulated, planning theories that are more than normative or prescriptive in nature cannot be formulated. Thus, the definitions that exist do not offer much assistance in transforming the art of planning into the science of planning. If choosing a definition of planning is risky, perhaps it is possible to find consensus on the planning process itself.

PLANNING PROCESS

On examination, most definitions of planning reveal some form of logic and formal procedure for engaging in planning. Two definitions illustrate this. Kahn's definition is implicit. He states: "Planning is policy choice and programming in the light of facts, projections, and application of values."[26] Dror's definition states that "planning is a process of preparing a set of decisions for action in the future, directed at achieving goals by preferable means."[27] A study of these definitions and the authors' explanations of them reveals a specific statement of the planning process that has largely been accepted by the planning profession and its theorists. The process is the same whether it is described as a two-step process[28] or a twelve-step process.[29] In the two-step process, the planner analyzes the situation and then simultaneously plans and implements those plans. These two steps may be expanded into finer divisions. Starting with the initial step of problem identification, the process proceeds through clarifying the causes of the problem, collecting and analyzing data with reference to the causes, stating alternative goals, and establishing projects with value connotations explicitly stated, followed by identifying work programs, strategies, timing, funding patterns for implementation, and ending with measurement and evaluation procedures. The cycle in all of these processes, except for the former preoccupation with absolute master plans by city planners, becomes continuous and, thus, subject to change.

However, while the steps in the planning process may be the same, regardless of whether they are reduced to two steps or expanded into twelve, there are variations of emphasis that should be considered. These are (1) the starting point of the process, a distinction between problem-oriented and goal-oriented planning; (2) the emphasis on means or ends; and (3) the relationship of the plan to its implementation.

Starting Point

The problem-oriented process begins with the problem. Implicit here is the understanding that the system lacks equilibrium and, through some adaptation, it can be brought into balance. The solving of the problems involves (a) an emphasis in the planning process on incrementalism because new systems are seldom recommended; (b) a means orientation as alternative to the current dysfunctional way of dealing with the problem; (c) usually an acceptance of the systemic ends or goals of this entity; (d) an emphasis on efficiency of these proposed solutions by trying to get the best results for the least cost; (e) feasibility of converting the plan and its objectives into solutions acceptable to the electorate and its elected leaders, regardless of whether or not the feasibility leads to a better solution; and, finally (f) a heightened preoccupation with methodology or how the problem should be studied in order to arrive at the alternatives for consideration by the decision makers. Essentially, a problem-oriented starting point is both conservative and reactive in nature. It does not lead to fresh or creative paths of analysis and thereby limits the degree of innovativeness that can be brought to bear on the problem. The foremost exponent of this type of planning is Lindblom with his emphasis on "disjointed incrementalism" in which planners or administrators limit their efforts in order to solve the immediate problem at hand in the most expeditious manner without regard to how that solution will affect other systems or actors in the system.[30] Unfortunately, Lindblom and other theorists acknowledge that most planning is done this way in real life. This leads to an end result of Darwin's "survival of the fittest" orientation in which actors are concerned only with their own self-interest.[31]

On the other hand, the goal-oriented starting point has a different set of characteristics. It is assumed that the system might require the creation of a completely new system, such as the antipoverty agencies that replace or compete with the voluntary welfare agencies. From this flows an alternative set of planning process emphases. Both means and ends are given strong consideration, because neither are given or accepted as is. The process is likely to be innovative with greater attention to the alteration of the system's social structure or its complete obliteration, such as the demise of the antipoverty and model cities programs. Less attention is paid to feasibility and more to effectiveness in improving the quality of life in some dramatic new way, as through a negative income tax or children's allowance plan as alternatives to welfare assistance. The costs of the programs are less important than finding ways to enhance the function of a society or some aspect of it. Methodology is less important than discovering new insights to identify alternatives to the present goals and objectives under study. Policy is emphasized rather than alternatives identified by sophisticated or rationally oriented.planning methods. This innovative planning style Friedmann refers to as "transactive planning."[32] Its emphasis is more on action (getting things done) than with the niceties of developing a plan to guide that action. Action and plan making go on at the same time so that the rationality of the planning process is less important than the results encountered from improving society in some basic manner.

Emphasis on Means and/or Ends

Friedmann and Mayer emphasize means and/or ends in their works on planning theory. A means-oriented planning process stresses those steps, especially analysis and the use of economic analytical methods, such as cost-benefit analysis and input-output analysis, to determine the most efficient alternative to achieve ends or goals that are either stated explicitly or strongly implied. The key question is not with the goal but with the most efficient means of achieving it. There is little consideration for whether the most effective goal is guaranteeing everyone a standard health care package. No thought is given to whether education on smoking or changes in the environment to reduce pollution and psychological tensions in everyday living might be goals that would be a greater asset to individuals' health than rendering them assistance after they become ill. The means emphasis is more on how to maintain a balance in the allocation of existing resources for given objectives and their programs than on how to foster new ones. It is, as Friedmann asserts, an essentially conservative orientation to the problems with which the planning process is supposed to deal. This is what Friedmann refers to as allocative planning.[13] Its essential feature is maintenance of the system in contrast to innovative planning that stresses an action orientation toward changing the system or replacing it with another one. Ends orientation is essentially task- or change-oriented. It is reformist in nature and is primarily concerned with the implementation steps in the planning process, and the strategies and resources for achieving a creative set of ends.

Relationship of Plan to Its Implementation

A plan is a guide that sets forth a direction, values, and general strategies for achieving goals and/or solving problems. Most plans that are means-oriented make a distinct separation between the development of the plan and its implementation. Most of New York City's public agencies, for example, acknowledge this separation by dividing the agencies into a planning arm and an implementation arm. Seldom do the two arms work together in either planning or implementing programs. For this reason, most of the plans developed by the planning arm are either not implemented or, if they are implemented, they are implemented in such a distorted fashion that they bear almost no relation to the plan on which they were based. Levine devotes an entire book to this issue:

> The thesis of this book is that public programs in the United States have not worked well in the past, nor do they in the present. The major reason suggested for this outcome is that programs designed to fulfill policy objectives are laid out by planners for operation by administrators, with the administrators fulfilling the plan by following a hierarchy of rules . . . ordinarily they [the original policies or plans] are changed around not by malfeasance but by honest attempts at interpretation, with each attempt a little bit off and the cumulated result far from the intended objective of the public program.[34]

It is this separation of plan from implementation that often leads to a planner's frustration when he or she observes the plan resting dormant on some decision maker's or administrative implementor's shelf. This is associated more often with means- than with ends-oriented planning.

Friedmann, on the other hand, deliberately reduces the plan and the action associated with it to an integrated whole to be carried out by the same agency. The planning process then emphasizes the constant adjustment, or integration, of planning ends to actions and resources. It is this principle that Edward Logue, the famous city planner who helped renovate

New Haven, Connecticut, and later Boston, Massachusetts, insisted upon before accepting any position.

Thus, while the planning process may be largely accepted by most planners, the emphases bestowed on different aspects of that process can have important implications on the nature of the plan produced. More often than not, the emphasis tells much about the value system and personality/structure of the planner/planning agency involved. It also illustrates how complex even an accepted concept of the planning process becomes.

PLANNING MODELS

While Kaplan offers a full explanation of six types of models,[35] in this section models will be used to help organize characteristics into a system of relationships. The conceptual model is based on the social system articulated by Warren.[36] He defines a social system as

> . . . a structural organization of the interaction of units which endures through time. It has both external and internal aspects relating the system to its environment and its units to each other. It can be distinguished from its environment, performing a function called boundary maintenance. It tends to maintain an equilibrium in the sense that it adapts to changes from outside the system in such a way as to minimize the impact of the change on the organizational structure and to regularize the subsequent relationships.[37]

In addition to its boundary maintenance and its tendency toward preserving its equilibrium, the social system has two other basic functions: (1) attempting to achieve the goals of the system or organization, and (2) maintaining the coherence and positive sentiment of the members of the group toward each other. In organization theory, the first is called a task function and the second a maintenance function. Social system theory is a general enough body of concepts to permit analysis of several types of organizational models. These organizational types can be perceived as ideal types that may or may not exist in reality. Both Warren and Friedmann identified two typologies, one related to interorganizational field theory and the other to the planning field. The two are so similar that, if each was done without knowledge of the other (Warren's was published first), the importance of the social system concept, its applicability to both organization and planning analysis, and explanation would be indicated.

According to Friedmann, there are different patterns identified with different planning models. These are based on the power and/or authority of the decision maker with whom the planner is associated. Friedmann refers to these models as allocative planning styles. By allocative, he means, "the distribution of limited resources among a number of competing users,"[38] which he states many feel is the major and only proper function of central planners. The emphasis of allocative planning is on the maintenance function of a social system. The four styles Friedmann identifies are (1) command planning, the greatest degree of power and authority in decision making, usually located at the central executive level of an organization or system; (2) policies planning, a centralized source of power, but weaker than in command because several units are involved in the implementation of centrally issued planning directives; (3) corporate planning, fragmented authority in which each autonomous unit comes together with others to agree in some narrow way on what to do, but leaving each unit to determine whether it is done or how it is to be done; and (4) participant planning, the weakest form of centralized control in which each unit determines for itself what it will plan and implement. Friedmann notes that these four styles are linked to each other in various ways, based on a continuum of power with the strongest at the top and the weakest at the bottom. On this continuum, it is elitist decision making, "top down" planning, that dominates.

Warren also identifies four typologies based upon different types of organization power and the relationship of the subunits to the central decision-making unit.[39] The unitary style of organization has the greatest authority, which resides at the top of the hierarchy. This is similar to Friedmann's command style. Next in power and authority is the federative style (somewhat similar to Friedmann's policies planning) with some power at the central level of the hierarchy, but with most authority residing in the units that make up the federation. The coalitional style of organization (somewhat simliar to Friedmann's corporate planning) has no formal central decision-making unit, but the autonomous units collaborate on specific issues. Each unit maintains complete authority within its own system. The relationships are primarily informal, and any group that comes together is ad hoc in nature. It dissolves when the issue is solved or no longer interests the participants. The lowest order of organization is a nonsystem, which Warren calls social choice (similar to Friedmann's participant planning). This is the economic marketplace concept in which each organization does its own planning without consultation, formal or informal, with any other unit. The difference between the social choice and unitary styles is that, like Friedmann's participant planning, the social choice actors have little power and/or authority to implement their plans.

They are dependent upon the power of the unitary or command unit for resources to implement goals.

In order to avoid the confusion inherent in using a classification not exactly fitting the models of health planning to be used in this study, it seems desirable to develop new terminology. In so doing, the author recognizes an indebtedness to the classifications of Warren and Friedmann. In Table 4-1, the four models on which planning agencies may be patterned are identified. The planning models are differentiated based on the various characteristics listed in the left-hand margins. For example, on the characteristic of decision making, the systems model shows that it is controlled at the top, while in the alliance model it is controlled by each of the actors involved in the project. On a second characteristic, primary roles of health planner, in the partnership model, are in coordinating, researching, and advising roles, while in the individual action model, the planner serves in advocate, resource-gathering roles.

Table 4-1   Typology and Selected Characteristics of Models of Planning Agencies

	Models of Planning Agencies			
Characteristics	Systems	Partnership	Alliance	Individual Action
Decision making	Located at the top—concentrated	Authority resides in independent organizations, some delegated to top	Each organization retains its own authority; agrees to act in concert on issues of mutual interest	Each organization acts in its own self-interest, but holds few resources of its own
Main direction of agency	Plan, implement, and evaluate program outcomes	Set general policies, maintain status quo among organizations involved in health planning	Work toward some common goal; develop plan, implementation, or monitor action of others	Achieve limited action goals
Primary roles of health planner	Main emphasis on functional specialty requiring technical expertise	Secretariat, coordinating, researching, and advising roles	Organizing, coordinating mediator roles	Resource-gathering, advocate roles

	Models of Planning Agencies			
Characteristics	Systems	Partnership	Alliance	Individual Action
Center of influence	In governing body (including chief executive officer of planning agency)	In governing body of agency with external forces influencing it	In committees or ad hoc bodies of agency's governing body with external forces influencing committee decisions	In independent actors (staff, governing body, committees or external actors) concerned with achieving self-interest goals
Strategies for goal achievement	Collaboration or contest w/ tactics of persuasion, inducement, agreement on ends and means	Collaboration w/ tactics of education, persuasion, and compromise; agreement on ends, but not on means	Voluntary collaboration w/ tactics of education, agreement on ends and means	Collaboration w/ reciprocity, contest with tactics of inducement and various forms of conflict, means not differentiated from ends
Commitment toward goals	Very high, except if controls on staff are too rigid or authoritarian	Modest	Variable according to actors involved, from high to low	Very high

From the typology and the illustrations given, it can be seen that these models are based on the degree of control held by the health planning agency over resources to plan and implement planning goals, especially in the light of potential resistance to such planning and goal implementation. The systems model assumes greatest control and the articulation of comprehensive and integrated socioenvironmental-medical delivery goals. At the other extreme, the individual action model assumes a narrow-based, homogeneous group of actors with narrow interests in program implementation and little concern about the impact such implementation may have on other medical programs. It is the typical ad hoc project planning that normally occurs in health agencies bent on making incremental improvements in programs and systems delivery of services. As such, it is mostly adaptive.

The partnership and alliance models have some characteristics of the systems and individual action models but to lesser degrees. The partnership model takes its name from the Partnership for Health Act, which establishes a federation as the basic authority structure. The alliance is based on the concept of goal-oriented voluntarism. Each actor voluntarily participates with others in order to achieve a specific objective. Each actor has a different input of resources and hopes to gain something different from the outcome. Unlike the partnership in which the actors give up some of their autonomy for the general good of its members, those involved in the alliance give up none of their autonomy. As a result, the alliance is less likely to be a permanent, enduring organization than the partnership; it is more likely to break up and restructure itself with new members or with different roles played by the same members for each new project or goal.

Each of these models with their related characteristics is an ideal planning agency construct. Because they are ideal models, it is unlikely that, in reality, any health planning agency can be found that conforms perfectly to any of the typology patterns. As such, they are subject to empirical testing and will require modification or rejection based on the closeness of fit to reality. To illustrate the relationship of these characteristics, the systems and individual action models are discussed in detail.

Systems Model

Decision Making

In this model, decision making must reside in the hands of one or a few persons who sit at the top of the organizational hierarchy. Any decision that a unit within the organization or system wishes to make either must have the approval of the top decision maker or be formulated in some rule or regulation approved by the chief executive officer. In the systems model, control is assumed over planning decisions as well as resources needed to implement planning goals and objectives. There are no known health systems agencies (HSAs) that have been organized where such power and control of resources reside in the hands of the chief executive officer or a select group of members of the agency's governing board. However, outside of health planning, Edward Logue, at the time he was the chief executive officer of the Urban Development Corporation of New York State, held such decision-making power and control over resources.

Main Direction of Agency

The primary emphases of the systems model are to develop plans with long-range goals and short-range objectives, to create work programs for purposes of implementing the objectives, and finally to evaluate the outcome of these programs. The staff of the systems model would use the rational approach to planning discussed earlier in this chapter.

Primary Roles of Health Planners

Except for the administrative officers of the systems model agency, the hired planners and other professionals would be expected to possess highly developed abilities in one or more specialties of planning. Each task would be highly structured and linked to the work of other professionals so that the individualized specialties of the interdisciplinary team could be integrated. The outcome of this process would be a goal-oriented plan. The primary emphasis of the chief executive officer and the governing body of decision makers would be on accomplishing tasks in the most efficient manner and setting time schedules so the entire project could proceed as planned.

Center of Influence

The main center of influence resides in the chief executive officer and the most influential members of the governing council of the agency. This is essential so that control can be maintained over the complex variety of tasks that must be performed by staff and committees of the governing body. Only through tight control and an explicit awareness of the goals to be accomplished can the many strands involved in the planning, implementing, and evaluating processes be coordinated to produce the desired results. In essence, an elitist, almost authoritarian form of influence would prevail in a systems model. Only rarely would an outside actor exert strong influence over the decisions and orientation of the central decision makers.

Strategies for Goal Achievement

There are two basic, general strategies that can be utilized to achieve the goals of the systems model agency. Collaboration strategy assumes agreement on ends, but requires some negotiation with respect to means or tactics required to achieve these ends. Contest strategies, on the other hand, assume a difference of opinion on both means and ends. Within the systems model agency, the ends are determined at the top. Only the means or techniques for achieving these must be agreed upon and orchestrated by the administrators. Thus, collaborative strategy and its tactics of education, persuasion, and use of rewards can be used to gain consensus on the means to be adopted. However, with respect to the relationship of the systems agency to external actors (legislators, other autonomous public agencies, or independent health agencies), both collaboration and contest strategies are used, depending on the agreement or disagreement between the agency and the external actors over means or ends. Even when the systems model agency has control over the planning and many of the resources to implement the plan's goals, it still must gain a degree of compliance from autonomous agencies and individual actors to implement those plans fully. For example, the construction of new health facilities in previously all residentially zoned areas would require approval from the appropriate citizens and municipal boards with the authority to change zoning designations. Likewise, to develop a pest control program, approval from a housing authority and cooperation with the municipal or county sanitation department would be required. In general, there is less need for the systems model to develop cooperative relationships with external actors than is true of the other planning models, because of its near self-sufficiency of, and control over, resources and sanctions required to plan and implement goals.

Commitment to Goals

The commitment to the systems model's goals by staff and the governing body is generally expected to be quite high. Sanctions in the form of rewards (promotion, special recognition, and higher salary) and punishment (loss of job, demotion, or loss of influence) are sufficient to motivate and stimulate the efforts of all members of the agency toward goal achievement. If negative sanctions are used too frequently, however, the commitment will diminish and be replaced by an atmosphere of fear and distrust.

As a whole, it can be expected that, if these characteristics are found together in a health planning agency, then a systems model of planning is in operation. On the other hand, because of the close linkage of the variables to each other, if any are not found in this pattern, then it is likely that the system is operating in a dysfunctional manner. It would, therefore, be difficult for the system's goals to be achieved.

Individual Action Model

Decision Making

In the individual action model agency there is no one place where decision making is done. Nominally, the governing board and the chief executive officer have the authority to make decisions. Yet, in reality, a staff member, a committee, or an external agency participant actor may act to achieve some individual objective. The agency itself merely performs an official sanctioning, rubber-stamping function for the various actors both in and outside of it. As such, the agency as a unit possesses little power of its own and is acted upon by those who need an official forum to achieve their own ends. The individual action model operates on the principle of reciprocity in which the individual units inside or outside agree to support each other's requests.

Main Direction of Agency

Unlike the systems model, this agency model is mainly concerned with the promotion of numerous ad hoc, unrelated, usually small-scale projects of interest to some actor. Thus, for example, a review committee of the agency may be concerned with sanctioning individual projects as they come up without regard to the impact they may have individually or collectively on the resource allocation of medical services in the region or on the work of other committees in the agency. As a rubber-stamping, sanctioning body, the individual action model is mainly concerned with achieving limited project goals, objectives, or programs.

Primary Roles of Health Planners

Health planners play two basic roles in this model: (1) advocating in behalf of a project and (2) gathering resources to assist in its implementation. In the agency itself, the planner would normally be assigned to a specific committee and devote all of his or her time to promoting the interests of that committee. If the committee desires to have some specific legislation passed, the planner would gather the political, community, and legislative support to achieve the goal. If an outside group desires to gain the agency's approval of a medical project or federally funded program, that group's planner would advocate in its behalf with the appropriate agency committee and/or staff person to gain such approval. Planners may advocate for their own pet projects as well as for those of others.

Center of Influence

Unlike the systems model, there is no one center of influence. Influence is exerted by any individual and/or committee, inside or outside the agency, who has enough initiative and status to secure support for a project. The individual action model agency serves as the meeting ground of the host of actors primarily concerned with implementing their own private objectives and programs.

Strategies for Goal Achievement

The primary strategy in the individual action model would be collaboration when the actor involved has sufficient status or influence to provide reciprocity to those who must provide the official sanction required. Where the advocate for a particular project lacks this status, the strategy of contest is more likely to be used. Contest tactics, such as inducement, demonstrations, or other forms of overt conflict may be used, depending on the situation. External community health organizations without established credentials are likely to resort to various forms of contest tactics because they often lack the status and influence to affect some form of trade-off with those on the governing body or committees of the individual action model agency. Prestigious external medical organizations, such as medical schools, professional associations, and municipal agencies, all have the necessary status to provide such reciprocity when it is required. Subarea councils of HSAs, however, may in some instances have to resort to contest strategies to achieve acceptance and support for their projects from the central governing body.

Commitment to Goals

Those involved in advocating for a specific project or objective can be expected to have a very high commitment to it. This comes from the common values and intense energy the members devote to achieving a limited number of goals. This is unlike the systems or alliance models where motivation to achieve a number of projects simultaneously becomes diluted.

Analysis of Planning Models

From these two illustrations, it can be seen that, conceptually, a number of variables logically fall together to form integrated social systems. The partnership and alliance models can be examined in the same manner from the information given in Table 4-1. As noted earlier, all four models are on a continuum based on the agency's control over resources for planning and implementing goals. The models on the extremes of the continuum, the systems and individual action models, are readily distinguishable from each other, but the partnership and alliance models tend to differ only by degrees and, thus, blend into each other.

As Friedmann noted, allocative and innovative planning is determined by whether or not an attempt is made to alter the basic social structure (innovative). Because there are differences in the objectives, different aspects of planning are emphasized in the allocative and innovative forms. For example, little emphasis is paid to methodology used in analysis in innovative planning, while it is the major emphasis in allocative planning. Innovative strategies tend to be action-oriented, even conflictual in nature, compared to allocative strategies, which tend to emphasize collaboration and maintaining the integrity of the social system. Although one set of values is emphasized over another, both forms of planning utilize all the characteristics to some degree. The dominant emphasis of the characteristic determines the type of planning model an agency typifies rather than the nuances inherent to the agency. However, if the conceptual models do not seem to fit reality, then it can be expected that the form of planning, allocative or innovative, may help explain the variances that occur.

The planning process discussed earlier in this chapter is applicable to all four basic types of planning models. As in innovative and allocative forms of planning, different models may emphasize different phases of the process or even eliminate certain steps, but the process itself remains the same for all models. Even Friedmann's emphasis on reeducation in transactive planning identifies the following three steps in the relearning process: (1) the ability to question existing reality (problem identification), (2) the ability to draw general lessons from concrete experience (identifying alternatives based on experience), and (3) the ability to test these lessons in practice. Although he refers to this three-stage process as a behavioristic rather than a rational planning process, the same concepts apply.[40]

COMPREHENSIVE HEALTH PLANNING

The word *system* is a euphemism that is often used to characterize the functions of health care. In reality, as one authority states, "the most prominent characteristic of the existing community health system is its complexity," and, further, ". . . health care is characterized by a multiplicity of poorly coordinated subsystems, many of which operate almost entirely independent of each other."[41] Because of its complexity and the existence of numerous subsystems, health care is, in fact, disorganized, creating problems in the distribution and quality of health care and the inefficient use of the services that exist.

The usual method employed by health planners is first to define the term *planning* and then discuss the dimensions of health it embraces. One such planner defines planning as "an organized intelligent effort to develop a flexible pattern of action to meet the uncertainties of the future.[42] When applied to areawide planning, such planning appraises the overall health needs of a geographical area to determine how these needs can be met in the most effective and economic manner by existing and future facilities and programs. This is accomplished by determining the population at risk, its level of health, the availability of health resources, and the utilization of existing health services in order to identify unmet needs and develop programs to meet these needs. This definition and its clarifying statement emphasize the elements of a process by which health planning will be done, the need to coordinate the actors involved in determining the needs, the making of decisions by actors in a position to implement these actions, the future orientation of the planning, and its continuity with the next planning cycle.

Another planner defines planning as "the process of making coordinated decisions which have consequences far into the future, particularly beyond a one- or two-year time span."[43] Implicit in this definition is a process that takes into account study and analysis, decision makers' use of this knowledge, and action implementation at some future date. There is little difference between these two definitions as stated.

A third planner defines planning as "those activities required to organize and implement an intervention in current patterns of activities, with the purpose of achieving a different outcome than would have occurred if there had been no intervention."[44] Again, this definition is similar to those noted earlier. Its difference is in the explicit statement that some form of rational planning will produce a result different from the result without such intervention. Whether the difference would be a more positive one than that afforded by the marketplace theory is not honestly known. Yet, one must believe that the planning effort would be intended to produce a better result.

A final definition of planning is "a means of dividing tasks into manageable pieces, massing resources and providing for their application on an orderly and timed basis for the purpose of accomplishing complex tasks."[45] Again, there is a similarity to the previous definitions. All four of these definitions were written by persons with primary interests in the health care field. When one compares these definitions with those presented earlier, the same basic characteristics are seen. These are oriented toward the future; they have explicitly stated goals, continuous process, implied values as expressed by goals and objective preferences, and a decision-making process for action. All of these definitions are goal-oriented, implying that the allocative form of planning as defined by Friedmann predominates. This in turn implies that health planning is adaptive, conservative, and distributive in nature. A maintenance of the status quo is its main aim.

Domain of Health

Comprehensive health planning requires specifically defined boundaries in order to function. One of the ways this is done is to delineate by category what is to be planned. Checko indicates that the four basic elements in any health system consist of health education, personal preventive services, diagnostic and therapeutic services, and rehabilitative and re-storative services.[46] These four categories are further subdivided into eight other areas, the whole of which accounts for all the basic subsystems within the health field. He recommends the use of a systems approach for studying and making decisions regarding any weaknesses identified in the subsystems.

In an editorial in the *American Journal of Public Health,* the health field is divided into four separate triads. The first triad is concerned with identifying the problem areas of community health and includes attention to mental and physical ailments, environmental hazards, and health-related social problems. The second triad focuses on the kinds of resources available in terms of funds, personnel, and material (facilities, supplies, and equipment). The third triad identifies the three types of community constraints and initiatives as authorizations required, norms and standards, and attitudes about health care and utilization. The fourth triad concerns itself with the planning process in terms of administration— including the theory and practice of organizational management, scientific methods for study, and need for processed data. These four triads are interrelated concepts that "explain the meaning of comprehensive health planning as a systematic activity for allocating resources within the limits of community constraints, to meet the expressed demands and needs of the people, to help them achieve optimum social functioning. . . ."[47]

Barry and Sheps define their idea of a health system by identifying four major goals that, if achieved, would result in a healthy population. These goals are (1) positive health, (2) prevention of onset of disease and disability, (3) early recognition and treatment of disease and disability, and (4) prevention of severe disability, social isolation, and untimely death.[48] The latter three goals are further subdivided into eight additional goals. These are arranged in a hierarchy from well-being to ultimate death. This model was included in a major Cleveland study to foster an improved health system for that city. A most significant point articulated by these health planners was their inability to define what was meant by positive health, a real problem in a field that tends to view health from a disease and illness bias.

A fourth way of conceptualizing who is within the health system boundaries was suggested by Palmer. He divides the health field into three major components: facilities, services, and personnel. Within each of these categories he identifies all the different types of facilities (from hospitals to clinics to air pollution measurement centers), services (from preventive care to health education to air and water quality control), and personnel (physicians to technicians to public health engineers) that should be included within these categories. He then identifies a number of nonhealth systems that have health components, but are not included as part of the health system. Examples of these are correctional facilities, schools, war, crime and riot control, welfare assistance, faith healers, and naturopaths. As Palmer pointed out, some of these related, nonhealth components may have more basic consequences for the health of a people than do health services themselves.[49]

A New York State Health Planning Commission document defines comprehensive as "dealing with the totality of the system with which we are concerned," and later, "the full range of forces which impact in a significant way on the physical and mental well-being of people; including social factors which may not be considered part of the health system, per se, but are relevant because of their effect on health."[50]

Section 1502 of PL 93-641 and the 1976 national planning guidelines[51] are the most recent concepts used to define the boundaries of the health care system. Section 1502 denotes 10 national health priorities that, taken collectively, spell out the board boundaries of the health care system. In addition to their emphasis on an integrated approach to the provision of health care services, these priorities focus on elements of the system that were once considered peripheral but are now recognized as significant components of health care. These are promotion of health, prevention of disease, education, nutrition, and the environment. These concepts were amplified in the Bureau of Health Planning's *Guidelines Concerning Development of HSPs* [Health Systems Plans] *and AIPs* [Annual Implementation Plans], issued in December 1976. There the health system is composed of a set of seven different services: ((1) community health promotion and protection, (2) prevention and detection services, (3) diagnosis and treatment services, (4) rehabilitation and habilitation services, (5) maintenance services, (6) support services, and (7) enabling services. These services are to be provided in one or more of six different settings:

1. home
2. mobile
3. ambulatory
4. short-stay
5. long-stay
6. free-standing support[52]

Through an analysis of these services and their appropriate settings, HSAs and State Health Planning and Development Agencies (SHPDAs) were expected to determine the availability, accessibility, quality, acceptability, cost, and continuity of these services in their areas.

The interaction of these three components (Figure 4-1) has been used by HSAs and SHPDAs in the development of their comprehensive and systems-oriented plans.[53] (See Appendix to this chapter for definition of terms.) If only one goal resulted from an analysis of the intersection of these three components, e.g., the cost of community health promotion and protection services in a home setting, there would be a minimum of 252 such statements for physical aspects of health care and another 252 for mental health. In addition, when environmental issues are considered, it becomes quickly evident how complex a comprehensive systems plan can be. It is therefore not surprising that the first editions of the HSPs were often 400 and more pages with separate volumes for data and special studies that had been made in preparing the plans. Under the guidance of the Bureau of Health Planning, the boundaries of the health care system

Figure 4-1   A Conceptual Model of the Health System according to the Services-Settings-Characteristics Taxonomy

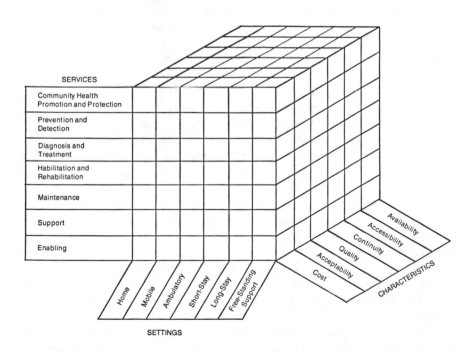

Source: Orkand Report, *Determining Manpower Requirements in the Planning Environment: A Report for the Bureau of Health Planning* (Health Resources Administration: Contract No. HRA 231-77-0083), January 15, 1979, p. 62.

have expanded, and their characteristics have been more explicitly identified. However, the boundaries of the health subsystems can be identified only by linking these components to desired end products. It is the role of the planning process to integrate these parts into a unified whole.

The Health Planning Process

PL 93-641 spells out the elements involved in the planning process in Section 1513, which calls for "improving the health of residents of a health service area, increasing the accessibility . . . , acceptability, continuity, and quality of the health services . . . , restraining increases in the cost of . . . health services, and preventing unnecessary duplication of health resources." There are four ways of meeting the purposes of the act. One is to identify local issues and develop solutions to them on an ad hoc and issue-by-issue basis. This has been characterized previously as a disjointed incremental method of planning. A second way is to analyze the availability of medical resources within the taxonomy (see Figure 4-1) and plan both to fill in the gaps and to reduce duplications and inappropriate distributions of resources. This method, usually referred to as resource planning, is based on estimating the demand for various types of services by settings and then supplying that amount. Both the disjointed incremental and resource planning processes are conservative and status quo-oriented; both assume the system is meeting the needs of all the people who really need services. Occasional dysfunctions of the system may require corrective action, such as supplying more physicians for an underserved area or reducing the number of beds for the care of acute illness in another.

The third method is concerned with meeting the needs of all the people residing in a health service area. Primarily a challenge to improve the health status of the population, it is referred to as population-based planning. It focuses on the causes of disease, but more importantly tries to determine the nature of health and to promote good physical and mental health. As such, it is far more innovative in its planning, seeks solutions outside the health care system (e.g., improved housing, jobs for all persons, a decent income to ensure that basic social needs will be met) as well as inside the system. Thus, this method extends the health systems planning boundaries beyond the limits noted in Figure 4-1 to include other systems.

The final approach to planning is the combined or balanced method, which integrates the best features of the other approaches into a comprehensive plan. Thus, the population-based approach might be used to identify a number of potential solutions for raising the health status of segments of the population. Part of the solution may call for an analysis of the medical care system to determine the medical resources needed to meet the population's needs. In this process, a more detailed study of various factors, such as ability to pay for medical care and accessibility to the handicapped and elderly, may be undertaken, and the recommendations resulting from this study may be incorporated into the systems plan as objectives to be achieved.[54] The planning guidelines of the Bureau of Health Planning encourage this balanced form of planning, but they also make clear that the analysis should center on the health needs and status of the population rather than on the problems of the medical care system. Thus, changes in the medical care system are predicated on their capacity to improve the health status of various segments of the population. As the guidelines state,

> in population-based planning, a specific population is analyzed to determine its health problems. The health system is then studied to determine how it must function if those problems are to be addressed. Population-based planning can be contrasted with demand or resource-based planning, which begins by examining the capabilities and/or utilization of the health system prior to consideration of the needs of the area's population. Population-based planning will help the HSA identify underutilization as well as overutilization of services. It is recognized that much developmental work needs to be done in establishing techniques for population-based planning and that, for the present, a population-based approach cannot be completely used.[55]

PL 93-641 identifies the following steps in the planning process it expects HSAs and SHPDAs to follow:

- study of the health status of the population and the medical system serving it
- identification of the gaps between the needs of the population and the services available to meet them
- setting of goals and objectives
  - —use of health status indicators
  - —use of health system indicators
  - —ranking of goals and objectives
- recommendation of alternative actions to achieve goals/objectives
- identification of resources for service development
  - —facilities
  - —personnel
  - —equipment

- evaluation of goal achievement through periodic assessments of services required by the appropriateness review function

These steps in the act's planning process are similar to those of the traditional/rational planning process advocated by most planners. Unlike most planning processes, however, the act calls for a two-tier process requiring the development of two types of plans, the HSP and the AIP. The HSP sets the goals and priorities for the long range, while the AIP indicates how many of the long-range goals can be achieved in the first year and each succeeding year thereafter. In medical parlance, the HSP is concerned with the diagnosis and treatment plan, while the AIP focuses on implementation. In previous federal planning efforts, most plans stopped at the HSP level. This is the first health planning legislation that includes implementation of the plan as a basic function of a health planning agency.

> HSAs are charged by the Planning Act with a leadership role in producing basic changes in the health care system. To meet this formidable challenge, they must define goals for health status and health systems improvement, including cost control in their plans. They must then: 1) develop a clear understanding of the issues which influence the accomplishment of those purposes; 2) define that set of changes necessary to produce improvement; 3) produce a community understanding and commitment to desired change; 4) undertake a defined set of implementation activities and regulatory recommendations sufficient to accomplish required changes; and 5) promote linkages between physical and mental health systems.[56]

The HSP is the basic blueprint of detailed goal statements that describe the desired level of health status, a healthful environment, and the health system appropriate for an area. It details the changes needed in the amount or type of an area's health services in order to contain costs and prevent unnecessary duplication of health services. It is a long-range plan, having at least a five-year planning horizon. Goals are defined by the national guidelines as "statements of desired levels of health status, desired performance of the health system, or desired levels of resources."[57]

It is not enough to develop a statement of health status and health system goals. These goals must be quantified so that they can be measured. Measurable indicators are often used as proxies of goals because they reflect the health status of the population or how well the health system is performing. Examples of health status indicators are infant mortality rates and the incidences of various medical disabilities, such as cancer or heart disease; examples of health system indicators used include the time required to get to a health facility (indicator of availability of service) and the cost of a medical service (indicator of financial accessibility or affordability of a medical service). Health system indicators generally refer to one or more of the six basic systems characteristics noted in Figure 4-1, i.e., availability, accessibility, continuity, quality, acceptability, and cost of health care services. Quantified goals or their proxy indicators are necessary to determine what changes, if any, are occurring in the population's health status or the medical care system.

Long-range objectives must also be part of the HSP. These are "quantified statements of desired health status or health system performance expressed as a level to be achieved within a specified time period."[58] Since goals cannot always be achieved within a specific time frame because medical technology has not yet solved a problem or the causes of a problem are unknown, partial levels of improvements, based on limited knowledge and existing treatment technologies, must be described. Thus, even if the true causes of heart disease are not known, through half way technologies such as medication therapy and surgical procedures or preventive measures such as changes in diet and eating habits, it may be possible to reduce the number of people who die of heart disease. An estimate of the number of persons who can be educated to change their life style or take medication becomes a five-year objective that can be stated in quantifiable terms, such as "to reduce the percentage of mortality in males 45–54 from 205 per 100,000 to 185 by 1985." In this way, desirable goals are converted into measurable objectives to be achieved within a defined time limit.

The strategies required for long-range objectives must be defined in the HSPs. These strategies are referred to as long-range recommended actions. Usually, two or more actions, either individually or collectively, are expected to achieve the objectives. With respect to reducing the mortality rate of those with heart disease, for example, one action may be persuading people to change their diets while another action may be improving the emergency medical system so that persons who suffer heart attacks obtain treatment more rapidly. Typically, the description of the actions should include who is involved, what improvement is expected, and an evaluation of its technical or administrative feasibility.

Finally, the resources required to carry out the actions should be specified. Resources are normally considered to be the costs of facilities, personnel, equipment, and training. Sponsors of resources, their location, whether new, or reallocated, and their potential benefits in relation to the costs should be specified. Through spelling out the costs of each alternative action, the planner will be able to determine which may be most effective in achieving the objective at the least cost.

An HSA's regulatory function becomes an essential component of the implementation phase of the recommended actions. Certificate-of-need project review and review of proposed uses of federal funds are crucial mechanisms for achieving long-range objectives. Appropriateness review, in fact, serves as an important evaluation tool. This procedure, which must be carried out every three years on all existing health care services, permits an HSA to determine which existing services should be closed, renovated, combined with another service, expanded, or converted to a new service.

Finally, the HSP planning process must link together the goals, objectives, actions, and resources. It is this linkage that stamps the plan as a system rather than a collection of miniplans that may or may not collectively achieve the plan's goals and objectives. For example, it is important to know whether an increase in the number of home health care services will reduce the need for nursing home beds, hospital beds, or mental health facility beds. It is important to determine whether the extra nurses, home health aides, physical therapists, and occupational therapists will leave an insufficient number of these professionals available for hospitals and nursing homes. It is important to ask whether short-term gains in the medical care system should be sacrificed for expected long-term benefits in the development of nonmedical services, such as environmental improvements. It is through asking significant questions and making difficult and usually painful decisions that the impact of one part of the system on another is revealed.

Systems planning helps to predict the consequences of efforts to implement HSP goals, including those that would not be anticipated in problem-oriented or disjointed incremental planning. Thus, the flow of logic, as the guidelines refer to the effort to link the parts, must be analyzed and taken into account in the development of an HSP.

The AIP is quite similar to the HSP except that its time frame is generally limited to one year, and it specifies a series of objectives that can feasibly be achieved within that period. The AIP objectives are directly linked to the long-range recommended actions of the HSP. Thus, if the five-year objective is to reduce the accident rate among 18- to 25-year-olds by 50 percent by 1985, alternative long-range recommended actions might include a) reducing the number of penalty points for driving infractions from 12 to 6 before a person loses his or her driver's license for one full year by 1985 and b) eliminating dangerous highway and urban street driving conditions in 50 percent of the recognized danger points by 1985. The AIP objectives would translate these recommended actions into one-year objectives. The first AIP objective might read: To reduce the number of penalty points required to lose one's driver's license for six months from

12 to 10 for all persons under 45 years of age. This would achieve a part of the five-year recommended action by reducing the number of penalty points by two in the first year and limit this to all persons under 45 instead of only to those under 26 years of age. The proportion of those who commit driving infractions that result in injury to the driver or another vehicle would be reduced by those who formerly were able to drive with 11 penalty points. The second AIP objective might seek to reduce the number of road impediments by 20 percent in the suburban and rural areas and by 10 percent in the two largest cities of the region. In this way, the five-year objectives would be partially achieved. The two actions, taken together, may result in a 10 percent reduction in the accident rate for the 18- to 25-year-old age group.

Unlike the HSP recommended actions, which only generally identify the strategies to be undertaken, AIP actions must be described in specific detail. In some instances, the HSA either provides technical assistance to those involved in the actions or itself drafts detailed project plans to show how the actions will be implemented. Together with an analysis of the resources required to carry out the actions, the SHA should conduct cost-benefit analyses to determine the most effective actions at the lowest costs among the various alternatives.

Thus, the steps in this planning process are the same as those outlined in the earlier section on planning. The only difference is the focus on health care. A planning process is essential, whether it is a four-step sequence as outlined by Williams (the survey, analysis, design of a complete plan, and implementation of the plan)[59] or the eight-step process outlined by Palmer with a well-designed systems approach that relies on a simulation predictor model requiring the use of a computer or some other version.[60] A real issue in these models of the planning process is whether the voice of decision makers can alter or affect the process, or whether the decisions are based on technical studies, cost-benefit analysis, or other allocative methodologies. In reality, the nature of decision making in the implementation of health plans necessitates existing health service agencies to carry out these decisions. This automatically ensures health providers of a major role in the entire planning process and thus in the governing process of the HSAs. Kissick underscores this point when he states that "system analysis without the social instruments of implementation will not be sufficient to develop comprehensive health care systems. Understanding of the system must be accompanied by the authority to act."[61]

A second issue affecting the rational planning process is the scope of the planning being considered. The wider the scope, in terms of geography or the number of health components being considered in the planning, the more general the plan is likely to be. A five-year plan would be more concerned with the general directions health care should take, based on changing values and the aspirations of society. These would be comprehensive in scope, similar to the master plans of city planners. They are policy plans and, as such, set a framework within which a narrower aspect of planning, often referred to as project, program, or operational planning, takes place. The combination of the HSP and AIP serves this dual function by setting forth a policy framework within which specific objectives and actions are detailed. This type of plan emphasizes the action or implementation factors in the planning process and is based on a set of priority objectives that is selected to carry out one or more of the goals in the policy portion of the HSP.

This type of planning suffers from some defects. In a cogent, thoughtful article, Arnold points out that program planning assumes that with "adequate knowledge man can control nature, or at least meet it on an equal basis."[62] Yet, she challenges that man has this capability because in very few instances has man had a sufficient scientific understanding of nature to control it. This means that planning decisions cannot be made by strictly scientific methodologies based on accepted canons of scientific theory. It must then be made by political consensus or result in segmental planning rather than total planning as implied in the comprehensive health planning legislation. The planning process, therefore, does not become local or lead to rational conclusions, but rather is partisan, with choice usually based on the self-interests of those most influential and most affected by the need to resolve a problem according to Lindblom's "disjointed incrementalist" approach. It becomes irrational, although the hope is that the decisions of each self-interested party eventually offset the negative consequences of decisions made by other partisans and that a new equilibrium by "mutual partisan adjustment" is established. It is the total of these mutual adjustments that leads to a semblance of rationality and maintains the health "system" in a more harmonious state. Thus, the planning process is ultimately more dependent on political—juridical—regulatory factors for implementation than on the alternatives offered by the sophisticated economic and mathematical methods of analysis that are supposedly predicated on scientific theory.

Finally, the planning process and the comprehensiveness of the health plan is dependent upon coordination for its potential implementation, especially if the combined effort of more than two actors is required to put it into effect. The danger of coordination is that it reduces innovation and stifles new approaches to health care. Arnold writes that "coordination reduces uncertainty for agency decision makers, but in so doing it also reduces the field of operations and the innovative alternative actions that might evolve were the larger system considered."[63] The "larger system" refers to the impact of decisions on other health components or on other societal systems. For example, the decision for women to use "the pill" to protect themselves against unwanted pregnancy has seriously affected the spread of venereal diseases among youth because of the reduced use of condoms by males. Had family planning units and health departments, which teamed to educate the public on the use and safety of birth control pills, also involved the subsystem of health educators, social workers, and churches in the potential consequences of an increased incidence of venereal disease, then steps could have been taken earlier to alert the public to this serious side-effect.

Coordination is merely the function of maintaining the balance among health actors within the health environment as stable as possible. Innovations in health care can seriously disturb this equilibrium. Yet, in many instances a disturbance in the system may be required to bring about major changes and improvements to whole segments of the population. Thus, while comprehensive health planning is concerned with both coordination and innovation, the weight carried by influential actors in the planning process and the methodologies used tend to emphasize the coordination aspect and, thus, the maintenance of whatever stability exists among the independent actors who make up the health environment.

In the final analysis, the rational planning process starts out with a strong emphasis on technical methods used by HSA planners. In the end, however, it is the decision makers who convert these alternatives into a series of priority choices, even though they are usually motivated by highly subjective values that may or may not take into account the carefully worked out technical decisions of the planners. For rational planning to be feasible, it must integrate the technical objectivity of the planner with the subjectivity of the decision maker.

NOTES

1. Abraham Kaplan, *The Conduct of Inquiry* (San Francisco: Chandler Publishing Co., 1964), p. 295. Chapter VII gives a detailed analysis of theory and its various types, functions, and validations.

2. *Ibid.*, p. 313.

3. John W. Dyckman, *Introduction to Readings in the Theory of Planning, The State of Planning Theory in America,* mimeographed (circa 1960).

4. *Ibid.*, p. 2.

5. *Ibid.*, p. 4.

6. *Ibid.*, p. 43.

7. *Ibid.*, p. 45.

8. Andreas Faludi, *A Reader in Planning Theory* (New York: Pergamon Press, 1973), p. 6.

9. *Cf.* Dahl and Lindblom, *Politics, Economics and Welfare* (New York: Harper & Row, Publishers, 1953); Marris and Rein, *Dilemmas of Social Reform* (New York: Atherton, 1969); Meyerson and Banfield, *Politics, Planning and the Public Interest* (Glencoe, Ill.: The Free Press, 1955); Altschuler, *The City Planning Process* (Ithaca, New York: Cornell University Press, 1965); and Kahn, *Studies in Social Policy and Planning* (New York: Russell Sage Foundation, 1969).

10. John Friedmann, "A Conceptual Model for the Analysis of Planning Behavior," and Richard Bolan, "Community Decision Behavior: The Culture of Planning," in Faludi, *Reader in Theory*.

11. Bolan, in Faludi, *Reader in Theory*, p. 386.

12. Friedmann, in Faludi, *Reader in Theory*, p. 368.

13. *Executive Office of the President Circular Number A-82*, revised December 18, 1967 (Washington, D.C.: Bureau of the Budget).

14. Doris Holeb, *Social and Economic Information for Urban Planning* (Chicago: Center for Urban Studies of the University of Chicago, 1969), p. 11.

15. John Friedmann, *Retracking America: A Theory of Transactive Planning* (Garden City, New York: Anchor Press, 1973), pp. 53–54.

16. Alan A. Altschuler, *The City Planning Process, A Political Analysis* (Ithaca, New York: Cornell University Press, 1965), p. 299. Specialist and functional plans and planners are to be considered as interchangeable concepts. City planning has the same contextual characteristics as comprehensive planning except that its geographical boundary is limited to the city lines whereas comprehensive boundaries are determined by the size of the area being studied.

17. Edward C. Banfield, "End and Means in Planning," *International Social Science Journal* 10 (1959): 361–368.

18. Paul Davidoff and Thomas A. Reiner, "A Choice Theory of Planning," *Journal of the Institute of Planners* 28 (1962): 103–115.

19. Faludi, *Reader in Theory*, p. 1.

20. Friedmann, *Retracking America*, p. 19.

21. Yehezkel Dror, "The Planning Process: A Facet Design," in Faludi, *Reader in Theory*, p. 330.

22. Friedmann, *Retracking America*, pp. 11–12.

23. *Ibid.*, p. 245.

24. Robert R. Mayer, *Social Planning and Social Change* (Englewood Cliffs, N.J.: Prentice-Hall, Inc., 1972), p. 132.

25. *Ibid.*

26. Alfred Kahn, *Theory and Practice of Social Planning* (New York: Russell Sage Foundation, 1969), p. 16.

27. Dror, in Faludi, *Reader in Theory*, p. 330.

28. Friedmann, *Retracking America*, p. 16.

29. Herbert H. Hyman, "The Social Planning Process," mimeographed (New York: Hunter College, Dept. of Urban Affairs, 1970).

30. Charles E. Lindblom, "The Science of Muddling Through," *Public Administration Review*, Spring 1969.

31. Faludi, *Reader in Theory*, pp. 151–170.

32. Friedmann, *Retracking America*, Chapters 7–9.

33. *Ibid.*, Chapter 3.

34. Robert A. Levine, *Public Planning* (New York: Basic Books, Inc., 1972), p. V.

35. Kaplan, *Conduct of Inquiry*, Chapter 7.

36. Roland L. Warren, *Community in America* (Chicago: Rand McNally and Co., 1963), Chapter 5.

37. *Ibid.*, p. 135.

38. Friedmann, *Retracking America*, p. 5.

39. Roland L. Warren, "The Interorganizational Field as a Focus of Investigation," mimeographed (Waltham, Mass: Brandeis University, 1967).

40. Friedmann, *Retracking America*, p. 232.

41. American Society of Planning Officials, *The Urban Planner in Health Planning* (Washington, D.C.: U.S. Department of Health, Education and Welfare, Public Health Service, 1968), p. 9.

42. Jack C. Haldeman, *Planning for Better Health Service* (New York: Health and Hospital Planning Council of Southern New York, Inc., May 1970), Appendix D.

43. Boyd Z. Palmer, et al., *An Advanced Health Planning System* (Springfield, Va.: National Technical Information Service, U.S. Dept. of Commerce, 1972), pp. 7–9.

44. Rick J. Carlson, *Planning and Law* (Minneapolis, Minn: Health Services Research Center, Institute for Interdisciplinary Studies, American Rehabilitation Foundation, 1969), p. 2.

45. James D. Williams, "CHP: An Organization Means for Transition," *American Journal of Public Health,* January 1969, p. 49.

46. George Checko, *The Recognition of Systems in Health Service* (Arlington, Va.: Operations Research Society of America, circa 1969).

47. Editorial, "Concepts of CHP," *American Journal of Public Health,* June 1968, pp. 1011–1013.

48. Mildred C. Barry and Cecil G. Sheps,"A New Model for Community Health Planning," *American Journal of Public Health,* February 1969, pp. 226–236.

49. Palmer, et al., *Advanced Health Planning,* Table 1, System Boundaries, p. 21.

50. New York State Health Planning Commission, "The Development of a State Comprehensive Health Plan," mimeographed, April 1973, p. 1.

51. U.S. DHEW, *Guidelines for the Development of Health Systems Plans and Annual Implementation Plans* (Hyattsville, Md.: Bureau of Health Planning, February 23, 1979).

52. *Ibid.*, pp. 30–33.

53. Donald S. Orkand, Nancy McGraw, and Martha Guthrie, *Determining Manpower Requirements in the Planning Environment: A Report for the Bureau of Health Planning,* Contract No: HRA 231-77-0083 (Silver Spring, Md.: The Orkand Corporation, January 15, 1979), p. 62.

54. Boyd Z. Palmer, *Data and Techniques: Implications of Plan Development Approaches,* workshop given September 17, 1976, in New York City (Syracuse, New York: ALPHA Center).

55. U.S. DHEW, *Guidelines for Health Systems Plans,* p. 5.

56. *Ibid.*, p. 1.

57. *Ibid.*, p. 9.

58. *Ibid.*, p. 12.

59. Williams, "CHP," p. 48.

60. Palmer, et al., *Advanced Health Planning*, pp. 38–39.

61. William L. Kissick, "Organization of Health Services" in *The Recognition of Systems in Health Services*, ed., George Checko (Arlington, Va.: Operations Research Society of America, circa 1969), p. 69.

62. Mary F. Arnold, "Basic Concepts and Crucial Issues in Health Planning," *American Journal of Public Health*, September 1969, pp. 1686–1697.

63. *Ibid.*

Appendix 4-A

Categories of Health Services[*]

Community Health Promotion and Protection

Those services directed at the community level toward improving the personal health behavior of residents and improving the quality of environmental factors affecting their health.

Prevention and Detection Services

Those services delivered to individuals in order to promote optimal physical and mental well-being, including protection from the development of disease and ill health, or those services that identify disease or ill health at the presymptomatic or unrecognized symptomatic stage.

Diagnosis and Treatment Services

Diagnosis and treatment services are those which identify and/or alleviate specific diseases and conditions of their symptoms once they have become symptomatic.

Habilitation and Rehabilitation Services

Services designed to assist the ill, injured, or disabled individual to achieve, or be restored to the fullest physical, mental, social, vocational, and economic usefulness of which that individual is capable.

Maintenance Services

Services provided to individuals with chronic physical and/or mental conditions in order to prevent deterioration of those conditions, as well as services provided to those in need of assistance in activities of daily living. The purpose of such services is to enable an individual to participate in the community to the fullest degree of which that individual is capable. Maintenance services do not include habilitation or rehabilitation services, since the primary purpose of the latter services is to *increase* functional ability rather than maintain an existing level of function.

Source: Appendices to this chapter are from U.S. DHEW, *Guidelines for Health Systems Plans,* Appendix, pp. 30, 32, and 33.

Support Services

Services provided to assure adequate management of medical care resources and patient care environment, which assist the delivery of services without the provision of direct patient care (as in pharmacy, tissue, and social services) and which contribute to continuity of care (as in referral and discharge planning services).

Enabling Services

Organized activities designed to influence the means by which health system services are delivered. These may include the concerns of

1. health planning (such as data assembly and analysis, goal determination, action recommendation, implementation strategy);
2. resources development (manpower, facilities, equipment);
3. financing (third party reimbursement, public grants, and expenditures for services);
4. regulations (Certificate-of-Need and 1122 agreements, manpower and facility licensure, rate and insurance regulation); and
5. research (biomedical, behavioral, technological, organizational, and services delivery).

Appendix 4-B

Settings in Which Health Services May Be Delivered

Community Setting

Settings in which community health promotion and health systems enabling services, rather than personal health care services or patient-related support services, are provided.

Home Setting

Settings in which health care services are provided in the patient's residence with the result that the patient does not travel in order to receive services.

Mobile Setting

Providing health care services at temporary locations (selected for their convenience to a geographically selected target population) using a movable vehicle or facility, or providing health care services during transportation of patients.

Ambulatory Setting

Providing health care services to patients who travel to the provider to receive services. An ambulatory setting has no regular provision for patients to stay overnight.

Short-stay Setting

Providing health care services to patients who stay overnight in the institution, 50 percent or more of whom return to their normal place of residence within less than 30 days of entering the institution.

Long-stay Setting

Providing health care services to patients who stay overnight in the institution, 50 percent or more of whom remain in the institution 30 days or longer. A long-stay setting may be the usual place of residence of some or all of its patients.

Free-standing Support Setting

A location where health services are provided to support the delivery of personal health care services without providing direct patient care, and which is not a component of an organization which delivers personal health services in another setting. Free-standing support settings include: (1) medical laboratories; (2) dental laboratories; (3) pharmacies; (4) tissue banks; and (5) health information centers.

Appendix 4-C

Characteristics of the Health System

Availability

The supply and types of health services that can be produced, given the supply and feasible alternative allocations of resources (personnel, equipment, facilities, and finances) to produce those services.

Accessibility

The ability of a population or a segment of a population to obtain available health services. This ability is determined by economic, temporal, locational, architectural, cultural, organizational, and informational factors, which may be barriers or facilitators to obtaining services.

Continuity

The extent of effective coordination of services provided to individual patients and the community over time, within and among health care settings.

Acceptability

The level of satisfaction expressed by consumers of services and providers of services with the availability, accessibility, cost, quality, continuity, and courtesy and consideration of the health system.

Quality

The degree to which services provided are properly matched to the needs of the population, are technically correct, and achieve beneficial impact. Quality can be considered in three dimensions: (1) the structural aspects of resources and services; (2) the process of producing and delivering services; and (3) the outcomes of services on health status, environment, and/or behavior.

Cost

All expenses incurred in producing and delivering health services.

Chapter 5

Health Planning Methodologies

Pursuant to the enactment of PL 93-641, millions of dollars were expended to identify and discover health planning methodologies that would be relevant to plan development, project review, appropriateness review, and other activities for which the Health Systems Agencies (HSAs) and State Health Planning and Development Agencies (SHPDAs) were assigned responsibilities. In all, seven basic functions have been defined by federal guidelines.[1] In this chapter, those that pertain to plan development will be discussed.

A review of the four basic planning models (see Chapter 4) to which the health planning agencies could conform reveals that they each focus on different aspects of planning. The systems model places its emphasis on plan development and implementation; the partnership model, on general policy formation and support; the alliance, on specific policy issues and possibly some program plans and implementation; and the individual action model, on program plans. Since these planning models are ideal constructs, it is not likely that, in reality, any one can be found in its pure form.

To counteract differentiation among the HSAs nationwide, the Bureau of Health Planning has issued performance standards that the HSAs and SHPDAs are expected to meet in carrying out their basic functions. Periodic assessments of these agencies are made to determine their compliance with the standards. In spite of this move toward standardization of agency performance, it is expected that each agency will continue to focus on what it considers to be the most relevant functions for its areawide responsibilities. This means that, while there will be some conformity to the federal standards, lip service will probably be paid to some of the mandatory functions, and, as in the past, those functions that are most consistent and comfortable to the planning agencies' orientation and patterns of operation will be emphasized.

What this means is that whether orientations and authority structure of the health planning agencies follow an evolutionary development from less complex to more complex planning and policy analysis, as Meshenberg believes,[2] or whether they arrive full-blown at a way of operation that is conducive to their style and accepted by community health forces, different planning methods will be required. For example, Meshenberg points out that in a health planning agency's first stage of development, "mostly organizational, public contact, administrative, and general planning" skills are required, whereas in the third of his three stages different and more highly developed skills are needed, a "variety of special skills: planning, policy analysis, research, and public contact."[3]

On the other hand, other writers have noted the relationship of specific types of planning methods to the type of authority structure required to implement the methods. Warren and his colleagues note the need for a central decision-making authority structure to implement systems analysis and program budgeting.[4] Bolan agrees with Warren as he notes that systems analysis and cost-effectiveness methods require strong central decision making for their implementation.[5] Wildavsky notes the same relationship, that systems analysis requires centralized decision making while cost-benefit analysis is based on less stringent centralized control.[6] In other words, the various planning methods are not equally applicable to all types of health planning agencies. They must be used selectively according to the primary orientation of activity and the authority structure of the agency.

Two organizing principles can be used to set the parameters of a methods discussion. First, methods can be separated according to whether their main function is linked to plan development, including needs analysis and goal setting, or plan implementation, including resource development, community support, and program coordination (Table 5-1).[7] Second, each of the methods can be related to the planning model in which it appears to be most feasible. Some methods are applicable to more than one planning model. Table 5-2 reveals that the systems model of planning is likely to use the more recently developed planning methods of systems analysis, operations research, and cost-benefit analysis. There is no single method utilized by all the planning models. While policy analysis has the widest use, it is applicable to the individual action model. The alliance model is indifferent to all methods, although it occasionally involves policy analysis and community organization methods. The individual action model places its greatest emphasis on the methods of ad hoc opportunism and community organization with some use of the other methods. Thus, the chart reveals that different methods are related to different planning models and their corresponding authority structure.

Table 5-1   Relationship of Methods to Plan Development and Plan Implementation

PLAN DEVELOPMENT	
Methods	*Techniques*
Needs analysis	
	Key Informant
	Social Indicator
Policy analysis	
Information systems and health indicators	
Systems analysis	
	Cost-Benefit
	Cost-Effectiveness
Forecasting	
	Delphi
	Buzz Groups
	Brainstorming
PLAN IMPLEMENTATION	
Operations research	
	Simulation
	Gaming
	PERT and Critical Path
Ad hoc opportunism	
Community organization	

PLAN DEVELOPMENT METHODS

In this section, five plan development methods will be discussed: (1) needs analysis, (2) policy analysis, (3) information systems and health indicators, (4) systems analysis, and (5) forecasting. For three of these, there are alternative techniques. There will be no attempt here to get involved with the actual computations of the methods. These are better done in numerous other volumes and articles specifically related to those methods. Several of these articles and texts will be cited. Readers are advised especially to read *Basic Health Planning Methods,* by Spiegel and Hyman.

Needs Analysis

Current health planning has dramatically shifted its emphasis from resource to population-based planning, which calls for an assessment of

Table 5-2 Relationship of Methods to Planning Models[8]

Methods	Planning Models			Individual Action
	Systems	Partnership	Alliance	
Systems analysis	Yes	No	No	No
Operations research	Yes	No	No	For improving existing program
Intuitive forecasting	Sometime	Yes	No	In developing new ideas
Information systems and health indicators	Yes	No	No	In very limited way
Ad hoc opportunism	No	No	No	Yes
Policy analysis	Yes	Yes	Sometime	No
Community organization	No	Sometime	Sometime	Yes
Needs analysis	Yes	Yes	No	No

the health care needs of the population, both as a whole and as a set of special subpopulations, in a health service region. It is no longer sufficient to describe who demanded and used services or whether there were sufficient resources to meet this demand. For a variety of reasons—inability to afford a service, inability to obtain transportation to a service, provider discrimination toward certain types of prospective patients, or patient rejection of perceived inferior quality services—persons with legitimate needs for medical and health services may not demand them or even perceive the need for them. Methods have been developed to estimate the number and location of these people. None of the needs assessment methods are applicable to all situations, and all possess characteristics that limit their validity, reliability, or accuracy. There is a basic trade-off among the methods; for example, some have the capacity to define the population in need with precision, but lack the data to determine the need. Others can use available data, but can estimate need only in gross terms. Because of the high costs involved in generating the data required by the more sophisticated needs assessment methods, health planning agencies have tended to use the simpler methods that rely on routinely collected data. Key informant and social indicator methods are only two illustrations of the numerous needs assessment techniques that can be used to determine the needs of a population.

Key Informant

Developed by Warheit and his associates to determine the mental health needs of a population,[9] the key informant technique is applicable to any general or subpopulation. The steps in the process call for

- stating the objectives of the research with as much precision as possible in order to ensure that the key informants focus on the issue at hand. For example, the key informants could be asked how many persons 12 to 18 years old have received treatment for a mental problem of a certain type during a specified period of time in a particular community. This provides the sharp delineation that would be lacking in a more generalized question, such as how many persons were treated for mental illness in the past.
- listing those key informants who would be in a position to know something about the issue. In mental health, these would include police officers, social service workers, teachers, camp counselors, members of the Parent-Teacher Association (PTA), as well as the usual community mental health staff. Such an array of persons would be aware of those who have been treated and those whose behavior in normal settings might indicate that they need mental health services.
- developing a list of questions linked to the issue. With respect to this example, questions would be designed to elicit answers that shed light on who received help or failed to, to whom they went for assistance, the duration of symptoms before service was sought, attitudes about asking for help, and constraints such as cost, location, or sense of shame that may have interfered with their asking for assistance.
- arranging personal interviews. While the questions might be used in telephone surveys or as a mailed questionnaire, the personal interview permits probing, clarification of statements, and uncovering unanticipated facets of the issue.
- tabulating the data, analyzing them, and comparing answers. The needs of the population under examination are identified and a report submitted to the relevant committee of the health planning agency.
- reaching a consensus of what the data mean and the priority to be given to the issue at hand. These are then written in a final report to be used by the plan development committee and its staff to determine the needs of the population and the goals and objectives required to deal with any unmet need, lack of resources, or inaccessibility to services.

This technique has some obvious advantages. It is quick, easy, and relatively inexpensive. With this technique, a gross estimate of the range of unmet need can be established by those in a position to know. The technique sometimes uncovers facets of the issue that previously received little or no attention. Finally, it sets a climate for future involvement of those involved in the survey.

This method generally lacks reliability, however. A second group of key informants or even a group that includes some of the original informants may produce different estimates of need. If key informants are selected from a narrow band of a wide range of orientations to the issue, then the bias of those selected will affect the estimate of need, and the needs of some may be excluded. For example, the mental health needs of the overly quiet, good child who causes no problems at home or school may be overlooked while those of the child who misbehaves may be disproportionately represented.

Given the probability that the federal-state-regional health planning system will not in the foreseeable future have the funds available to carry out the extensive surveys required to determine health needs on a continuing basis, a needs assessment that depends on the expert judgment of key informants becomes a feasible alternative, in spite of its disadvantages.

Social Indicator Technique

The use of social indicators in health planning has been perfected by the National Institute of Mental Health; this technique is used to identify geographical areas where many people are likely to need mental health services.[10] It is based on the assumption that certain descriptive data (vital statistics, census) can be used to identify the needs of a population and to estimate the degree of need. The steps in the technique call for developing an ecological picture of the geographical area in question through analysis of four factors:

1. housing arrangements of people and the facilities they use
2. sociodemographic characteristics of the people in the areas including sex, age, income, marital status
3. degree of social stability and well-being of the people with reference to mobility, work stability, crime, school attendance, welfare assistance
4. general social conditions, including degree of overcrowding, type of housing, availability of social, educational, and recreational services

These factors, taken together, form an environmental picture of the area and how the people live. It then becomes possible to focus on the specific objective that concerns the health planning committee. Are the committee members interested in identifying the rate of infant mortality in the area or the morbidity related to heart conditions, cancer, or hypertension, or are they concerned about a specific population grouping such as young adults, children, or the elderly? By being as specific as possible, the planning committee can highlight those descriptive indicators that provide further insight into the populations at risk for certain conditions.

For an objective dealing with heart disease, the committee would examine data describing nutrition, percentage of persons on welfare with large families, overcrowding, unemployment, school drop-out rates, and juvenile delinquency. These data deal with environmental and psychological stress, as well as behavioral manifestations that are likely to be associated with tension and possible heart disease.

The data collected should be related to the outcome sought. If there is a concern about the degree of hypertension among white school-age children, 10 to 18 years old, who live in three different residential levels of the region, then planners would collect morbidity information on, for example, hypertension, percentage of families with health insurance, number of ambulatory visits to physicians per year for those families and/or their children 10 to 18 years old, the unemployment rate, and the mobility of the families. These data, taken together, may highlight the need for hypertensive services. It is essential to determine the unit of analysis before collecting the data. In this situation, there might be two levels of analysis: the individual children or the family with such children if it were not possible to obtain data on the children themselves, and/or the geographical area, which might include a health area, a census tract, or a block. Data from smaller subdivisions within a larger area would make it possible to isolate areas of need where data from the general area would indicate no such problem. Because several types of data are needed, data may be obtained from the health department, the welfare department, the city planning commission, and the department of economic development.

Finally, after the data have been collected, analysis can be done through charts, use of map overlays, tables, and so forth to compare how the geographical areas differ from some acceptable norm, such as a national average, urban median, or state standard. Through this analysis, social indicators would be identified to show how the geographical areas rank with each other and, thus, areas of potential need.

Advantages of this technique are that data are usually available from public sources, are inexpensive to obtain, and can be manipulated to meet different types of planning needs. Further, it is fairly easy to update the data and determine trends.

It must be kept in mind that indicators are proxies, or indirect measures, of the real objectives. Without careful thought and analysis, data that are not validly related to the objective may be collected. Because data often come from different sources, the way in which data are collected may not be consistent from one source to another. Thus, the department of health may group data on young people according to age ranges of 5 to 14 and 15 to 20, while the welfare department may show three-year increments, i.e., 9 to 12, 13 to 15, and 16 to 18; this makes it difficult to accept the reliability of the data between the different bases. Another limitation is that the products of this technique apply to collective cohorts of children, rather than individual children. Finally, this technique relies heavily on census data. Unfortunately most of these data are old and inaccurate, especially near the end of a decade. In spite of these disadvantages, the social indicator technique does permit a general comparison and ranking of need among several subareas of a health service area of a state.

Needs analysis is most relevant for the systems and partnership planning models since both are concerned with determining a population's health status and relative needs. The systems model requires more quantitative data, while the partnership model is satisfied by relative ranking of a population's health status, regardless of whether ranking is based on measurable factors. For this reason, the social indicator technique is more likely to be used in the systems planning model, while the key informant technique is more often applied to the partnership model. Since the objectives of the alliance and individual action planning models are usually stated before planning is begun and the scope of action and implementation encompass a rather narrow slice of the population's health status at any one time, neither model is involved in determining a population's health needs.

Policy Analysis

As defined by Wildavsky, policy analysis is "the sustained application of intelligence and knowledge to social problems."[11] He calls policy analysis an "art form" because there are no precise procedures for doing it. The aim of the analysis is "to reduce obscurantism by being explicit about problems and solutions, resources and results. The purpose . . . is to raise the level of argument among contending interests."[12] Rein generally concurs with Wildavsky's concept as "accounting for the development of public policy and explicating the choices and assumptions underlying present and anticipated programs, without necessarily attempting to alter the direction of policy or make specific and detailed choices."[13] He deliberately distinguishes policy from planning by noting that planning is concerned with transforming policies into concrete programs for implementation.

It is the analysis of policy issues that helps uncover the values implied so that they can be set forth clearly for others to consider and make choices. Policy analysis is concerned with (1) the political aspects of public decision making, (2) the search for new and possibly innovative policy alternatives, (3) qualitative rather than quantitative methods, (4) long-range thinking, and (5) a systematic approach, although flexible, to clarifying the means-ends relationship, the multichoice of criteria that are applicable for policy, and the tentative nature of policy choices and their underlying values.[14] In health, policy analysis might be concerned with the provision of health services for everyone through health insurance. The analyst may consider the criteria of the individual's freedom of choice as paramount and may then suggest the use of credit cards or the direct payment of providers through a tax-supported money pool. However, the individual may not be able to obtain the necessary services because they are not available in that individual's neighborhood. To ensure services, the analyst may emphasize the value of an individual's access to health services at the expense of freedom of choice by suggesting that a system of health clinics be built through prepaid health insurance. While there may be a choice of physicians within the clinic, the individual's choice of clinic would be limited. In this way the analyst, through policy analysis, would present health planning agency boards with a series of alternative policy recommendations to solve the health issues with which they are confronted.

Policy analysis is most relevant for the systems and partnership planning models, in which alternatives are extensively analyzed before policy choices are made. The systems model agency implements its policy choices, whereas the partnership model agency sets policy but expects others to implement that policy because it usually lacks the required authority to mandate implementation. The policy analysis method is unlikely to be used by either of the other planning models because of the ad hoc nature with which they make and implement decisions.

Health Information Systems and Indicators

Although health information systems and health indicators are not methods that are used by planners, they are important tools for analysts and decision makers. Both are almost mandatory in the development of and continued maintenance of a systems approach to planning and implementation.

Health Information Systems

A health information system provides the data needed in the procedures of other planning methods, such as operations research or cost-benefit analysis. Health indicators are generally considered a part of the information system; the system collects data to permit planners to monitor whether or not the health indicators, themselves proxies for health objectives, point toward improvement of these objectives. As Deshaies and Seidman state: "Health Information System is designed to be a base for planning, implementation, and evaluation programs."[15] The crucial variable for both the information system and health indicators is the decision maker's capacity to identify the goals and objectives for which data are needed. In addition, the objectives should be specific enough so that the program data and the interrelationships among the programs can be stated in such a way that both quantitative and qualitative data can be isolated and collected in order to monitor how the objectives are faring. For example, an objective that calls for increasing annual health checkups in a neighborhood by 20 percent is amenable to the collection of quantitative data, i.e., the number of those actually coming in for such health examinations. The output or end result of such an objective might be the capacity of the health system to diagnose and treat potential diseases in the early stages of their development. Qualitative data might be collected to ascertain the attitude of the population toward such health examinations and obtain a description of the general robustness displayed by people in the neighborhood compared to a period preceding the inception of preventive health examinations.

The problem is to know what to collect. Noble points out that the information requirements for health planning agencies "are so extensive and overwhelming in their implications for data collection, processing, interpretative analysis and publication" that priorities and limits have to be set "lest they dissipate resources and energy in a frenzy of research activity."[16] Because the development of data for various objectives can be very expensive and time-consuming, the Department of Health and Human Services (HHS) encourages planning agencies to serve as clearinghouses for data collected by other agencies and, in a sense, to become the repository and coordinator of health data used in the community and needed by various health agencies for planning.

There are two types of data required by health planning agencies: (1) general demographic and health-related data and (2) specific data that are geared to particular objectives and can only be obtained in special studies. Most health information systems are based on general health data. Deshaies and Seidman identify five types of general data that should be collected and link these to various categories of health indicators.[17] These are

1. data related to the status of community health, which is linked to such widely accepted indicators as mortality rates, disability rates,

and incidence and prevalence rates of specific diseases
2. utilization of health services data that are related to such health indicators as hospital admissions per year, discharges per year, and annual number of visits for ambulatory care
3. general population and housing characteristics that are related to such indicators as median income of population in a specified community, percentage of population below the officially recognized poverty line, the education level of the population, and the percentage of dwelling units that are below accepted federal housing standards and their rate of overcrowding
4. inventory of health facilities and health personnel related to such health indicators as number of hospital beds per 1,000 population in a specified community; number of physicians, nurses, and dentists per 1,000 population; and the ratio of auxiliary staff to physicians in a hospital
5. status of community environment, which is related to such indicators as degree of air pollution, rate of rat bites per 1,000 children, and general sanitary conditions in the community as judged by garbage and refuse debris, dirt in the streets, and graffiti on private and public dwellings

Health information systems can also be designed with other classifications. For example, they can be based on (1) health activity, e.g., personnel, facilities, services, environment, and research and development; (2) the auspice of the federal agency providing health services and/or funds, e.g., Civil Service Commission, and U.S. Soldiers Home; (3) type of service activity, e.g., prevention of disease, normal development of the population, treatment of illnesses, and control of chronic conditions; or (4) program budgets for health, e.g., provision of health services for special beneficiary categories, such as migrants, the elderly, and Indians; the improvement in quality and organization of community services, such as training of health personnel and improvement in health facilities; research of health issues and problems; and health protection and prevention of communicable diseases, injury control, emergency health activities; and regulation and inspection of health facilities and services.

The summarized enumeration of the types of general information on health that is available and required and the alternative criteria that can be used to classify the data offer some idea of the complexity of designing a health information system. It requires interpretation and analysis, which in turn depend on identifying relationships that offer deeper insights into the planning goals established. One of the major criticisms of most health information systems, such as the data collected by the National Center for

Health Statistics of HHS' Health Resources Administration is that it is aggregated at too high a level of generalization and fails to show interrelationships of the variables. Thus, information on specific populations, e.g., the elderly, the urban populations, females and males in different age brackets is masked. It is for this reason that some experts suggest that data be collected at the lowest level of geographical population and then aggregated so the relationships can be determined and the planning agencies can plan for different population segments in their areas.[18] It would permit them to pinpoint the health needs and services required for different geographical areas and for different population groups within these areas.

Yet, even if the generalized information were collected in a manner that can elicit relationships of significant variables and at a level of geographical and demographic specificity that can be useful for a planning agency concerned with a limited sector of its area, special studies are required to clarify ways to achieve agreed upon goals and objectives. An information system linked to goals and objectives still requires a decision maker to know what the alternative ways of reaching the goals are. Is the goal of guaranteeing basic health services met by providing tax-supported insurance to certain categorical groups, such as the poor and elderly; by providing a national health insurance for everyone, regardless of ability to pay; by providing free health services that are publicly supported and operated; or by responding to different self-interest groups whose health needs are manifest? A health information system can provide data on costs, number of people needing health services, the facilities available, etc. The special study would relate these data to various alternatives for meeting health needs. Yet, still necessary would be a study to determine whether a higher priority should be given to prevention, treatment, or long-term care.

An example of the complexity of collecting data is offered by the matrixes the New York State Health Planning Commission designed to help them achieve seven basic goals. Exhibit 5-1 is the matrix concerned with the goal of developing an effective health care delivery system responsive to human needs. The commission identified eight service elements, such as facilities concerned with prevention or long-term care; twelve desired characteristics (only six of which are appropriate to the matrix in Exhibit 5-1) that are applied to these various service elements, such as flexibility in use of service or accessibility to services; and, finally, indicators already developed or being developed for each of these characteristics, such as population ratios, travel time, and outcome. Each empty box is eventually filled with specific objectives that take into account the service element, the desired characteristics, and the indicators. As a general design to help the planner and decision maker keep track of the

Exhibit 5-1 Development of an Effective Health Care Delivery System Responsive to Human Needs

Desired Characteristic	Indicators	Service Element							
		1 Pre-vention	2 Primary Care	3 Emergency Care	4 Acute General Care	5 Acute Specialty Care	6 Long-Term Care	7 Home Care	8 Rehabil-itation
Availability	Population ratios								
Accessibility	Travel time; schedules; fee structure								
Quality	Outcome; PSRO evaluation								
Freedom from financial barriers	Coverage by insurance; provision without charge								
Flexibility									
Coordination	Formal and informal relationships with other services								

Source: New York State Health Planning Commission. Undated, *circa* 1972.

numerous issues involved in health, the matrix is very useful and can be applied to any geographical area health population. Only if the data base and the indicators were similar in each of the health planning areas could comparisons be made as to whether the objectives were being reached. Unfortunately, the wide range of objectives and their corresponding indicators make it difficult to design a health information system that permits comparison of one health area or subarea with another. Thus, while the design of health information systems is an essential tool for system planning, it is also complex, costly, and not guaranteed to provide the basis of comparison through the use of health indicators.

Health Indicators

With respect to health indicators, there is growing criticism that the current indicators are too limiting and no longer relevant for measuring the dynamic changes that have taken place in the health field in the United States.[19] The national health indicators measure longevity, disability, and access to medical care. Examples of specific indicators are death rates, infant mortality rates, days of disability by type of disability, patients in mental hospitals, incidence of acute conditions, or persons injured.[20] Elinson and Austin state that such indicators, and especially the use of mortality rates, are becoming insensitive in the United States "where there is little to suggest that the increase in health services over recent years has resulted in improvements in the level of health."[21] The reason for the insensitivity of mortality indicators to the changes occurring is that the relationship between mortality and morbidity has not been made clear. The difficulty in interpreting the cause of mortality when multiple health conditions contribute to it, and the cause of nonfatal conditions, such as arthritis, that are contributing factors to the cause of death are seldom recognized in the statistics.

The health indicators tend to emphasize negative rather than positive health conditions. Critics of negative health indicators recognize the difficulty in stating what positive health indicators should be. It is for this reason that Elinson believes indicators should be sociomedical in nature, i.e., indicators that take into account a person's capacity to perform basic social roles as worker, father, mother, student, community volunteer, etc. To this, Stagner would add psychological indicators that take into account degree of satisfaction with health services, environmental conditions in a person's neighborhood, or sense of satisfaction with accomplishments at work, in the home, or at school. Emphasis on factors other than physical health would lead to enlarging indexes of positive health to include population growth, progress toward eliminating deficiencies in housing, community or environmental health conditions that relate to well-being, and satisfaction with use of health services. Recently, there has been more awareness of the deficiency of the present biomedically oriented health indicators. The *Health United States* series has included indexes dealing with obesity, smoking among teen-agers, air pollution, consumption of alcohol, weight control, and preventive immunizations. In one way or another, these indexes concern personal behavior and environmental determinants of health status. They represent a major step toward providing a comprehensive description of the total range of determinants of health.

It is the influence of health planners that has overcome the past resistance to acceptance of these sociomedical indicators. Elinson notes that "since they represent operationally defined and measurable expressions of social goals [they] must inevitably exert some influence on social policy and social action. To measure is to point the way to policy."[22] This boils down to a political issue that most planners and academicians prefer not to engage in overtly, since it requires a confrontation with those administrators, physicians, and associations already strongly linked to the current health indicators and what they represent. However, the demands on the health planning agencies to develop plans based on the systems approach inevitably lead to the development of new health indicators that are linked to the developed objectives. It may become evident that the general biomedical indicators are inadequate measures of health trends. A look at some of the indicators developed by the New York State Health Planning Commission confirms the new direction. They use such health indicators as travel time, Professional Standards Review Organization (PSRO) evaluation, formal and informal relationships with other services, information flow, patient attitudes, fragmentation, gaps, responsiveness to changing physical, social, and political environments, and cost per capita. These indicators open up new territory that has been previously untapped. Data for them are almost impossible to secure, since collection requires a whole range of special studies. It also places great pressure on any type of health information system that is developed. Thus, the systems approach to health planning is forging into new territory and challenging the comfortable and formerly meaningful health indicators.

With respect to the relationship of health information systems and health indicators to the planning models, it appears that they most logically are related to the systems model of planning, with its strong emphasis on systems planning and strong centralized authority structure. It is less likely to be used in the other models where the emphasis is on policy development that is more politically derived than technologically influenced (partnership and alliance models) and on highly specific objectives and programs that require a narrow range of information and indicators related uniquely to these concerns (individual action model).

Systems Analysis

Systems analysis is an approach to viewing problems that involves established procedures. Enthoven, Assistant Secretary of Defense under Robert McNamara, states that it "is nothing more than quantitative or enlightened common sense aided by modern analytical methods."[23] Wildavsky characterizes the systems analyst as a "chochem, a Yiddish word meaning 'wise man' with overtones of 'wise guy.' His forte is creativity."[24] It is an art form that presupposes large doses of wisdom and intuition on the part of the analyst. The reason for this is obvious, when one becomes aware that systems analysis does not start out with given objectives. Rather, the objectives have to be discovered in the course of the analysis. This discovery process requires the rigor of a scientist and the creativity of an artist. Nevertheless, systems analysis does have a framework and a process that helps guide the analyst.

The elements involved in systems analysis are the following:

1. There is a need to examine the entire operation and structure of the system under study. Forrester calls this a "closed-system boundary." He states that the "boundary must be established within which the system interactions take place that give the system its characteristic behavior."[25]
2. A model of the system should be developed. A model is a representation of reality. It should include only the relevant variables that require study and analysis and should be presented as simply as possible.
3. The system or its model concept must be goal-oriented with an explicit statement of the objective(s) considered important by decision makers.
4. There should be alternate ways to reach the goals. It is this aspect of analyzing alternatives that often requires the use of the technique that is referred to by various terms, i.e., cost-benefit, cost-effectiveness analysis, or program budgeting. The distinction among these various methods is noted later in the chapter.
5. A time horizon should be established so the incremental steps toward achievement of the goal and the degree of success can be set forth with some specificity on a year-by-year basis. Characteristically, systems analysis has a long-range time horizon, five or more years.
6. Finally, systems analysis requires an interdisciplinary team to work on various facets of the problem.

The following characteristics must be taken into account in the process of systems analysis as outlined by Akman and Gordon: (a) a statement of objectives or ends to which planned action is directed, (b) a statement of alternatives to the objectives, (c) identification of the costs for achieving each alternative, (d) creation of a model or description of relationships between alternatives and what they achieve and cost, and (e) specification of criteria for selecting alternatives.[26]

This process appears to be fairly close to the rational planning process discussed previously. This similarity identifies one aspect of systems analysis, namely, that it is a systematic analysis of a problem, the same as the rational planning process. The difference is that systems analysis also assumes that a system of some kind exists that can be analyzed, whereas this is not required in the rational planning process. From this perspective, systems analysis is an analysis of a system. It becomes necessary to identify the boundaries of that system and the interacting parts within it. What is essentially being changed is the system's structure. Figure 5-1 shows a generalized health service system based on Palmer's conception.[27] The system is based on inputs of staff, facilities, equipment, funds, knowledge, interaction of these resources according to an organized pattern of relationships, and outputs of products that can be measured and provide the basis for an evaluation of how well the system is doing.

Knowing the general characteristics of the system does not really tell a health planner what to look for, where the problems are located, or what to improve if the system is not working effectively. The system does not spell out what happens in the interaction among the components of the input elements. This is the reason systems analysis is considered an art, requires imagination, and necessitates a scientific investigation of how the system is operating.

Uses of Systems Analysis

It should be obvious from this discussion that systems analysis is difficult to define because it is characterized by looseness. A consequence of this looseness is that the analyst cannot rely on past experiences to determine what should be done with subsequent health planning problems. Each problem must be considered on its own merits. Therefore, as several analysts have noted, one of the most important considerations of systems analysis is structuring the system in its totality and taking into account the constraints (such as regulations, administrative procedures, and legislative limitations) that affect its operation.[28] Unlike previous problem-solving methods, it forces the planner to look at the whole picture.

Systems analysis forces planners to discover and understand the general goals and specific objectives of the health system they are studying. Too

Figure 5-1   General Health Services System Representation

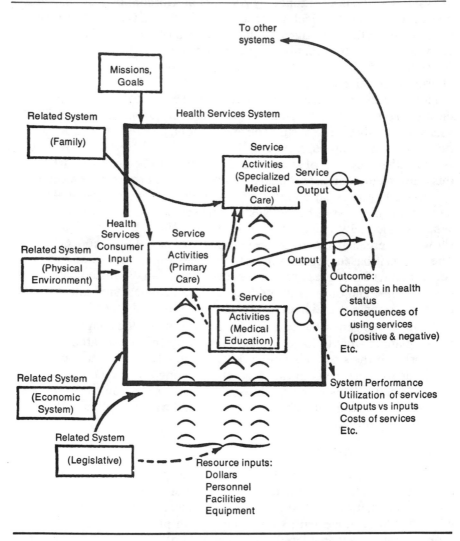

often, the officials who direct the programs that comprise the health system have forgotten what they are interested in achieving. There has been a subtle shift from emphasis on the goals of the organization or system to a major concern about its maintenance. The goals are taken for granted and in time lost sight of by administrators and policy board members who are more concerned with the fiscal health and day-to-day operations of the system.

A corollary that flows from the preceding point is that, in order for systems analysis to be meaningful, it must involve the chief decision makers of the system. In the case of the agencies, this means the mayors of large cities, the city managers, or the county leaders. It also means involving the key executive officers of the major health components within the geographical area, which are often autonomous, but which represent the subsystems that form the area's health care system. This is necessary because any changes in goals or structure of the system recommended by the planning agency boards will be inoperative without this approval.

Planning by its nature is future-oriented. Systems analysis is helpful in structuring the system and using planning techniques that can identify how various alternative objectives will fare at some future time. By making it possible to predict the future rather than abandon it to chance, systems analysis reduces uncertainty and future risks. Forrester has noted that simulation models are needed for this, and he defines a model as "a theory describing the structure and interrelationships of a system."[29] However, he cautions that models can be useful or useless, depending on how accurately the theory on which the model is predicated is correlated to reality. Through the use of computers and valid scientific means for testing the models, it may be possible to determine in advance how well the model fits reality. Wildavsky believes that one of the major goals of systems analysis is dealing with uncertainty in a more effective manner.[30] Although he states systems analysis cannot lead to more effective ways of dealing with issues, it can at least identify wrong assumptions and ineffective programs proposed or already in use. This is a major gain when one considers that millions of dollars are associated with federally funded programs and health planning agency jurisdictions.

Techniques

A technique is a specific tool that can be used to solve a problem or a series of problems through its proper application. Because systems analysis is a generalized concept, such methods as cost-benefit analysis and cost-effectiveness analysis may be considered techniques of systems analysis. These submethods have their own vast literature and specific techniques.

In hospital facility planning, Stewart discusses a technique he refers to as *QUEST*.

QUEST stands for Question, Understand, Evaluate, Select, and Together. We continue questioning until we have all available facts. We try to understand the options within a generalized rather than particularized framework. We evaluate the subsolu-

tion against specific criteria for the problem at hand. We select
and proceed with the solution that best meets the goals. We do
all this together as a team with the client and other consultants.[31]

The author described how QUEST was used on a hospital expansion plan.
Stewart analyzed the hospital's operating system and the problems related
to its expansion. Alternatives were considered, using criteria to determine
which alternatives were most effective for the objectives sought. The use
of the computer facilitated the determination of the advantages and disadvantages of each alternative. In the end, the hospital officials, both staff
and board members, had to make a choice from among several alternatives.
At all points in the process an interdisciplinary team analyzed the impact
of one solution or another on the existing and future hospital system. The
solution chosen was one that permitted the most rapid construction at the
lowest cost. Other examples of the application of systems analysis to
health problems have been presented by Harvey Adelman (study of New
York City's Health Department), Allan Akman and Jerome Gordon (general model of urban improvement, including health component), Whitney
Murphy (study of health facility planning), Morris Schaefer and Herman
Hilleboe (study of health personnel needs), Harold Smalley (hospital facility planning), and Boyd Palmer (goal-oriented simulation model of health
systems planning).[32] A review of the subjects studied indicates the wide
range of problems to which systems analysis can be applied.

Relationship of Systems Analysis to Authority Structure of Health Planning Models

The systems approach to health planning by its very nature requires the
involvement of all decision makers who control funds, facilities, services,
or knowledge. PL 93-641 stresses the involvement of all relevant actors,
including a majority of consumers, concerned with health care. Although
Palmer views the health system as integrated in his simulation model, he
recognizes the autonomous nature of its components. He handles this by
noting that, in the marketplace, consumers and providers interact in such
a way that the independent parts normally provide the health care services
required by people. If the marketplace always worked to the benefit of
both consumers and providers, the need for comprehensive health planning would be minimized or eliminated. Since this is not the case, and the
costs of health care have been escalating out of proportion to the rest of
the economy, great pressure has been brought by Congress to make the
system more efficient in the use of its resources and more effective in
assisting the population with its health care needs.

Since the health planning agencies have areawide jurisdiction, they must deal with the numerous public, voluntary, and proprietary health care services involved in their geographical area. The systems approach to health tells nothing about the level at which the planning is directed: the entire area; specific cities or towns in the area; neighborhoods of the cities or towns; individual health care components, such as clinics, private physicians, hospitals, or medical schools; or a subsystem of one of these system levels. Consequently, it is important to identify at what level the system planning is directed. Regardless of the level of planning, the systems analyst must work with a central decision maker who has both the power and authority to implement what is planned. This means, for example, working with the hospital board and administrator in changing the hospital as a whole or one of its subsystems; the chairman of a college department and the dean to alter a health planning course; a commissioner and mayor for changing a health department, etc. It is unlikely that the systems model of planning is applicable at the areawide level because there are too many powerful decision makers with control over independent health resources. This makes it difficult to implement any comprehensive plan because the potential losers of power, resources, status, and funds will not forego these symbols of success without a struggle. At the areawide level, the partnership planning model is most applicable because it is possible for the various decision makers to agree on general policies and goals without coming to any decisions on specific objectives, timetables, or programs. It is at this level of specificity where most conflicts erupt. This issue highlights the classic dilemma Bolan refers to as the tensions between the political system and the requirements of comprehensive planning.[33]

Since systems analysis is predicated on the ability of a centralized decision maker to make informed choices among alternatives that can be transformed into active health programs, the lack of centralized authority or power means that systems analysis cannot be applied. It is applicable for the partnership planning model only as long as the planning is stated in general policy or goal terms. If more specific objectives are identified and agreed upon by an agency's planning board in this model, autonomous health care subsystems cannot ordinarily be required to implement them. Such compulsion would destroy the federation and the consensus upon which that health planning model is built, erupting into conflicts between the health planning agency and the health subsystem being pressured to implement the objectives.

In a nationwide survey of methodologies used by health planning agencies, Kennedy made the following observations:[34]

. . . the mind-set of the actors within the planning process tends towards solution of problems at the component level and not at the system level.[35]

. . . strategic planning implies that there is a small group of decisionmakers (the corporate board) that have the responsibility and authority to decide and to see that the plans when adopted are implemented. The community health system has no counterpart in which is vested the requisite responsibility and authority.[36]

In essence, Kennedy is stating that health planning agencies do not generally have the authority structure to undertake systems or what he calls "strategic" planning. Even if they did, the agencies would not have a staff competent to undertake such analysis. According to the survey, most of the professionals were person-oriented and spent their time trying to obtain consensus among actors to solve subsystem level problems.

Disadvantages or Limitations of Systems Analysis

Although systems analysis is not relevant for areawide systems planning, in various forms it is being used for specific subsystem analysis and solution. Until such time as health planning agencies have the requisite authority and power to undertake systems analysis, health planners should be aware of the limitations and disadvantages in the use of this important method.

Systems analysis requires the collection of data that are directly related to the variables of the system being studied. All too often, there are vast amounts of data available, but they have little reference to what is being studied. Thus, there is a shortage of pertinent data with which analysts must contend.

One of the basic requirements of systems analysis is the specification of objectives and alternatives. Since this is a task for decision makers the value differences of the various decision makers make agreement on and identification of specific objectives difficult. No one is willing to be worse off once the objectives are implemented. Arnold offers three reasons for this difficulty. (1) Decision makers who have traditionally thought in terms of budget lines and inputs are now being asked to consider the impact of these inputs. This shift will be difficult and often confusing until it is absorbed and integrated into the existing agency operations. (2) The conflict in values among the several groups represented in a health planning agency makes it difficult to decide whose objectives to use. Should ambulatory clinics be decentralized and controlled by local community leaders, or should they be located in hospitals and under the jurisdiction of the hospital board? The answers to such questions result in benefits for one group and costs to the other. Owing to the unbalanced costs and benefits, health planning decision makers are often reluctant to render decisions that will subvert an existing health program, even if it is beneficial to the general public. (3) Because decision makers find it important to point to goals they have achieved, they are cautious about setting objectives that cannot be achieved. Lack of achievement leads to a loss of credibility in the eyes of those responsible for the position of the decision makers. Decision makers will be inclined to support traditionally popular and successful programs and promote their extension into areas of need or favor minimal adaptations to make such programs more efficient and effective rather than risk new or unproved approaches to health problems.[37]

Systems analysis requires ongoing involvement between the decision makers and the systems analysts. Unfortunately, the time frames, the different orientations in thinking between the decision maker and analyst, and the technical complexities of systems analysis, especially if it requires the use of computers and mathematical computations, tend to set up barriers between the two. Systems analysis has not proved itself in spite of President Johnson's order back in the 1960s that all federal departments present budgets based upon systems analysis. It failed to have the same success in other departments as it did in the Department of Defense under Secretary McNamara. Wildavsky analyzed the differences that resulted in success in the Department of Defense and failure in other departments. These differences were not perceived at the time the executive order was given.[38] The subsequent lack of success has resulted in much disenchantment with the concept and its use in the federal government.

Systems analysis requires theory upon which to base its models. Most analysts are skilled in model building, but weak in knowledge of the social and behavioral sciences, as well as the theory upon which the models must rest. This requires a wedding between the two disciplines of social science theory and methodology. In spite of the fact that systems analysis has been characterized as interdisciplinary, there are few illustrations of how such teams have operated together or whether they can. Howard analyzed the basic orientations of program planning and budgeting and noted the desirability of a linkage between the two. Yet, he concluded that the analyst and the budgeteer cannot make the necessary marriage because of their inherent differences in background and orientation.[39] The same applies to the model builder and the social scientist. Unless the marriage of models and theory can be made, the models will be abstractions that test nothing. The models may be "useful or useless" in Forrester's words, depending upon whether or not they are based on testable concepts.

Systems analysis models generally require some form of quantitative measures that are comparable. However, it may not only be difficult to find the measures, but the most significant variables may also be excluded from the model because of the lack of valid measures on their nonquantifiable nature. It is for this reason that critics question the outcome of systems analysis. Hemmens and Lathrop stated:

> Current solution techniques, particularly mathematical programming, are limited to a small subset of the total spectrum of problems to which the process of systems analysis or rational planning might be applied, and in most cases operate under such restrictive assumptions and oversimplifications as to make the solution obtained only of general relevance to the problem.[40]

Forrester's awareness of these simplifications has led to the development of his complex system to deal with urban problems. Yet, these complex systems are, for him, counterintuitive, insensitive to changes in many system parameters, resistant to policy changes, and often conflicting in response to long-run policy change as opposed to short-run policy change, as well as likely to result in a low performance.[41] The solution for Forrester is to organize "the information that exists into a structure that represents the structure of the actual system and, therefore, has an opportunity to behave as the real system would."[42] But others have criticized even Forrester's more complex systems approach as too simple to reflect the wide range of behavior that must be taken into account to model adequately the urban scene or even the smaller health service system.[43] These comments serve only to show the limitations of systems analysis, not to refute the effectiveness of its general approach.

Systems analysis is a tool and not a solution to a problem. In the first flush of its widespread use, it was too often seen as a way of solving complex problems that did not require the intervention of a decision maker. The solutions were handed to the executive officer who was expected to implement them. In fact, there were many decision makers who uncritically accepted their staff's conclusions. Gross refers to two of the directors of the Council of Economic Advisors as "lazy executives" because they left "PPB [Programming, Planning, and Budgeting] largely in the hands of the 'backroom boys' borrowed from McNamara and The Rand Corporation."[44] Almost all knowledgeable supporters of systems analysis perceive it primarily as a tool to aid the decision maker in the selection of the best alternative at the time. Hemmens and Lathrop sum it up well:

> SA [systems analysis] does not offer a complete cure for the difficulties of the decision maker. It does not replace intuition,

experience, or judgment. . . . Secondly, SA is not something that is done to handle a problem in (a mechanical way) . . . it is a way of organizing decision making which calls for the rigorous use of scientific tools. Finally, SA is not done for a decision maker. It is done with a decision maker.[45]

Cost-Benefit/Cost-Effectiveness Analysis

Cost-benefit analysis was an outgrowth of the federal government's desire to determine under what circumstances it should intervene in what had been traditionally considered private sector issues. It was based on the convergence of two economic developments. The first was the recognition that "economists found it increasingly uncomfortable to assume that the basic structure of the economy was that of free competition in which government activities represented only a minor aberration from universal private decisionmaking."[46] The federal government accounts for about 20 percent of the gross national product, which is no "minor aberration." Under these circumstances, the government has been intervening in the lives of the nation's population. The second development was the government's interest during the 1950s and 1960s in identifying criteria by which it could decide how best to use its limited resources for the benefit of the less developed nations. Parallel with these two developments was the growing chorus of voices among decision makers within the federal government for improved policy analysis. As Gross has noted, Keynesian economics was primarily concerned with macroeconomics or major bundles of federal programs, such as national defense or health, welfare, and labor.[47] There was still a need to discover ways for deciding which programs should be funded to meet the broad goals of these major bundles of national programs.

Welfare economics was developed to assist the federal government in determining when it should intervene in the market economy and to provide "guidance for the choice of instruments to accomplish social objectives."[48] The basic thrust of economic analysis is that of economic efficiency. Conceptually, if the ratio of the costs of a program to its benefits exceeds one, then it is considered beneficial to undertake the program. This model, which came from the orientation of private firms to maximize its profits, was first used by the federal government in water resources projects.

In general terms, cost-benefit analysis has been variously defined as providing more explicit and logically organized information on the effects, or outcomes, of specific programs or projects,"[49] or as an attempt "to secure an efficient allocation of resources produced by the governmental system in its interaction with the private economy,"[50] or "as a process whereby a public agency in pursuit of economic efficiency allocates its resources in such a way that the most 'profitable' projects are executed and developed to the point where marginal benefits equal marginal costs."[51]

These definitions have in common the attempt at discovering better ways to use limited resources, linking the use of these resources to some goals, coordinating a wider range of information or data in a systematic way on the goals being sought, and finally identifying when a decision point for use of the resources has been reached. The motivation for the use of cost-benefit analysis is derived from the imperfection of the marketplace and the limited resources necessitating choices. The concept of efficiency becomes important when there are too few resources to meet all needs. It is here that cost-benefit analysis serves to provide alternatives. This process analyzes choices when the costs and benefits of each possibility can be stated in monetary terms, preferably dollar figures. The merits of widely different objectives can be compared.

When only one objective is given and the aim is to find the best way or alternative (at the lowest cost) for achieving this objective, the analyst reviews nonmonetary information as well as monetary data. This type of analysis is referred to as cost-effectiveness analysis. Thus, it is possible to establish an objective that will realize the greatest benefit at the least cost, but not both at the same time. These techniques are referred to in the planning and budget systems of government as PPBS (planning, programming, and budgetary system). When incorporated into a PPBS program, cost-effectiveness analysis is used to identify either the most effective objectives and programs for realizing basic goals, or the least costly programs for achieving stated objectives.

The Process of Cost-Benefit Analysis and Its Uses

There are four steps in the process of cost-benefit analysis:

1. A statement of program objectives should be made. Does the planning agency want to improve the ambulatory care and/or the referral system for low-income residents, and/or the reduction of hospital costs?
2. Once the objectives are specified, the output for the program becomes necessary. Is the concern how many persons a clinic handles per year, or how many are kept well enough to perform normal functions at work, home, and school? Or is the concern how many low-income persons receive various types of health care or the manner with which the health care is offered?

3. After the various objectives and the outputs of the program have been identified, the estimate of the total costs of the program for both the first year and several years thereafter should be undertaken. The first year expenditures for an ambulatory health system will be costly, since they include both capital expenses and maintenance costs. After the facilities have been constructed, renovated, and equipped, the operating costs may be lower. For this reason, the costs should be considered over the life of the project or a suitable time period.

4. Finally, it is necessary to analyze the alternatives to determine which have the greatest impact in accomplishing the various objectives or which achieve a given objective at the least cost. Thus, an analysis could be made of how best to spend a billion dollars of new public funds: should it go all to ambulatory care, a referral system, or a reduction of hospital costs? Or should it be spent on some combination of these? The analysis should help determine on which single objective or combination of objectives to spend the billion dollars. On the other hand, if the objective is to improve health services for the ambulatory patient, then the question becomes one of economics or how such a program can be offered at the least expense. Such alternatives as issuing credit cards so that each individual may seek his or her own health care provider, or building clinics to offer direct service in convenient locations, or purchasing hospital-based mobile health units would require evaluation.

Through feedback evaluation techniques, it becomes possible to measure the effectiveness of the objectives and programs chosen. In this way, cost-benefit analysis becomes a cyclical process that strives to improve the health system through these techniques.[52] To carry out cost-benefit analysis, the indirect side-effects, or externalities as economists refer to them, of the program must be taken into account. These side-effects may be positive or negative. Thus, a side-effect of building ambulatory health clinics in poor communities may result in pressure by the community leaders to take over the policy role of operating the clinic; it may also result in more jobs for local residents, and it may raise the wage levels of local businesses so they are not able to compete with the higher wage structure of the tax-sponsored health facility. There may thus be benefits to local residents and harm to local businesses.

A second aspect of cost-benefit analysis that should be considered is the effect of time on the program, referred to as discounting. Discounting is the assignment of a value or discount rate to the present value of the programs so that it is possible to compare different programs by their costs and benefits at any future time period. For example, the current value of someone agreeing to pay $100 in one year is around $95 because if one were to deposit it at a 5 percent interest rate tomorrow, it would have earned $5 in one year to return a total of $100. All future costs and benefits should be discounted to their present values.[53]

Finally, the cost-benefit analysis should be based on the increments to the existing projects that are being considered rather than the total project, because what is being compared are the additions or increments to the existing programs. Thus, the cost-benefit analysis a $10,000 increment to an existing $100,000 clinic program is based on the benefits that are conferred from that $10,000, not from the total $110,000. If it is a brand new program, then the total costs are computed and compared to the total benefits. A second way of comparing programs is to subtract costs from benefits to attain the net benefits. This method is preferable when different programs or objectives with different values that cannot all be put into a dollar figure are compared. A third method of comparing costs and benefits is the use of a ratio. A ratio would be used, for example, in determining whether a higher rate of satisfaction with services rendered and a subsequent higher rate of kept appointments were achieved by the use of indigenous outreach workers or by the physician making the appointments.

Cost-benefit analysis is used for three major reasons, First, it forces the analyst to prepare for the decision maker alternative choices and background analysis in the use of scarce resources. Like systems analysis, cost-benefit analysis is a tool to aid decision makers, not to replace them. Second, it is an excellent tool for conflict management. With many competing interests, proponents of different objectives and programs would be faced with a method that enabled the decision maker to assess their demands, gain perspective, and support the decision. While the political or value factors are not eliminated, the decision maker acquires additional technical knowledge on which to base a decision. Finally, it is used in PPBS to help integrate the planning-budgeting process by proposing alternatives based on technical analysis and greatly improves the analytical capacity required in the planning-budgeting process.

Limitations of Cost-Benefit Analysis

A number of limitations already noted in the discussion of systems analysis are also applicable to cost-benefit analysis. Among these are the difficulty in identifying a common measure, in finding agreement on objectives because of the varying values applied to them, and in dealing with important intangible values because they cannot be quantified or measured to permit comparison.

In addition, Akman and Gordon note that there is a great difference between the statistical accuracy of predicted behavior of important variables and the ability to predict what will happen to a variable in the real world.[54] Statistical probability might point out that an expansion of ambulatory health clinics will find them operating at capacity for the next ten years based on population projections. Yet, for reasons unforeseen, the clinic operates at only 50 percent of capacity in ten years, since the neighborhood has lost its ability to hold its population. But, in all other neighborhoods, the prediction of the forecasts may turn out to be accurate.

A further limitation of cost-benefit analysis is that during the implementation process it is difficult to know when actions taken will produce results. This is so because of the numerous constraints that are placed on action, such as physical constraints (inability to find a facility in which to locate a clinic), legal constraints (difficulty in changing civil service rules to permit the hiring of community residents without the usual education or experience requirements), administrative constraints (lack of sufficient time to train local residents for their positions in the clinic), or political constraints (the time required to work out an agreement that would permit local residents and health officials to work together on the clinic's policy board). These constraints and others such as financial, social, religious, and distributive can delay the implementation of a program.[55]

Another important limitation is that cost-benefit analysis cannot be taken to mean that a "cause-effect" analysis has been undertaken. This is what Galloway meant when he said that "using cost-analysis in capital investment decisions will not indicate the best of all possible courses to follow, but only which is the best choice among those analyzed."[56] A thorough examination of all the major and minor contributions to a problem is not usually attempted because of the time required. Solutions are usually based on the experiences of experts, or what was successful elsewhere, rather than on an analysis of the problem.

While these limitations to cost-benefit analysis must be considered, the method remains a valuable tool for the decision maker. It serves to enhance his or her already well-developed intuition, experience, and knowledge.

Relationship of Cost-Benefit/Cost-Effectiveness Analysis to Planning Models

Cost-benefit analysis is most conducive to the systems model of planning because it assumes a central decision maker who can select among the alternatives presented. Cost-benefit deals with specific objectives that are for the most part quantifiable for measurement purposes and, therefore, are specific enough to be transformed into program terms. Both partnership and alliance models of planning do not assume that degree of specificity of its goals nor are they concerned with the comparisons of various goals. The alliance model especially assumes a collectivity of actors who are in general agreement about some general goal and define their part in the fulfillment of it. Its members are not interested in considering alternative goals or objectives. If another goal is decided upon, it may very well result in a break up of the alliance because some members with little interest in the new goal would drop out and others would become antagonistic if it challenged their basic interests. In most instances, it is doubtful that the actors involved in the individual action planning model have either the technical expertise or the interest in undertaking cost-benefit analysis to determine their objectives. These objectives grow naturally out of the needs of the community and the pressing problems with which community leadership strives to cope. Consequently, this method is primarily a tool of a centralized authority structure such as the systems model.

Forecasting

Forecasting as a method has been used for many years, especially by business firms and governments as they have attempted to assess sufficient taxes for the coming years to meet expected expenditures. Planning is a forecast of anticipated goals and objectives that society or some group within it hopes to achieve. Forecasting, which has become a discipline in its own right, is being practiced by more and more analysts and is receiving attention and use by scientists, government, the military, and business. Jantsch, who has made a detailed study of forecasting, has counted more than 100 forecasting techniques or elements of techniques.[57]

Definition of Forecasting

Technological forecasting is "the forecast of the invention, innovation or diffusion of some technology."[58] It is more an art than a science and must take into account social and economic factors, which are normally interrelated. It is a viewpoint about something in which an analyst or decision maker is interested. Forecasting helps bring out significant factors and/or interrelationships that might have been overlooked. Systems analysis and operations research are also concerned with eliciting significant factors and interrelationships. In the health planning field, the inventions and innovations alluded to in the definition could refer to inventing authority structures that could replace the present fragmented, pluralistic health care system; to finding new ways of keeping people healthy without medical interventions; or to using computers to identify alternative solutions to planning issues that minimize consumer and provider participation. These concepts are merely illustrations of potential new inventions or innovations that might arise during the process of technological forecasting.

Forecasting is also concerned with how fast new inventions, once adopted by an official body, are diffused to the general population. New ambulatory family clinics sponsored by the federal government have not been diffused very rapidly beyond the funding capacity of the government itself. However, the use of computers for many hospital activities has had wide and rapid diffusion; prepaid health care plans have had very slow diffusion since their inception. Forecasting would attempt to predict the dispersion of these health concepts by geographical area, by social strata, and by their rate of acceptance. To do this would require both a knowledge of the behavior of different subgroups of people toward new concepts that affect their health as well as the economic capacity of the public sector, in interaction with the private sector, to finance such ideas.

It is because forecasting is so complex that Jantsch states that forecasting techniques "have been developed for a 'man-technique dialogue' and are very sensitive to man's knowledge and his capacity for imaginative thinking, technical and value judgment, and synthesis."[59] It is for this reason that the technological aspects of forecasting, which are still in too limited a state of development, must rely equally as much on human forecasting. Forecasting cannot take the place of the decision maker, but the results of forecasting techniques serve as an auxiliary aid in decision making.

The essence of forecasting is the extrapolation of base line data to the future. The trends are then modified by taking into account other known factors that affect them. Thus, forecasts project the known into the unknown. Where the projection is for a short time span (one or two years), the forecast takes on an incremental change in the status quo, similar to much of the planning that takes place in firms and hospitals. Where the time horizon is longer or covers a wider aspect of the environment (a larger geographical area or a concern with several variables simultaneously, such as social, education, or health characteristics), more intuitive forecasting techniques come into play.

Techniques of Forecasting

Jantsch identifies three intuitive techniques of forecasting: brainstorming, buzz group sessions, and the Delphi technique. These techniques are used either when there are no data from which to extrapolate the past into the future or when there is no model that can be used to simulate the current reality. Intuitive forecasting springs fresh from the minds of people, based on their own experiences, fantasies, or aspirations. It is an uninhibited type of mental exercise. Of these techniques, Delphi is receiving increasing attention. The procedure for this technique has been fairly well formulated.

First, a panel is established; it is composed of six to ten experts in the area or subject matter of the forecast: future trends in hospital use, the impact of pollution on extended health care facilities, or the physician-patient relationship as the consumer becomes more knowledgeable about health care. Second, each member of the panel is requested to make an estimate about the subject without contact with the other experts. Third, the mean and standard deviations of the estimates are then computed. Fourth, a report of the results is made and given to each member of the panel. Those members of the panel whose estimates were outside the central range are asked either to alter their estimates or to explain why they hold to their original estimate. Fifth, the revised estimates and written rationales are collected and a new mean and central range are computed. They are again distributed with anonymous justifications attached. Again, the experts are asked to alter their answers or provide justification. It is expected that the mean and central range will be narrower. The process is repeated until no further movement takes place. Usually, four estimates will result in a final judgment. The important factor here is the consensus reached by anonymous experts about the state of the future, in which a judge, planner, or analyst plays the role of catalyst or mediator among the panel members, none of whom are identified to each other.

Buzz groups are similar to Delphi with the basic exception that the panelists sit around the table and are subject to each other's direct behavioral influence. However, there are usually several tables "buzzing" about the same topic. The main ideas from each of the tables are discussed in turn in open sessions. Their ideas are supported, opposed, or amended through this open dialogue. After a lengthy discussion, the central areas of agreement and disagreement emerge. Eventually, the sponsors of the meeting terminate the debate as a consensus forms around some of the issues initially presented. More typically, the sponsors conclude the discussion after each table has presented and defended its views. Out of the discussion, the sponsors attempt to identify the ideas that have received the greatest acceptance.

Brainstorming usually takes place in larger groups. Members of the audience are encouraged to say whatever comes to their minds about the subject, until a series of alternatives is cited. From these, a consensus is formed, through a process of rating. This technique is a compromise between Delphi, where anonymous panel members influence each other through rational written arguments, and buzz sessions, where members influence each other directly and engage in a dialogue until some consensus is reached. In brainstorming, the members occupy the same room, but those in one part of the room are unknown to those in another part. Only their ideas are discussed. Thus, the personal interaction and its influence are diminished.

The two major uses of forecasts at this time are (1) the exercises that enable decision makers to obtain greater insights into the nature and interrelationships of influencing factors, and (2) the development of specific alternative solutions that otherwise might not have come to light.

Limitations of Forecasting Techniques

Like all methods discussed thus far, forecasting often cannot be done because of the lack of appropriate data. Second, theory that explains the conditions needed in order for the predicted changes to occur is often lacking. In the absence of theory, Schon points out that "forecasting relies on the projection of trends related to a small number of variables, modified qualitatively by intuitive judgments."[60] Third, while some data may be available there may be insufficient information to offer a basis for predicting the rate of diffusion that is usually so important to forecasts. Finally, forecasts themselves may serve as self-fulfilling prophecies by setting the psychological atmosphere so that no one can take an opposing position. The dire predictions of the American Medical Association (AMA) that a socialist form of medical practice would take place in the United States similar to that of England or Sweden had such a strong hold on people that it was many years before the most innocuous form of national health insurance for the poor, the Kerr-Mills amendments, could be passed. Even with the passage of Titles XVIII and XIX of the Social Security Act, providing medical coverage for the elderly and the medically indigent, AMA's predictions have not come to pass. Instead, a new threat unanticipated by the AMA has arisen. The specialization of medical practice has been driving physicians into various forms of group practice or hospital-based practice and thereby undermining the sanctity of the physician-patient relationship and diluting the influence of the AMA on its members.

Yet, in spite of these limitations, Schon noted the need for forecasting. Policy makers in health planning agencies "look to them [forecasts] for insights rather than answers . . . and guard against the public use of forecasting as self-fulfilling prophecies."[61]

Relationship of Forecasting to Planning Models and Functions

It would appear that the less technological forecasting techniques of Delphi, brainstorming, and buzz sessions are highly conducive to the partnership planning model where greater emphasis is placed on locating the general consensus of health issues through human forecasting. Policy makers in partnership-oriented health planning agencies are often selected as experts to assist in the implementation of the Delphi technique. In addition, buzz sessions and brainstorming techniques would be used by these agencies when the emphasis is on policy issues rather than on comprehensive planning.

Intuitive forecasting techniques would also be useful with systems planning models in the efforts of policy boards to arrive at general policy alternatives and goals that might be included in a comprehensive health plan. Brainstorming and buzz sessions would also be applicable as a means of uncovering a wide range of goal alternatives, while Delphi techniques would be more useful in identifying the interrelationships of the goals. Those involved in the alliance planning model are too action-oriented and committed to specific issues to find forecasting tools useful. While this is also the case with the individual action model, there are times when its members reach a point of stagnation with respect to what changes in the health system should concern them. At these strategic points in their history, forecasting techniques may prove useful. Except for the systems model, it is unlikely that the other planning models would utilize the more technological forecasting techniques.

PLAN IMPLEMENTATION METHODS

Operations Research

Operations research is defined by Ackoff and Sasieni as "the application of scientific method by interdisciplinary teams to problems involving the control of organized man-machine systems so as to provide solutions which best serve the purpose of the organization as a whole."[62] Its three main characteristics are those of system orientation, interdisciplinary teams, and application of scientific methods to problems of control.

Although it is based on systems theory and accepts the assumption that the behavior of any part ultimately affects every other part, it differs from systems analysis in three ways. First, systems analysis is characterized by an uncertain environment. Operations research requires a known system. It is taken as given. Second, systems analysis has unknown or conflicting objectives. Operations research starts out with known objectives. Third, systems analysis deals with a large number of elements, as Forrester's emphasis on complex systems revealed. Operations research can deal with only a few elements at a time, usually tactical problems that are characterized by short-range solutions, involving a small part of the organization, and primarily concerned with means rather than ends.[63]

Operations research has been most frequently applied to problems of business and the military. Only recently have operations research techniques been applied to the health field, but even then they have been used primarily with problems quite similar to those found in industry. Young, one of the keynote speakers in a major conference called by the Operations Research Society of America in 1969 to relate how these techniques are applicable to health planning and health systems, stated that "OR [operations research] has generally failed the health services . . . no really significant developments have yet occurred in health through the use of OR techniques."[64] Examples of the application of operations research techniques were cited in the better use of nurses in obstetrical hospital units, the development of special facilities for victims of heart disease, the efficiency and effectiveness of Pap smears in reducing mortality from cancer of the cervix, the use of automotive engineering to reduce accidents on highways, and the more effective queuing of patients through an ambulatory clinic.[65] Yet none of these examples are related to comprehensive health planning, but primarily to hospital systems that have many of the characteristics of the business firm. Ackoff and Sasieni recognize that operations research can most effectively deal with only one of their three patterns of planning, the optimizing pattern. This pattern is mainly concerned with adapting and adjusting problems of segments of an organization system to its environment and goals, and with maintaining the status quo rather than with growth or change. In this respect, it differs from the adapting pattern of planning, which seeks to change the system or suggest new systems. Operations research is unable to deal with this type of planning in its present stage of development.[66]

Operations research makes great use of computers and models. Models are representations of reality. There are three basic types of models. The iconic models are small-scale representations of reality such as maps, drawings, or photographs. Analogue models substitute one form of property to represent another, such as contour lines to represent the elevations of land on a map. Symbolic models substitute symbols for reality such as mathematical equations. Symbolic models are the most precise and most utilized in operations research.[67]

Operations research usually requires five basic steps in solving problems: (1) formulating the problem; (2) constructing a model, usually a symbolic model; (3) finding a solution from among the alternatives; (4) testing the model and evaluating the solution; and (5) implementing and maintaining the solution. It is restrictive in the size of the problem it can handle. If the problem is large, it must be broken down into several problems and each handled in sequence. There must be two or more courses of action, one of which is preferred by the actor or decision maker, and the solution must have some chance of success.

Techniques and Uses of Operations Research

Operations research has a number of uses and specific techniques have been developed for solving problems.

Simulation. One technique for experimenting with models is simulation. Whereas models represent reality, simulation imitates it. Simulation ". . . is a way of manipulating a model so that it yields a motion picture of reality, usually involves large amounts of computation."[68] A model is a static structure of a real system, a hospital, a clinic, or the transportation paths to health facilities. Simulation is the dynamic process that enables an analyst to experiment with the system, using the model in successive trials until the best solution to a problem is found. Because these experiments can become fairly complicated, the use of a computer is an important tool in testing various solutions.

Simulation, while used for a variety of problems, is primarily associated with queuing problems such as Flagle's use of it in an experiment with an outpatient clinic to devise a way to reduce the waiting time of patients going through the clinic.[69] In his example, he showed that by combining two clerical functions, the registration of patients and the patient's paying for services, he could reduce the waiting time. Flagle stated that simulation was most useful in experimenting with subsystems of hospitals such as laboratories, operating rooms, or outpatient clinics. Simulation is also useful in understanding the dynamics of interim states as a system moves from the current situation to a planned new one in the future. Through simulation it is possible to identify problems that may come up in the expansion of a clinic or a change in the system and, thus, be in a position to confront obstacles as they arise.

Gaming. A technique that is used in situations of uncertainty is gaming. "Its objective has been to convert the uncertainty type of situation into a certainty type."[70] This is done by assuming rationality on the part of the two or more players so that they will each attempt to benefit as much as possible ("maximize his minimum gain") or reduce his losses as much as possible ("minimize his maximum loss"). According to Ackoff and Sasieni, "A game is a situation in which two or more decision makers choose courses of action and in which the outcome is affected by the combination of choices taken collectively."[71] Each player knows and accepts the rules of the game and understands the possible courses of action available. There is an outcome that ends the game, such as a win, loss, or draw. The payoffs to the players are known in advance. If real decision makers are used, it is called operations gaming.

The main uses of gaming are to help develop a decision model, to help find the solution to a model that has been developed by gaming, and to help evaluate proposed solutions to problems modeled by the game. Whereas simulation is primarily involved in problems dealing with structures and systems, gaming deals with human beings who are involved with these systems and for which there is little theory upon which to construct behavior models. Gaming is a heuristic device to help discover this behavior. Consequently, as Ackoff and Sasieni state, "gaming is essentially experimentation in which the behavior of decision makers is observed under controlled conditions."[72] While gaming is being used more in industry, its applications to comprehensive health planning have not been identified. Like most operations research techniques, gaming does require a specification of the rules and a statement of objectives being sought. In health planning, it is seldom that the rules are explicitly known or stated in advance or that the real players, or decision makers, know what the objectives of health planning are or will be. As Ackoff and Sasieni state, "The fundamental weakness of current gaming is the inability to draw strong inferences from the play of the game to decisions in the situations that the game models."[73] In other words, it is difficult to know why the players made the plays or decisions they did based on the game that was set up to simulate reality. Reality is extremely complicated, whereas a model to be useful must be simple. As Gross noted earlier, observing the actions of the players does not mean that an observer can draw a cause-effect relationship from these actions. Other factors that were not modeled by the game may have been involved, such as a player trying to trick or throw off the real intentions of his or her strategy by making a seemingly false move.

PERT and Critical Path Techniques. Program Evaluation and Review Technique (PERT) is a tool used in planning for "mapping out interdependent program steps so that planning can follow a more rational and objective course."[74] It is used in scheduling, costing, redirecting, and evaluating health programs. It can be used in such public health programs as immunization, processing data, and charting the steps involved in the promotion and passage of health legislation. It is most effective in the implementation and evaluation stages of the planning process; less so during the problem analysis-goal setting phase.

The steps involved in PERT are (1) identification of the network of events and activities (time and resources needed to move from one event to another) that make up the whole program; (2) the arrangement of the events in sequence so that no event can be started before the preceding event is completed; (3) the assignment of time values to the activities; (4) determination of the critical path through the network to the completion of the task's objective; and (5) selection of the work processes. The critical path is "the longest path, in terms of time, through the network from the beginning to the ending event."[75]

Diagrams are usually made detailing the network, the time values for each activity leading to the final objective, and the critical path. The aim of this technique is to provide the most efficient use of scarce resources to achieve a specific, identifiable system objective.

Limitations of Operations Research

Operations research suffers from many of the same limitations cited with respect to systems analysis and cost-benefit analysis. It requires large amounts of data that are not often available. It requires a statement of objectives to which the techniques can be applied to solve the problems that interfere in the system's achieving its objectives. Where these are known and accepted by the decision makers, many operations research techniques can prove very useful. Where there is uncertainty about the objectives, they are less applicable. Operations research is a limited tool that requires the decomposition of complex system problems and their solutions in a logical sequence. Often problems cannot be solved through the reduction of a whole to its parts, and it is this deficiency that limits operations research as a method for planning, which requires a more holistic view of health planning issues. Thus, it is more feasible for subsystem problem solving than for system solutions. It requires the input of the decision makers in the application of operations research especially if the analyst hopes to implement, monitor, and control the solution to the problem. However, the language and technical backgrounds of the manager as decision maker and the analyst often create a communication gap and an attendant loss of commitment by the decision maker to the work of the analyst. Young noted that operations research is not understood or accepted by physicians, many of whom conceive it to be a form of efficiency study.[76] Chamberlain notes that an end result of operations research is to produce a higher degree of routine or automation in the activities of workers. This reduces them to robotlike activities, undermining their sense of worth and contribution to the objectives of the organization.[77] In spite of these limitations, operations research as an aide to decision makers can reduce their uncertainty in making decisions about the future while complementing their intuition and experience, both of which are essential in making nonroutine decisions.

Relationship of Operations Research to Planning Models

The operations research method is most applicable to the plan implementation and evaluation phase of a systems model of a health planning agency. It is only after the plan design and goal-objective setting phases have been completed that the techniques become relevant, because operations research requires a statement of goals and objectives. It is then in a position to help identify the alternatives to the achievement of those goals. However, as noted earlier, operations research assumes that the analyst or planner can identify the health system and its interrelationships and model it. If no such system exists, whether it is structurally under the authority of one decision maker or whether it acts in an autonomous system, it is not possible to apply the techniques of operations research except to some minor components of one of the subsystems in the health field. Since only the systems planning model assumes such an integrated health system under one decision-making body, it is the only planning model to which these techniques are applicable. The same arguments that were advanced for the lack of applicability of cost-benefit analysis to other forms of planning models are also relevant to operations research.

Humanitarian-Oriented Implementation Methods

Humanistic orientations to plan implementation include ad hoc opportunism and community organization. These methods emphasize political approaches to solving health problems although policy science analysts may well argue that their method is as much imbued with the scientific method as operations research. While this may be true, the emphasis of these methods is on action, such as organizing a community, influencing legislators, proposing alternative solutions to a health issue, etc. The technological methods assist the decision maker in diagnosing a problem and recommending a preferred solution. They also may suggest strategies for implementation. Their essential strength is on the diagnosis-solution aspect of planning; they are weak on implementation. In contrast, the humanistic approach is weak on diagnosis and strong on plan implementation.

Ad Hoc Opportunism

Ad hoc opportunism is a method proposed by Bolan that has received little research or attention in the planning field, yet it is widely used in practice. As Bolan states:

> . . . the method is as follows: operating within certain predetermined rules of the game, opportunities to move toward some

> highly generalized goal are seized as circumstances permit. No
> particular program point is articulated nor is any definite
> schedule set. No preconceived notions or detailed goals are set
> forth and, consequently, particularized goals may vary consid-
> erably over time.[78]

This is a pragmatic form of action within generalized goals that Bolan
perceives as operating within neighborhoods and supported by local
groups. An example would be the Lower East Side Health Council block-
ing of the planned expansion of a backup hospital to the Gouverneur
Hospital. The council used its opposition to the backup hospital to
illustrate Gouverneur Hospital's need to have its own surgical unit, which
was not included at the time it was constructed. The council seized this
opportunity after the hospital was officially opened to note the low occupancy rate, about 50 percent in Gouverneur, because so many of its
patients were being transferred to the backup hospital for surgical procedures. It used this opportunity to strive for the conversion of Gouverneur
into a complete community hospital. The council wanted a hospital that
offered all basic services to the community and reduced dependence on
the backup hospital over which it had no influence in determining what
and how health services would be provided to the community. In the end,
the backup hospital won on its proposal to expand its facilities as planned.
Yet a compromise was reached. Gouverneur Hospital was also granted
permission to open a small surgical unit to perform the more routine
surgical procedures needed by people in the community. The council and
its supporters had to appeal to the health planning agency in New York
City, the Health and Hospital Corporation of New York City, and the
Health and Hospital Planning Council of Southern New York to gain
approval for the addition of the surgical suite. Nonetheless, a few years
later, the Health and Hospital Corporation, citing the fiscal constraints of
its budget, closed the hospital as a community facility and converted it to
another medical use. Just as the neighborhood group used its influence at
an opportune time to obtain a commitment to open the surgical unit, the
corporation used a later opportunity to reverse the result.

Community Organization

Community organization has been defined by one of its foremost theo-
reticians, Ross, as

> . . . a process by which a community identifies its needs or ob-
> jectives, orders these needs or objectives, develops the confi-
> dence . . . to work at these needs and objectives, finds the re-

sources . . . to deal with [them] . . . , takes action in respect to them, and, in so doing, extends and develops cooperative and collaborative attitudes and practices in the community.[79]

Community organization has been treated by the social work profession as one of its three major methods of practice. Ross' definition emphasizes the planning aspect and suggests a process of implementing action through collaboration. However, since Ross' theoretical exposition in 1955, there have been numerous advances on the method of community organization so that it has become a very complex field of practice, requiring the integration of several social sciences.

Thus, political science has brought forth the concept of conflict and the strategies required to deal with it, the concept of influence and the various types required in order to promote a group's goals, and the theoretical issue of pluralistic versus authoritarian forms of government. These concepts are particularly relevant to health planning agencies since they have had to organize themselves into viable bodies and create subarea councils to deal with small geographical territories. In New York City alone, 33 subcouncils have been developed, and conflict, resources, uses of influence, and the type of authority structure to be developed have been very real issues to the participants.[80]

Sociologists have advanced ideas related to social systems theory, roles played by community organizers and self-interest groups in their community activity, and the nature of the structure of community organizations at various levels of government. These concepts are often related to concepts of political power and influence. Two books of community organization readings have elaborated on strategies, conflict management, social analysis, and theory and organizational structures.[81] In both texts, the influence of the recent strivings for opportunity, equality, and justice have been major values espoused by community organizers in their work with minority groups. Community organization has been moving into the mainstream of political activity, and the literature related to self-interest groups and advocacy reflects this. The use of these concepts indicates how far this method has developed since the presentation of Ross' advanced concepts. The importance of this generalized statement of the various and complex characteristics related to community organization is to suggest some of the complexities health planning agency staff can be expected to encounter as they organize their health constituencies to implement health plans.

Major Use of Implementation Methods

Community organization is concerned with the implementation strategies that can result in the achievement of the more specific objectives and concrete programs that are embodied in these policies. As such, it is concerned with arousing elite or broad-based support for the objectives, utilizing whatever resources of influence are available to the groups involved. Typically, a health planning agency board tends to involve communitywide decision makers or community leaders and use their influence to accomplish its objectives, while the subarea council tends to rely on grass roots support of community groups, each with its own leadership and special interests, to achieve the implementation of its objectives and the concrete programs desired in the community. Ad hoc opportunism more typically is utilized in subareas under the jurisdiction of health planning agencies as they press for programmatic implementation of felt needs. As such, it is a more action-oriented activity that will be played out by interest groups with representation on the agencies' subarea councils or as autonomous bodies attempting to influence the subarea councils to support the programs in which they have an interest.

Noble has stated that health planning agencies are consensus-oriented organizations that must emphasize strategies of collaboration and cooperation.[82] While this may be their emphasis, it can be taken for granted that they will have to deal with numerous conflicts. Some of these conflicts will be between members of the health planning board itself. Others will arise between the board and other health service boards, such as those of hospitals and clinics, over suggested changes in the direction of policies and/or programs. To ensure that the changes are made requires what Banfield calls control of the actors who have the requisite authority to do as the actor (the health planning agency) desires. Adoption of an action can take place when all actors who have control over necessary requisite actions come under one decision maker's control. That decision maker is then said to have centralized control of the action, and the adoption of the action is assured.[83] The range of influence strategies that can be used is wide and includes such tactics as persuading, deceiving, inveigling, rewarding, punishing, and inducing others to do one's bidding. The resources to use these strategies successfully include such means as votes, political or social status, control of funds, authority over official actions, or control of some aspect of mass media.

A description of these techniques of persuasion and resources to influence others underscores the potential health planning agencies have toward coercion. The problem is in knowing how to apply these strategies to achieve goals. It is here that community organization is effective in determining which are the feasible techniques. Almost all theorists and writers on planning state that technical or policy planning must be tied to the decision maker if goals are to be transformed into reality. Wildavsky states that the "first requirement of effective policy analysis is that top management want it."[84] This top management may be the board of a health planning agency, the legislative leadership, or a corporate firm.

Because these methods—ad hoc opportunism and community organization—are not as rigorous in their technical and data demands as operations research, systems analysis, or cost-benefit analysis and because they are more oriented toward actions involving human relationships, they are apt to be most emphasized during the initial years of health planning agencies' development. Once the agencies are well established and plans have been fully developed, the methods continue to be important, but are used on a par with the technical planning methods discussed earlier. Whereas the technical methods are more rigorous in their procedures, these methods are less procedurally defined and depend as much on art as on science for their execution. In fact, it can be expected that, as these methods grow more complex as time passes, they will be even less susceptible to the niceties of rigorous procedures that are being developed for operations research and cost-benefit analysis. Yet, these methods will continue to be highly relevant in the work of health planning agencies.

Relationship of Implementation Methods to Planning Models

Ad Hoc Opportunism

The most significant application of ad hoc opportunism is to the individual action planning model, as Bolan himself asserts. "None of the actions are taken as part of a predetermined plan, but are decided with the people of the neighborhood as opportunities present themselves."[85] Since the emphasis is on program implementation rather than the achievement of explicit and accepted goals and objectives, this planning model is ideally suited to this method. It may have some relevance to the alliance model if the coalition stays in business long enough to continue to seize opportunities as they arise. However, the nature of a coalition is such that it generally goes out of business once its immediate objective has been achieved. It is thus unlikely that in too many instances this planning model will use this method. Ad hoc opportunism has little relevance to the other models.

Community Organization

Community organization is a method that has relevance for all the planning models except the systems model. Community organization, with its emphasis on political strategy, general policy formulation, the gathering of resources, and the involvement of many levels of support for actions desired, is used in various forms and at different times by these models. The primary emphases for the partnership planning model are on (1) the development of the board and later its subarea councils, (2) the deliberations that lead to a statement of general policies, and (3) the mobilization of support in legislatures and other bodies for their implementation. With respect to the alliance model, the community organization method is used to maintain the cohesion of the cooperating autonomous bodies as they strive to achieve a specific objective. It is assumed that members of the coalition already have sufficient resources to implement the objective collectively, but should this prove not to be the case, then community organization methods are applied to secure the essential resources needed. With respect to the individual action model, applications of the methods are needed primarily to obtain community support and resources for the achievement of its programs.

DATA SOURCES

There are numerous sources of data that health planning agencies can tap to obtain the information they need. PL 93-641 specifically prohibits health planning agencies from developing their own data. Rather, they are to serve as depositories of data for the state and regional levels of planning. A full- or part-time librarian, when a health planning agency can afford one, is becoming increasingly valuable to ensure the acquisition, control, and dissemination of data. A special manual has been developed by the Bureau of Health Planning to guide health planning agencies in carrying out this important function.[86] Among the items considered essential in health planning agency libraries are the following:

Core Materials

1. Basic Subscriptions
   American Journal of Public Health
   Center for Health Planning Newsletter
   Council of Governments Newsletter
   Data User News, Bureau of the Census
   Federal Register, General Services Administration
   Health Care Week
   Health Planning, National Health Planning Information Center
   Health Planning Developments, American Health Planning Association

Health Resources News, Health Resources Administration (HRA)
Hospitals, American Hospital Association (AHA)
Journal of Human Services Abstracts, Project SHARE, Rockville, Md.
Medical Care, J. B. Lippincott Co.
Monthly Vital Statistics Reports, National Center for Health Statistics
Morbidity and Mortality Weekly Report, Center for Disease Control
Nation's Health, American Public Health Association
News of the Cooperative Health Statistics System, National Center for Health Statistics
PSRO Selected Information Services, Health Care Financing Administration
Public Health Reports, HRA
State Department of Health Bulletin
State Hospital Association Journal
State Medical Association Journal
State Morbidity and Mortality Report
2. Secondary Subscriptions
American Medical News, AMA
Commitment, HRS
Family Health, Family Media, Inc., New York
Health Planning and Manpower Report, Capital Publications, Inc., Washington
Health Perspectives, Consumer Commission on the Accreditation of Health Services Inc., New York City
Health Policy Advisory Center Bulletin, New York
Health Services Research, Hospital Research and Educational Trust, Chicago
Health Systems, Morris Associates, Inc., Washington
Health Values: Achieving High Level Wellness, Charles Slack, Inc., Throfare, N.J.
Hospital Week, AHA
International Journal of Health Services, Baywood Publishing Co., Farmingdale, N.Y.
Medical Care Review, University of Michigan, School of Public Health
Topics in Health Care Financing, Aspen Systems Corporation, Rockville, Md.
Urban Health, Urban Publishing Co., Atlanta, Ga.
Washington Report on Medicine and Health, McGraw-Hill

3. Reference Works
    Stedman's Medical Dictionary, Williams & Wilkins Co., Baltimore
    A Discursive Dictionary of Health Care, Government Printing Office (GPO)
    Catalog of Federal Domestic Assistance, GPO
    Statistical Abstract of the United States, GPO
    Code of Federal Regulations: Title 42 (Public Health)

Government Publications

1. General Public Health Service
    Catalog of Publications (HRA)
    Forward Plan for Health, GPO
    Papers on the National Health Guidelines, HRA
    Health of the Disadvantaged, Chartbook, HRA
    Vital and Health Statistics: Techniques of Community Health Analysis, Center for Disease Control
    Algorithms for Health Planners Series (Hypertension, Infant Mortality, Breast Cancer Mortality, Heart Attack Mortality, Preventable Death and Disease), Bureau of Health Planning, HRA
2. National Center for Health Statistics
    Health United States Series, HRA
    Selected National Data Sources for Health Planners, HRA
    Vital and Health Statistics Publications Series, each dealing with a separate topic including data from:
        Series   10: Health Interview Survey
                  11: Health Examination Survey
                  13: Health Resources Utilization
                  14: Manpower and Facilities
                  20: Mortality
                  21: Natality, Marriage, and Divorce
                  23: Family Growth
                 117: Hospital and Surgical Insurance Coverage
                 118: Disability Days
                 120: Acute Conditions, Incidence and Associated Disability
    The Nation's Use of Health Resources
    Health Resources Statistics
3. National Center for Health Services Research
    Nurse Practitioner and Physician Assistant Training
    Changes in the Costs of Treatment of Selected Illnesses
    Impact of State Certificate-of-Need Laws on Health Care Costs and Utilization

      Analysis of Physician Price and Output Decisions
      Controlling the Cost of Health Care
4. National Health Planning Information Center
      Health Planning Information Series
        Trends Affecting the U.S. Health Care System
        Guide to Data for Health Systems Planners
        A Guide to the Development of Health Resource Inventories
      Health Planning Methods and Technology Series
        Health Manpower Planning Process
        Guide to Financial Analysis and Introduction to
          Economic Impact Analysis for Health Planning
        A Taxonomy of the Health Systems Appropriate for
          Plan Development
      Health Planning Bibliographic Series
        Consumer Participation in Health Planning
        Selected Bibliographic References on Methodologies for Community Health Status Assessment
        Women and the Health System
5. Bureau of Community Health Services
      Promoting Community Health
      Child Health in America
      The National Health Service Corps
6. Social Security Administration
      Compendium of National Health Expenditures Data
      Work Disability in the United States: A Chartbook
      The Size and Shape of the Medical Care Dollar: Chartbook

Other Publications

      Health Insurance Source Book, Health Insurance Institute, Washington, D.C.
      Accreditation Manual for Hospitals, Joint Commission on Accreditation of Hospitals, Chicago
      American Hospital Association Resource Catalog, Chicago
      AHA Guide to the Health Care Field
      Hospital Statistics: Data from the AHA Annual Survey Plans; Health Systems Plans; State Health Plans; state plans involving drug abuse, mental health, alcoholism, maternal and child health; plans from the council(s) of government relating to health

This array of documents and materials provides the health planning agency with the basic data needed to plan, develop, and carry out their basic functions:

- socioeconomic information
- health status, including mortality, morbidity, natality, marriage, divorce, and disability
- capacity and staffing of facilities
- services and their utilization
- payment for services
- quality of care
- ambulatory care
- mental health
- insurance coverage

These data are generally available at the national, state, and regional levels, but they are not usually found at the subregional levels unless they are vital statistics or census data. A further restriction is that only fragmented data on specific functional medical elements, such as drug abuse, home health care, health education, or emergency medical services, are available. This makes it difficult to undertake a systematic analysis in plan development in order to set goals, objectives, and priorities. Statements on resource requirements are even more difficult to develop. Most of the readily accessible data are oriented toward health systems (facilities, resources, personnel, equipment) rather than toward health status (morbidity, mortality, disability) or its determinants (genetic, behavioral, or environmental factors). Consequently, while the data base is being enlarged to place more emphasis on health status and its determinants, health planning agencies are currently caught in a dilemma. They are unable to carry out those special studies and surveys that would provide the data needed to make statements in the areas of health status and its determinants, both because the federal funding on which they are largely dependent is too limited and because they are expressly forbidden to use the funds in this manner without HHS' prior approval. They can make statements on medical system changes, but these may have limited effect on the population's health status.

It should be noted that the federal government has funded an extensive number of special studies that take into account almost every aspect of health planning. Computer searches and bibliographic services, often at little or no cost, are readily available from a number of governmental and private sources.[87] The most important of these are:

- National Technical Information Service (NTIS), Department of Commerce, Springfield, Va. NTIS offers a variety of computer search services from its more than 1 million titles of technical reports from every branch of government and foreign countries. Through its

Selected Research in Microfiche service (SRIM) it provides a current update on 500 subject categories, including health planning, at low prices for full text microfiche reports.

- National Health Planning Information Center (NHPIC), Bureau of Health Planning, Health Resources Administration, Hyattsville, Md. NHPIC was authorized under PL 93-641 to "facilitate the exchange of information concerning health services, resources, planning and resource development practice, and methodology."[88] It prepares monographs and bibliographies, provides reference and referral services, and a weekly announcement of new holdings. Its computerized information files contain abstracts of over 30,000 items. Services are primarily available to components of the health planning system developed under PL 93-641.
- Medical Literature Analysis and Retrieval System (MEDLARS) National Library of Medicine, Bethesda, Md. MEDLARS is a system that links more than 900 universities, medical schools, hospitals, government agencies, and commercial organizations to the National Library of Medicine's extensive holdings. The three retrieval systems that have the most importance for health planning agencies are
  1. *Medline,* which contains 600,000 reference items of biomedical journals for the current and two preceding years
  2. *Catline,* which contains some 200,000 references to books and serials cataloged since 1965
  3. *Health Planning and Administration,* which has around 100,000 items on health planning, organization, financing, management, personnel, and other related subjects

In addition to these generalized reference services, there are other specialized clearinghouses. The most important of these are

- PSRO Information Clearinghouse
  Health Services Administration
  Rockville, Md.
- High Blood Pressure Information Center
  Bethesda, Md.
- National Clearinghouse for Smoking and Health
  Atlanta, Ga.
- National Clearinghouse on Aging
  Washington, D.C.
- Scientific Technical Information
  National Center for Health Statistics
  Hyattsville, Md.

- National Clearinghouse for Drug Abuse Information
  Rockville, Md.
- National Clearinghouse for Mental Health Information
  Rockville, Md.
- National Clearinghouse on Emergency Medical Services
  Rockville, Md.
- National Clearinghouse for Alcohol Information
  Rockville, Md.
- National Clearinghouse for Improving the Management of
  Human Services: Project SHARE
  Rockville, Md.
- Public Information Center/Library
  U.S. Environmental Protection Agency
  Washington, D.C.
- Health Law Center
  Rockville, Md.

These information clearinghouses, together with the information provided on a routine basis by federal, state, and local governments and private resources, should generally make available to health planning agencies the total range of articles, monographs, and books needed to carry out their functions, especially those relating to plan development, regulation, and plan implementation.

CENTERS FOR HEALTH PLANNING[89]

To assist health planning agencies in fulfilling their technical, administrative, and organizational responsibilities, Congress provided funds for the establishment of centers for health planning. At least five were authorized in the legislation, PL 93-641, but ten were developed, one in each HEW region. In the last two years, the ten centers have been reduced to four, mainly because of budget constraints and the desire to avoid duplication in the use of scarce center resources.

The law asks the centers to assist health planning agencies by "conducting research, studies and analyses of health planning and resources development, and developing health planning approaches, methodologies, policies, and standards . . ." (Sec. 1534(a)).

Since their inception in 1976, the centers have concentrated on improving health planning agencies' capacity for four vital planning functions: (1) plan development, (2) plan implementation/project review, (3) plan implementation/resource development, and (4) data management and analysis.

In the first two years, the most time was spent on plan development and data management. These two functions are not only closely linked but also essential to the creation of regional and state health plans. As these plans have become more highly developed and consistent with established federal guidelines, the focus has shifted to their implementation. Thus, more attention has been devoted to the two main strategies for plan implementation, project review and resource development.

Four major technical assistance strategies were generally used to assist the health planning agencies: (1) educational services, (2) materials development, (3) information services, and (4) consultations. Educational services include training of health planning staff and their volunteer boards. Examples of educational sessions include:

- developing regulatory strategies: the use of plans
- evolving improvement of plans
- financial analysis training workshop
- state planning guidance
- tools and tactics of implementation
- promoting competition as a regulatory strategy

In the first two years, such educational sessions were offered as regionwide meetings, group meetings that involved selected health planning agencies, or tailor-made educational meetings for a specific planning agency.

Materials development has been a second important center strategy. Using either their own staffs or consultants with expertise in the subject, the centers develop technical assistance materials, as well as the materials used in their training sessions and consultations. These materials are either surveys of the latest knowledge, methods, or policy alternatives on a specific subject or newly developed concepts and methods. As such, they bring the latest information on the state of the art and technology to the health planning agencies. Examples of materials developed are

- *A Health Planner's Guide to Planning and Review of Hospital Based Alcoholism Services*
- *Conditions on CoN [Certificate-of-Need] Approvals*
- *Recent Studies and Information on Long-Term Care Planning*
- *Plan Implementation*
- *Guide to Resource Estimation*
- *Priority Setting*
- *HSA Workshop for Review and Approval of Federal Funds*
- *Reshaping the Acute Care System*

When this list is compared to the types of seminars and educational sessions offered, it can be seen that the titles of the materials developed are quite similar to those of the educational sessions. All of these were developed to meet the needs of health planning agencies and to guide them in fulfilling the responsibilities thrust on them by federal initiatives.

Health planning agencies require information of all types, and centers attempt to provide information services either through giving the agencies the information directly or referring them to sources where the information can be secured. Centers also publish periodic newsletters that offer legislative information, discussions on policy and planning issues, upcoming center conferences and other important meetings, and special topic discussions.

In the first two years, consultations were in the form of group, region-wide, or individual sessions. With the reduction in the number of centers to four and the concomitant increase in the number of health planning agencies turning to each center, an individual consultation can now be provided only if the agency is able to pay for it. Centers have also offered consultation services to the Bureau of Health Planning and its regional offices. These have focused on clarification for the federal staff and written guidance for health planning agencies on the 1979 amendments to PL 93-641. Some of these consultations have taken place at the initiative of the centers; some, in response to the needs of the agencies or federal officials.

Of these four strategies, educational sessions and consultation services were given the most emphasis in the first two years of the centers' existence, while in the last few years there has been increasing attention on materials development and information services. Nonetheless, the first two strategies are still given the greatest emphasis by centers. For example, Table 5-3 shows how one center allocated its time during an 11-month period. Table 5-4 shows that it targeted 46 percent of its time on training (educational services) and consultation, while 54 percent was to be spent on information (communications and reference services) and materials development. Two years earlier, 58 percent was spent on education and consultation, and only 17 percent on information and materials development. The remaining time was spent on center administration. It becomes obvious from this information that the reduction in centers from ten to four has caused the remaining centers to devote less time to direct contact with health planning agencies and more time to developing the materials and information they require to carry out their responsibilities.

With the reduction to four centers, each of them became a lead agency to specialize in one topic of importance to health planning agencies. Subjects of specialization included data management and analysis, relationships of health planning agencies to mental health, project review, plan

Table 5-3 Analysis of Project Days by Health Planning Functions
(July 1, 1979– May 31, 1980)

Health Planning Functions	Person Days	Total to Date Percentage to Date	Annual Target
Plan development	153.25	14%	16%
Plan implementation/project review	133.50	12%	13%
Plan implementation/health systems development	195.0	17%	20%
Data management and analysis	157.0	14%	14%
Mental health specialty	78.25	7%	7%
Subtotal planning function days:	717.0		
Communications	115.0	10%	11%
Reference services	209.75	19%	19%
DHEW advisory meetings	75.5	7%	
Total project days:	1125.25	100%	100%

implementation, and legal information. However, after a year of this specialization, there was confusion about the dissemination, utilization, and relevance of the material developed for each specialty. Areas of special interest within each of these specializations may be important to health planning agencies in the region where they were developed, but not in another. This emphasis was consequently abandoned.

The basic purpose of the centers has been to improve the capabilities of the health planning agencies in their effort to carry out the goals and priorities of PL 93-641. There is no way to assess at this point what impact

Table 5-4 Analysis of Project Days by Mode of Service
(July 1, 1979– May 31, 1980)

Modality	Person Days	Total to Date Percentage to Date	Annual Target
Training	301.5	27%	27%
Consultation	175.5	16%	19%
Materials development	161.5	14%	15%
Communications	160.25	14%	17%
Reference services	243.25	22%	22%
DHEW advisory meetings	79.5	7%	
Total:	1121.25	100%	100%

the centers' work has had on the agencies. Nevertheless, issues have been raised by the centers' operations that require attention. Who is the primary client of the centers: the health planning agencies or the federal bureau and its regional branches which finance most of the centers' activities? Given limited resources, how do the centers determine their priorities: from their own assessment of the health planning agencies' needs, from the agencies themselves, or from the federal funding agency? Given the fact that center staff must be recognized experts in their areas of responsibility (in data, in plan development, in agency management or plan implementation, from where are these staff members recruited to ensure the respect, competence, and acceptance of the centers' clientele? The centers are expected to play a major role in improving the performance of the members of the health planning system. How do they do this when they have limited funds and large geographical territories to cover? Which of the four major strategies do they emphasize to carry out this assignment? When the centers have many competing claims on their limited resources and no clearly defined constituency, will the centers be able to offer the technical assistance and services needed with a minimum of conflicting pressures exerted on them? From these questions, it can be readily perceived that the role of the centers, while important, is fraught with problems for which there are no ready solutions.

NOTES

1. U.S. DHEW, "Health Systems Agency: Performance Standards Guidelines," mimeographed (Hyattsville, Md.: Bureau of Health Planning, February 1, 1977).

2. Michael J. Meshenberg, *Health Planning and the Environment: A Preventive Focus* (Chicago: American Society of Planning Officials, March, 1974), Chapter 4, especially Table 1, p. 18.

3. *Ibid.*, p. 18.

4. Roland L. Warren et al., *The Structure of Urban Reform* (Lexington, Mass: D.C. Heath and Co., 1974), p. 80.

5. Richard S. Bolan, "Emerging Views of Planning," *Journal of American Institute of Planners,* July 1967, pp. 239–242.

6. Aaron Wildavsky, "The Political Economy of Efficiency: Cost-Benefit Analysis, System Analysis and Program Budgeting," *Public Administration Review* 26 (1966): 292–310.

7. Readers interested in a wider selection of health planning methods can obtain them from Allen D. Spiegel and Herbert H. Hyman, *Basic Health Planning Methods* (Germantown, Md.: Aspen Systems Corporation, 1978). Methods in this text are linked to six steps that comprise the basic health planning process. Plan development and plan implementation are generic steps in this process.

8. The assertions made are those of the author. They are based on his knowledge and experience of where an agency is likely to place its greatest emphasis. They do not imply that the methods are not used where a "no" notation is made, but rather they are used infrequently and not given much attention by this planning model.

9. For further information, see George J. Warheit, Roger A. Bell, and John J. Schwab, *Planning for Change: Needs Assessment Approaches* (Washington, D.C.: National Institute of Mental Health, 1974); A. T. Kearney, Inc., *Population-Based Mental Health Needs Assessment Methodology for Use in HSA/SP* (Health Systems Agency of Southeastern Pennsylvania, December 1979), pp. II-4 to II-6; Allen D. Spiegel and Herbert H. Hyman, *Basic Health Planning Methods,* pp. 28, 29.

10. See Spiegel and Hyman, *Basic Health Planning Methods,* pp. 32–34. For a detailed illustration in the use of social indicator technique see Beatrice M. Rosen, "A Model for Estimating Mental Health Needs Using 1970 Census Socioeconomic Data," *Mental Health Statistics, Series C, No. 9* (Rockville, Md.: National Institute of Mental Health, 1974).

11. Aaron Wildavsky, "Rescuing Policy Analysis from PPBS" in *Public Expenditures and Policy Analysis,* eds. Julius Margolis and Herbert H. Haveman (Chicago: Markham Publishing Co., 1970), p. 463.

12. *Ibid.,* pp. 462, 463.

13. Martin Rein, *Social Policy* (New York: Random House, 1970), p. 5.

14. Based on Wildavsky, in Margolis and Haveman, *Public Expenditures.*

15. John C. Deshaies and David R. Seidman, "Health Information Systems," *Socio-Economic Planning Sciences* 5 (1971): 516.

16. John H. Noble, Jr., "Designing Information Systems for Comprehensive Health Planning," *Inquiry* 7 (4):35.

17. Deshaies and Seidman, "Health Information Systems."

18. Deshaies and Seidman, "Health Information Systems;" also Ross Stagner, "Perceptions, Aspirations, Frustrations, and Satisfactions: An Approach to Urban Indicators," *The Annals of the American Academy of Political and Social Science,* March 1970, pp. 59–68.

19. See Stagner, "Urban Indicators;" Michael Springer, "Social Indicators, Reports and Accounts: Toward the Management of Society," *The Annals of the American Academy of Political and Social Science,* March 1970, pp. 1–13; Jack Elinson, *Toward Socio-Medical Health Indicators,* mimeographed, paper given at International Conference of Medical Sociology, Warsaw, Poland, August 20–25, 1973; and Charles J. Austin, "Selected Social Indicators in the Health Field," *American Journal of Public Health* 61 (1971): 1507–1513.

20. U.S. DHEW, *Health United States 1976–1977* (Washington, D.C.: U.S. Government Printing Office, 1977), pp. 183–216.

21. Elinson, *Socio-Medical Health Indicators,* p. 1.

22. *Ibid.,* p. 14.

23. Alain C. Enthoven, "The Systems Analysis Approach," in *Program Budgeting and Benefit-Cost Analysis,* eds. Hartley Hinrichs and Graham Taylor (Pacific Palisades, Calif.: Goodyear Publishing Co., Inc., 1969), p. 160.

24. Wildavsky, "Political Economy," p. 298.

25. J. W. Forrester, *Urban Dynamics* (Cambridge, Mass.: MIT Press, 1972), p. 12.

26. Allan Akman and Jerome B. Gordon, "Systems Analysis and Occupational Health," *American Journal of Public Health* 60 (1970): 1749–1759.

27. Boyd Z. Palmer, *An Advanced Health Planning System* (Springfield, Va.: National Technical Information Service, U.S. Department of Commerce, 1972), p. 23.

28. Wildavsky, "Political Economy;" Forrester, *Urban Dynamics;* and Harvey Adelman, "Systems Analysis and Planning for Public Health Care in the City of New York," *Archives of Environmental Health* 16 (1968): 258–263.

29. Forrester, *Urban Dynamics,* p. 112.

30. Wildavsky, "Political Economy," p. 300.

31. Clifford D. Stewart, "The QUEST Approach to Design," *Hospitals* 46 (1972): 95–102, 196.

32. Adelman, "Public Health Care;" Akman and Gordon, "Occupational Health;" Forrester, *Urban Dynamics;* Whitney Murphy, "The Systems Approach to Planning," *Hospitals* 46 (1972): 111–114; Morris Schaefer and Herman E. Hilleboe, "The Health Manpower Crisis: Cause or Symptoms?" *American Journal of Public Health* 57 (1967): 6–14; Harold E. Smalley, "The Systems Approach," *Hospitals* 46 (1972): 50–54; Palmer, *Advanced Health Planning.*

33. Bolan, "Views of Planning."

34. F. D. Kennedy, "An Evaluation of Comprehensive Health Planning," mimeographed (Atlanta, Ga.: Department of Health and Social Service Planning, Atlanta Regional Commission, 1972).

35. *Ibid.,* p. 6.

36. *Ibid.,* p. 8.

37. Mary F. Arnold, "Use of Management Tools in Health Planning," *Public Health Reports* 83 (1968): 820–826.

38. Wildavsky, in Margolis and Haveman, *Public Expenditures,* Chapter 19.

39. S. Kenneth Howard, "Planning and Budgeting: Marriage Whose Style?" in *Planning and Policies: Uneasy Partners,* eds. Boyle and Lathrop.

40. George C. Hemmens and George T. Lathrop, "Systems Analysis, Politics and Planning," in Boyle and Lathrop, *Planning and Policies,* p. 129.

41. Forrester, *Urban Dynamics,* p. 109.

42. *Ibid.,* p. 114.

43. See David J. Berlinski's critique of General Systems Theory and Forrester's application of it in his article, "Systems Analysis," *Urban Affairs Quarterly,* September 1970, pp. 104–126.

44. Bertram M. Gross, "The New Systems Budgeting," *Public Administration Review,* March/April 1969.

45. Hemmens and Lathrop, "Systems Analysis," p. 144.

46. Margolis and Haveman, *Public Expenditures,* p. 5.

47. Gross, "New Systems Budgeting."

48. Margolis and Haveman, *Public Expenditures,* p. 4.

49. Gross, "New Systems Budgeting."

50. Wildavsky, "Political Economy," p. 293.

51. Morris Hill, "A Goal-Achievement Matrix for Evaluating Alternative Plans," in *Decision-Making in Urban Planning,* ed. Robinson (Beverly Hills, Calif.: Sage Publications, 1972), p. 186.

52. For full examples of cost-benefit analysis, see the illustrative cases in Hinrichs and Taylor, *Program Budgeting;* the cases in Margolis and Haveman, *Public Expenditures,* especially the case by Robert N. Grosse, "Problems of Resource Allocation in Health;" or for the layman with a limited mathematical background, George M. Galloway, "The Use of

Cost-Benefit Analysis in Analyzing Recreational Facilities Expenditures," mimeographed (Ann Arbor, Mich.: Symposium, University of Michigan, October 31, 1972).

53. Galloway, "Recreational Facilities Expenditures," pp. 17–20.

54. Akman and Gordon, "Occupational Health."

55. See Hinrichs and Taylor, *Program Budgeting,* pp. 13–14 for a discussion on constraints.

56. Galloway, "Recreational Facilities Expenditures," p. 24.

57. Erich Jantsch, "Technological Forecasting Techniques in Perspectives," in Robinson, *Urban Planning,* pp. 151–176. Most of the discussion in this section is based on Jantsch.

58. Donald A. Schon, "Forecasting and Technical Forecasting," *Daedalus,* Summer 1967, p. 759.

59. Jantsch in Robinson, *Urban Planning,* p. 155.

60. Schon, "Technical Forecasting," p. 766.

61. *Ibid.,* p. 769.

62. Russell L. Ackoff and Maurice W. Sasieni, *Fundamentals of Operational Research* (New York: John Wiley and Sons, 1968), p. 6.

63. *Ibid.,* Chapter 1.

64. John Young in George K. Checko, ed., *The Recognition of Systems in Health Services* (Washington, D.C.: Operations Research Society of America, 1969), p. 396.

65. See case illustrations of operations research in Checko, *Recognition of Systems;* Charles D. Flagle, "The Role of Simulation in the Health Services," *American Journal of Public Health,* December 1970, pp. 2386–2394; William J. Horvath, "Influence of Change," *Health Services Research,* Spring 1968, pp. 3–9; and Walter Merten, "PERT and Planning for Health Programs," *Public Health Reports,* May 1966, pp. 449–454.

66. See Ackoff and Sasieni, *Fundamentals of Research,* Chapter 17.

67. *Ibid.,* Chapter 3.

68. *Ibid.,* p. 96.

69. Flagle, "Role of Simulation."

70. Ackoff and Sasieni, *Fundamentals of Research,* p. 329.

71. *Ibid.,* p. 328.

72. *Ibid.,* p. 110.

73. *Ibid.,* p. 111.

74. Merten, "PERT and Planning," p. 449.

75. *Ibid.*

76. Young in Checko, *Recognition of Systems,* pp. 396–397.

77. Neil W. Chamberlain, *Private and Public Planning* (New York: McGraw-Hill, 1965), Chapter 2.

78. Bolan, "Views of Planning," p. 241.

79. Murray G. Ross, *Community Organization: Theory and Principles* (New York: Harper & Row, 1955), p. 39.

80. See for example Meyer Schwartz, "Community Organization" in *Encyclopedia of Social Work,* ed. Harry L. Lurie (New York: National Association of Social Workers, 1965), pp. 177–189. The author discusses a whole range of new studies and research related to development of the method.

81. See Ralph M. Kramer and Harry Specht, eds., *Readings in Community Organization Practice* (Englewood Cliffs, N.J.: Prentice-Hall, 1969), pp. 324–386; and Fred M. Cox et al.,

eds., *Strategies of Community Organization* (Itasca, Ill.: F. E. Peacock Publishers, Inc., 1970), Chapters 6, 7, 9, 11, 13.

82. Noble, "Designing Information Systems," p. 34.

83. Edward C. Banfield, *Political Influence* (New York: The Free Press, 1961), Chapter 11.

84. Wildavsky, in Margolis and Haveman, *Public Expenditures*, p. 473.

85. Bolan, "Views of Planning," p. 242.

86. U.S. DHEW, *Organizing and Maintaining a Document Collection in a Health Systems Agency: Suggested Resources*, Health Planning Methods and Technology Series, No. 9 (Hyattsville, Md.: Health Resources Administration, December 1978).

87. *Ibid.*, pp. 13–25.

88. *Ibid.*, pp. 79–81.

89. This section is based on reports from the ALPHA Center for Health Planning, located in Bethesda, Maryland; *Health Resources News*, published by HRA; and the Senate hearings on the Health Planning Amendments of 1979. Discussions with officials in the Bureau of Health Planning and the ALPHA Center also provided information.

Chapter 6

Functions, Goals, and Authority of Health Planning Agencies

In 1966 Congress enacted PL 89-741, the Partnership for Health Act, which called for "promoting and assuring the highest level of health attainable, for every person, in an environment which contributes positively to health for individual and family living." Almost ten years later, PL 93-641, the National Health Planning and Resources Development Act, reasserted this broad health policy goal by stating that the purposes of health planning agencies are to improve the health of the population they serve; to increase accessibility, availability, acceptability, continuity, and quality of the health care services to be provided; to restrain costs of health services; and to reduce duplication while increasing needed services. The law also describes ten priorities in Section 1502 and calls for the development of national guidelines and standards, as well as additional goal priorities. Thus, PL 93-641 has gone beyond its predecessor by presenting more detailed specifications of what is expected of health planning agencies in their development and implementation of plans. Health planning agencies are responsible not only for developing a set of goals and priorities, but also they have a number of other functions to carry out, several of which have a direct impact on their capacity to plan.

FUNCTIONS OF HEALTH PLANNING AGENCIES

Guidelines issued by the Bureau of Health Planning indicate that health planning agencies are expected to carry out seven functions:[1]

1. plan development
2. plan implementation/review activities
3. plan implementation/health system development
4. public involvement and education

5. agency organization and management
6. data management and analysis
7. coordination

The first four functions might be thought of as the core functions, those functions that are the purposes of the health planning agencies. The last three might be viewed as support functions, i.e., the activities that permit the achievement of the core functions. Of these seven functions, perhaps the first one—plan development—is the most important because the other functions depend upon its completion. Plan development is directly related to public issues and to the standards and priorities required to evaluate the numerous projects under review.

Plan Development

Federal guidelines describe plan development as follows: "The plan development function encompasses all agency activities related to developing the various health plans for which the [health planning agency] is responsible, including agency recommendations pertaining to the development of related State plans."[2] Health Planning Agencies are themselves responsible for developing or assisting other agencies in developing four types of plans:

1. a long-range five-year plan
2. an annual implementation plan
3. project plans for achieving AIP objectives
4. recommendations to the state on needed health facilities in the region

The first two plans are the primary responsibility of the regional health planning agency. The last two are collaborative efforts of local providers and the state health planning agency.

The plan should be flexible, involve community residents (including consumers, providers, and government officials), and be based on the needs of the community's population. The guidelines (see Appendix 6-A at the end of this chapter) require the agency to deal with the broad range of services, such as health promotion, diagnosis, and treatment, and the settings in which they are offered, e.g., home, mobile, and short-stay. Agencies must also take into account environmental conditions. Within this framework, the capacity of health services to raise the health status of subpopulations whose health status is particularly low must be evaluated. Goals, objectives, and priorities, together with strategies and costs for achieving them, are to be detailed. Finally, specific projects or work plans for implementing the high-priority objectives should be developed in conjunction with providers who have a direct interest in their implementation. Those goals and objectives that relate to changes needed in the region's health facilities are submitted to the state health planning agency for inclusion in its plan. To ensure a commonality among health planning agencies, planning formats should be developed collaboratively among health planning agencies at the state and regional levels.

During the life of PL 89-741, progress in the development of health plans was limited. Part of the problem stemmed from the fact that the agencies did not know what a health plan should encompass. This deficiency was corrected with the passage of PL 93-641 and the development of its planning guidelines. However, not all health planning agencies have adequate staff and a consensus among board members to develop at one stroke what federal guidelines expect of them. In an interesting critique of the organizational development of health planning agencies, Meshenberg sees the systems approach as the ultimate planning model.[3] However, there are two prior stages that must be reached before the sophisticated systems approach becomes feasible. There is first the incremental stage, where the emphasis is on organizing the agency to do planning and developing some initial general policy statements. Second, there is the strategic stage. This represents the arrival point where the agency has formulated its plan and priorities, has sufficient resources and a beginning staff of specialists, has some fairly well-developed institutional relationships, and begins to initiate studies and issues with which it is concerned. Thus, Meshenberg perceived these three levels to be a linear development in which a health planning agency has to go through one stage of development before it can attain a higher level. He implied an agency could be fixed at either of the two lower stages.

While it is possible to view the four planning models previously discussed in Chapter 4 on a continuum of development (similar to Meshenberg's three stages) the view taken here is that they are distinct, specific models having unique identifiable characteristics. Because of their differentiated characteristics, each planning model can be viewed as an alternative planning choice, one not being considered superior to the other but more appropriate for its sociopolitical environment.

With respect to plan development, Table 6-1 indicates levels of development a health plan can take under the various planning models. In the systems model, a fully developed health plan can be achieved using the systems, goal-oriented approach espoused by Palmer[4] and PL 93-641. In this approach, goals are clearly articulated, objectives and their indicators are identified, and a work plan with costs and timetables is fully developed for implementation. In this model, the centralization of power in the

Table 6-1 Plan Development by Planning Model

Planning Model	Plan Development and Implementation
Systems	Systems, goal-oriented plan with specific objectives and detail. Implementation highly possible.
Partnership	General plan and policy statement and goals, no detailed plan with objectives and priorities. Implementation problematic. Agency takes some initiative.
Alliance	Partial plan based on self-interest parts of agency, not related to general plan with goals. Emphasis on process of planning, not the substance. Implementation takes place when special interests desire it. Agency reacts to demands of outside bodies.
Individual action	No plan, process-oriented, emphasis on status quo except in crisis. Reacts to external initiative. Not advocate for implementing anything.

planning agency permits such planning and implementation to take place.

More of the recently developed health plans are approaching the degree of specificity, comprehensiveness and identification of system linkages called for by the systems planning model. Failure to meet these criteria in the past usually resulted from the difficulty of the board members in reaching a consensus on an issue; lack of available data, methodology, or standards; or limited resources. However, an impressive beginning has now been made to develop feasible health systems plans for the regions and states.

The Acute Care Section of the Nassau-Suffolk (located in Long Island, New York) health plan for 1978 illustrates the progress that has been made. This section deals with the scope of the issues, the resources available, a needs assessment, and a statement of goals/objectives and long-range actions. The resource discussion is concerned with general care services, including medical/surgical, pediatric and maternity services, and specialized services such as renal dialysis, burn care, computerized axial tomography (CAT) scanners, and ambulatory same day surgery. Based on its needs assessment of its medical/surgical beds, the agency set a goal to reduce the number of acute care beds between 25 and 246 for Nassau County and between 221 and 397 for Suffolk County by 1982. Its recommended actions generally state how this should be achieved. The plan calls for an 85 percent occupancy rate, an average length of stay of nine days, and an admission rate of 125/1,000 population. A second acute care goal calls for approved chronic renal dialysis programs to have a minimum of six machines that are used for at least 12 procedures a week. Other plan goals, which are not amenable to quantifiable statements, include defining and categorizing levels of care for burn care services and seeking the establishment of a consortium to maximize use of existing CAT scanners. In the partnership model, only very general plans with broad policy statements and goals that can be agreed to by all interests within the board are formulated. While implementation is possible, the lack of specific objectives and priorities usually makes it difficult for an agency to know what to advocate for implementation unless a crisis forces a stand on an issue and the development of ways to solve a health problem. Most agency goal statements are of the type that acknowledge vague health care provisions, such as supporting ambulatory health care closer to areas of need or supporting a system of health care payments, without specifying what is meant. It is difficult to quarrel with these types of broad general goals because they are subject to individual interpretation from supporters of the status quo to advocates of utopian changes. More often, such statements serve the status quo while seeming to favor change.

While all health plans have such generalized policy statements of goals, the development of new methodologies, the availability of additional data, and the analysis of those data to show areas of need, have made it possible to reach a political consensus more readily in order to adopt more specific, quantifiable statements of goals. Goals related to home health, health education, and health promotion are usually described in qualitative statements because neither the data base nor the methodology to determine needs or standards has as yet been developed.

The alliance and individual action planning models are at the same stage of plan development. Both are preoccupied with formal organization or interorganizational relationships and the need to cultivate a cooperative and harmonious atmosphere. With the emphasis on the maintenance of good agency relationships, actual planning receives token consideration. Ad hoc bits of arbitrary planning take place without regard for the total or comprehensive view. Such total planning would be too threatening to one or more of the participants involved in the agency. Seldom are health planning agencies based on this type of planning model, as advocates of specific changes, for implementation would mean supporting some additional power for one agency at the expense of another, which risks the sought after balance and harmony.

The corporate model would focus more on studies and issues concerned with some special interest within the agency, while the participant model would respond more to external pressures. This difference between the two models is exemplified by a statement made by an agency executive,

". . . we get requests from county legislators that we damn well better honor."[5] The individual action planning model would place less emphasis on studies and more on relationships.

Plan Implementation/Review Activities

The health planning agency has responsibility for at least the review and approval or disapproval of requests for federally funded health programs; the review of proposals for new institutional services, more commonly referred to as certificate-of-need requests; and the periodic review of existing health care services to ascertain their appropriateness. These reviews are made to ensure the proper development of the health system. Decisions made in the reviews should be consistent with the goals and priorities of the regional and state health plans.

The procedures by which the reviews are made and the substantive criteria by which the need for a health service is assessed must conform to certain standards designed to ensure that health planning agencies' reviews are fair and consistent. Review procedures include such factors as limiting the period of the review to 90 days, informing the applicant when the review has officially started, keeping the applicant informed of the progress of the review, and permitting public debate and hearings about the proposal and/or the decision rendered. Criteria require the evaluation of such elements as whether a need exists and for whom, the availability of personnel to carry out the service, and the existence of alternative and equally effective services as those proposed by the applicant. (See Section 1532 (b) and (c) of PL 93-641 for a complete list of the minimum procedures required and criteria that must be considered by health planning agencies.)

Health planning agencies are responsible for reviewing some 35 federally funded programs. A list of some of these shows the wide range of review responsibilities that planning agencies have: Migrant Health Programs, National Health Service Corps, family planning projects, community mental health centers, communicable disease control programs, and state public health and mental health services plans.

This function has been one of the major activities of health planning agencies since the passage of Section 1122 of the Social Security Act gave them the task of reviewing and commenting on the feasibility of any health facility addition, renovation, or service that cost $100,000 or more. Initially, the main difficulty in carrying out this function was the health planning agencies' lack of guidelines, standards, or an approved plan against which to evaluate proposals. Therefore, decisions were usually made on a subjective basis, with consideration given to duplication, the provider's capacity to carry out the project, the provider's fiscal ability to operate the program, and its effect on the quality of care and the health needs of the population. The few studies of review decisions have shown health planning agencies tended to approve 90 percent or more of the proposals.

The arbitrariness with which decisions were made has been reduced with the passage of PL 93-641, the development of standard procedures and criteria, and the completion of approved health plans. Further, the adoption of national guidelines and promulgation of standards on ratio of acute care beds to the general population, pediatric and obstetric services, use of CAT scanners, and renal dialysis specialized services have given the agencies a more specific set of benchmarks against which to measure the need for health services in their regions. Nonetheless, as noted in the discussion of the plan development function, none of the plans are so fully developed that a planning agency's review committee can make decisions solely on technical grounds. Thus, it can be expected that review decisions will be based on a blend of human and technical considerations. For example, few health plans specifically indicate which populations and subareas of a region may need a health maintenance organization (HMO), a community mental health center, or more home health services. When such services are proposed, seldom can a review committee approve or disapprove based on the true needs of a segment of the population. Rather, such proposals are usually approved because a need for such services has been demonstrated for the region as a whole, even though approval on this basis sometimes results in a maldistribution of services. Progress has been made to reduce bias in review decisions, but bias will not be totally removed even if health plans become more detailed, specific, comprehensive, and quantifiable.

Table 6-2 shows how the four planning models are differentiated in performing the review function. The criteria used are how decisions are made, the degree of technical input in the evaluation of programs and services, and the nature of external influence upon the decisions.

The importance of the approved plan is the key factor in determining which proposals are accepted by the systems planning agency. Where ambiguity exists in how the plan relates to the proposal, the agency relies on the technical specialists to determine what secondary effects the proposal will have on the efficiency, effectiveness, and cost factors of the health plan desired for the area. For example, planners will have to determine what impact a drug prevention program or a special heart disease clinic will have on the areawide family care clinic it plans to establish in which general services related to these two conditions will be provided. Will the new proposals dissipate the use of the center for these two services

Table 6-2 Review Function by Type of Planning Model

Planning Model	Review Function
Systems	Approved plan, policy statements, and accepted standards are determining factors in deciding whether to approve or to reject a proposal or facility.
	Heavy reliance is placed on technical inputs by an agency planning specialist with some assistance from the committee.
	Influence of external actors is generally minimized.
Partnership	Policy statements and values held by staff and committee determine how decisions are made.
	While some technical inputs are made, major emphasis is on judgments of staff generalists and lay citizens.
	Influence of external actors is an important factor.
Alliance	Decisions are made on the basis of trade-offs and consensus, if possible, of internal and external actors involved. Staff plays a small role in the absence of a planning document or policy guidelines.
	Only general technical inputs are needed and are probably ignored except to ensure that the process of agency research and development standards are carried out.
	Staff inputs are generally of a routine nature.
	Influence of external actors is very strong.
Individual action	Decision is based on arbitrary influence of external actors on agency staff and/or committee members to accept their proposal. Consensus is not essential. No plan or policy is available to guide the decision. Board approval is perfunctory or not sought.
	Technical inputs are made by external actors seeking approval of a proposal. Staff steers proposal through agency process on a routine basis.
	External influence is the major force in getting a proposal approved. Approval is automatic unless very strong opposition develops.

or will they provide essential specialized backup services? Technical analysis of the costs involved for the programs, how many patients the center can and will serve, the categories of patients it plans to serve, and accessibility to the services, both in terms of eligibility and transportation, are significant factors that will require evaluation before a decision is made. These technical factors and the plan priorities and objectives rather than the external influence of actors proposing the new programs are the guiding factors in the decision process.

In the partnership model, general policy statements replace the specific statements of the plan document as an influencing factor. However, since these policies are too general and probably too ambiguous, the subjective value judgment of staff and committee members and external inputs of the proposal's initiators are accorded a more important role. Technical inputs are made by staff who are generalists rather than specialists in the area under study. Consequently, they will not be too technical and will provide justification for the proposal's acceptance or rejection based on the wishes of the committee. For example, a general policy of an agency indicates that 4 beds per 1,000 population is an adequate standard to meet the needs of the general public. The proposal of a hospital to expand by 100 beds will bring the 3.9 beds the area has to the 4 standard desired. On this general policy basis, the hospital proposal meets the agency guidelines. However, the influence of the hospital director on the agency board and in-kind data analysis and computer services it offers are influential factors in determining the proposal's acceptance even though the expansion of a second hospital in an area of unmet needs would have been preferable.

Without policy guidelines or standards, the alliance and individual action models rely heavily on the dominant values of the group. The staff's major input is to ensure that the process of the review is carried out according to these values. They serve as expediters for the decision makers evaluating the proposals. Consensus and bargaining are the modus operandi of the alliance planning model, whereas the individual action planning model, with its lack of staff cohesion and its fragmented character, cannot risk seeking consensus on every proposal. The staff in the individual action model usually rubber-stamps all proposals, or they may be passed along without official board action. The staff's role in these two planning models is minimal, except to ensure that the process is carried out.

Plan Implementation/Health Systems Development

Those activities in which the health planning agency seeks the assistance and support of others in implementing its high-priority goals and objectives are part of the plan implementation/health systems development function.

This support may involve individuals, public and private agencies, and providers. In carrying out this function, the health planning agency may offer technical assistance and consultation to obtain another agency's cooperation. For example, it may assist a provider institution in preparing a proposal to start a new health service called for in the health plan, or it may recommend consultants who can assist the provider in evaluating present services with an eye to making them more efficient. When area health services development funds are made available to health planning agencies they will be in a position to offer seed funds to provider institutions to initiate new services consistent with the regional or state health plan.

Health planning agencies can also promote development of their regional health system by taking stands on key health issues. In recent years, planning agencies have pressed for greater availability of ambulatory services, especially HMOs, for underserved areas; for greater financial assistance to public hospitals serving the poor; and for a reduction in the use of high-cost specialized medical services except when need can be clearly shown. It is not clear how much influence a health planning agency can have on public issues, however. Roseman questions whether planning agencies can become seriously involved in public issues because they are a "meeting ground for these interests, but cannot shape an independent policy to which other agencies must conform."[6] The interests to which he refers are established agencies, such as hospital councils and the American Medical Association (AMA). This is especially true where planning that is not consistent with current medical practice cannot be undertaken. Most basic issues must raise questions about those practices, i.e., whether to approve or disapprove of them. Yet, Gustafson and Chewning found that health planning agencies spent more time on "crisis intervention" than on long-range or preventive planning.[7] Crisis intervention often calls for public involvement by the agencies either to take a position on the crisis or to act as mediators. Table 6-3 shows how the planning models differ on this function.

The differences with respect to public issue involvement are dependent upon whether the agencies get involved, and if so, how they get involved. Do they take the initiative, or do they respond to public outbursts? Is their position an outgrowth of their planning and policy studies, or is it based upon arbitrary self-interest? Are their positions founded upon technical knowledge or upon value judgments? Are the agencies willing to involve themselves in issues of a controversial nature?

Most agencies have been involved in public issues. It is one of their responsibilities. The question of how they become involved is more important. With respect to taking the initiative, only the systems model planning

Table 6-3   Plan Implementation Function: Public Issue Involvement by Type of Planning Model

Planning Model	Public Issue Involvement
Systems	Agencies get strongly involved, using their plan documents as the basis for taking positions.
	There is strong use of technical knowledge to support their positions.
	They are not overly concerned with public opinion or conflict about their positions.
	They initiate public issue statements; seldom take mediator roles.
Partnership	Agencies become ambivalently involved. Too dependent on other constituencies for support.
	If policy exists, it Is used to support their positions on issues.
	More reliance is placed on agency's values than on data to support a position, provided consensus on issue exists in agency.
	They are concerned with public opinion.
	They tend to mediate issues and set out alternatives without taking a stand if division exists in agency.
Alliance	Agencies become involved over ad hoc issues on which one part of agency (staff or committee) has a special interest and point of view.
	Their positions are not based on plans or policy.
	They are not concerned with general public opinion, but with special interest groups; ambivalent about promoting change in a conflict situation.
	They tend to respond to issues raised publicly by others except when trying to promote their own.
Individual action	Same as for first two points under alliance model.
	They promote social change through issues except with actors in their constituency. Not generally affected by public opinion.
	They promote issues quietly, defend them if others make them public issues.

agencies would have little hesitation in promoting a public issue. This is a logical outgrowth of their already having developed a planning document that has received public acceptance. This gives them the sanction for involving the public on those issues that promote the implementation of those aspects of the plan that demand attention. For example, a plan that calls for the closing of an outdated hospital in one geographical area and building one in another calls for periodic public attention by the agency to educate the public and promote its point of view, even in the face of conflict. To a more limited extent, the partnership model would use what general policy guidelines it has developed to support or defend a position, but would be less apt to take the initiative because its constituency is less strongly committed to the central mission of the agency. Many of its members must satisfy their own constituencies, whose point of view may or may not be similar to that of the agency. Roseman perceives the pluralistic nature of the forces that make up the health care field as contributing to the ambivalence of taking the initiative on public issues and thereby risking conflict and possible loss of support.

On the other hand, the alliance and individual action planning models have no plan documents or policy guidelines for determining whether they should be involved in public issues. Rather, they have their own special interests to promote, which have been adopted arbitrarily by some special collection of actors, either in the committee structure or among the staff. Both types would prefer to promote their special interests quietly, but are ready to promote or defend them if attacked and raised to the level of a public issue. For example, a few members of the committee and its staff members may be in favor of a drug prevention program for a certain geographical area that does not really need it. However, research-oriented hospitals desire this program in order to study factors that promote family stability. The external influence of hospital officials and the special interests of the committee collectively carry the program proposal through the approval circuit of the health planning agency. A small, militant body of health advocates from a low-income area that has a great need for such a program learns of the proposal and begins to escalate it into a public issue. The agency committee and staff can decide to promote and defend it, as the hospital desires to do despite public controversy, or to table the proposal temporarily rather than entangle the fragile structure of the agency board in a controversy for which there may be no consensus. If the committee, staff, and hospital officials were strongly supportive of the program, they would continue to defend it in the face of this opposition; they would represent a coalitional force that has a strong commitment to the proposal. If the committee was divided, the hospital officials would most likely apply pressure on the committee members favorable to its position while the committee as a whole would remain passive. This would be an example of the individual action model of planning at work within the structure of the agency. Unlike the systems and partnership models of planning, the alliance and individual action models would be guided more by their own self-interests and their arbitrary selection of issues to promote or defend.

The nature of the support for the agency position would also vary according to the planning model. The systems model would support its public position with technical, documented evidence and with authority of professionalism and expertise. These are the types of support that public interest corporations like Rand Institute, A. D. Little, or Greenleigh Associates, all consulting firms, might develop. While it is thought that the technical data influence the position the agency has taken, it is sometimes hard to distinguish whether or not the data were biased in order to support a previously held position of the agency. The partnership model of planning would tend to rely on logic and rationality to support its position, rather than on technical data. Many of the agency studies are of this type.

The alliance and individual action models would mobilize what data they could to strengthen their positions and would continue to rely on their value judgments, capitalizing on the authority and expertise the public believes is inherent in the agency.

The systems and individual action models would not hesitate to become involved in controversial issues, since both have positions to promote and little to lose in terms of constituency support. The systems model relies on the plan document for its sanction, while the individual action model relies on the homogeneity of its group's interest. On the other hand, both the partnership and alliance planning models have more tenuous constituencies, those not fully committed to the goals of the agency, as Warren notes in his paradigm.[8] If there is strong consensus on a particular issue by the members of either of these two types of planning models, then it is more likely they will support a public position in the face of controversy. If not, then they will either retreat to a mediator role, more likely in the partnership model, or to a neutral role, more likely in the alliance model. Their constituency composition is too fragile in most controversial issues to risk losing the greater benefits that the agencies derive by keeping the constituency intact.

It appears that there is a similarity in the potential behavior of the systems and individual action planning models, even though the systems model gets its backing from a previously approved public plan, while the individual action model gets its support from a like-minded self-interest group. This group may be located within the agency, such as in a committee or executive body, or it may be a pressure group outside the agency that, nevertheless, exerts great influence. The partnership and alliance models, in contrast, have weaker constituency support and are, therefore, more vulnerable to internal disunity and hostility that can paralyze the agency because of stands taken on public issues. Consequently, it is usually safer to do nothing or to take a moderator role. In other words, the organizational structure, the constituency, and the values its members hold are the crucial factors in determining the extent to which an agency gets involved in public issues.

Public Involvement and Education

"The public involvement and education function encompasses all agency activities related to developing and maintaining informed and effective public involvement and participation in the plan development and plan implementation programs" of the health planning agency.[9] This involves giving information to area residents and health care provider institutions, opening all agency records for public inspection and copying, encouraging comments from area residents on agency operations, and increasing area residents' knowledge of personal health care and appropriate use of the health system. In these ways, the public is kept informed of the planning agency's operation, its policy positions, its decisions on review proposals, and other agency matters. In opening its records to the public the health planning agency is also ensuring the broadest possible involvement of the public in the development and implementation of its health plans. Because of the open dialogue among consumers and providers, the views of selected interest groups are held up to public scrutiny. Furthermore, decisions made on controversial issues are more likely to acquire a supporting constituency to withstand internal or external opposition. More important, the development of this constituency permits the health planning agency to take stands on controversial issues that have already been aired and decided upon within its organizational structure.

With respect to the four planning models, the systems model would encourage the greatest public involvement in agency operations, particularly in decision making on policy and goal issues. By encouraging a discussion of conflicting views within the health planning agency, the agency can feel comfortable in promoting its policies and goals once decisions are made. Therefore, the systems model planning agency can be expected to make the most extensive use of newsletters, television, and radio to inform the public of its activities, positions, and approved decisions. At the same time, it would develop specialized material to meet the needs of individual groups for information and introduce it through conferences, meetings of various interest groups, and training sessions. All of these strategies would be used to obtain public involvement and support of agency policy, goals, and priorities.

In the partnership model, public information would take a more diluted form. Concerned about the fragile relationships among the constituencies that comprise its governing body, the partnership model of a health planning agency would be more likely to offer information to those established groups that have a general understanding and acceptance of the broad policies of the agency. The agency would provide general information to the public on changes that have already occurred in federal and state legislation, policy, grants awarded, and high level staff assignments. It would not provide information on conflicts that have not already been resolved within the agency's governing body. Finally, on those personal health practices that have been endorsed by established medical and public health groups, the agency would provide information to interested groups. Since the agency is mainly concerned about maintaining the tenuous balance among the disparate groups represented on its board, it would disseminate information only on those matters that have been settled and only to those external groups that are not a threat to its structure or policies.

Since the constituency of an alliance model of health planning is concerned generally with a few policy issues at any one time and has an active interest in achieving specific resolutions of those issues, this model agency would normally provide information and access mainly to those public interest groups that have expressed support of the agency's positions on these issues. The agency would resist providing information to those opposed to its point of view. It has little interest in promoting personal health education unless this happens to be one of the vital concerns of the agency.

As the most highly partisan of the planning models, an individual action health planning agency would oppose revealing its agency activities or providing information to any except the most enthusiastic supporters of its views. The public would have to threaten or litigate under the Freedom of Information Act to obtain information. Public involvement in its activities or promotion of its policies would be limited to those groups that strongly support them. Unless the agency were promoting a goal of improving personal health education, it would not take any initiative in this direction.

Table 6-4 summarizes the positions that would be taken by the four models of planning.

Table 6-4   Public Involvement and Education Function by Type of
Planning Model

Planning Model	Public Involvement and Education
Systems	Encourages involvement and openness of activities to general public. Provides information to public through newsletters, radio announcements, and television. Offers material to promote beneficial health practices through specially designed conferences, speeches, and discussions at meetings.
Partnership	Limits open communication to already established agency policies and plans. Disseminates general information about federal and state legislation, policy, grants, and staff changes. Limits direct community involvement to established groups whose views are largely consistent with agency's leadership. Concerned about dissident groups whose points of view and tactics may fragment delicate balance of its organizational leadership.
Alliance	Access to agency information limited mainly to those who actively support the agency coalition and the few issues in which the agency is involved at any one time. General public must ask for and fight to obtain information about agency operations except for those groups who support agency goals. General information about personal health care is not offered.
Individual action	No public information provided unless forced to comply under the Freedom of Information Act. Public involvement discouraged unless groups actively support agency positions. No effort to improve personal health care practices unless a goal of agency.

Support Functions

Health planning agencies are responsible for three support functions: agency organization and management, data management and analysis, and coordination. Support functions are necessary to ensure the implementation of the agency's substantive functions.

Agency Organization and Management

"The organization and management function encompasses all agency activities directly related to the organization and governance of the agency, the management of agency resources, and the provision of administrative and logistical support services required to maintain an effective health planning and resources development program."[10] Activities involved in this function include

- setting policy and developing an organizational structure
- developing a work program that allocates staff and other resources to the agency objectives
- managing the agency's resources and evaluating the results
- training and educating agency staff and board members to carry out their responsibilities

One of the real problems in agency management comes from the size of the board and the size of the staff that can be hired to support the work of the board. While PL 93-641 calls for a governing body of no more than 30 members, in fact many of the agency boards have 50 and more members. One agency in Region II has more than 120 members. When boards are so large, they become unwieldy; then the "director works to insure that the members 'neutralize' each other and let staff do the work."[11] This report, an evaluation of boards developed under PL 89-741, states that federal guidelines require full representation and therefore tend to require large boards. On the other hand, the report notes that boards with fewer than 30 members become "working" boards. Congress took this report into account when it included a provision in PL 93-641 that any health planning agency with a governing body larger than 30 members had to have an executive committee of 10 to 30 members. This ensures that all health planning bodies have active working boards. Further, PL 93-641 provides that all health planning agencies have a minimum of five professional staff members, even in regions with small populations, to ensure their capacity to carry out basic agency functions.

To operate efficiently and fairly, health planning agencies should have personnel policies and procedures that deal with hiring, promotion, resignations, vacation and sick leave, grievance procedures, and other factors to guide staff conduct. There should be a consultant policy that details when a consultant should be hired, method of payment, tasks and completion of products, and a method of evaluating the work. There should be a system of financial administration that spells out how the assets, liabilities, revenues, and expenses will be accounted for; accountability for receipt and expenditure of public tax funds; a bookkeeping system; and a means for financial analysis and certification of agency operations. An agency should also develop an annual work program and budget consistent with its goals and objectives, as well as a management reporting system that shows the progress being made in carrying out the annual work program. These should show major tasks, staff resources, and budget costs for each function. Finally, policies related to agency organization, governance, and operation should be developed. These should cover such items as agency bylaws, relationships with the general public, the roles and responsibility of the governing body, and its relationship to its executive committee.

A review of the 1979 work programs of 13 health planning agencies shows they gave their greatest emphasis to the following management matters:

- revise bylaws and operations manual
- monitor the progress of the work program
- train and orient staff and board members
- recruit staff and board members
- explain and adjust programs to new Department of Health and Human Services (HHS) guidelines
- develop and work with subarea councils
- develop financial reports and audits
- prepare grant applications
- improve mailing systems (newsletters, notices, etc.)

These reports reveal a concern on the part of most health planning agencies to improve their management practices and to keep them up-to-date. To do this, they tend to hire consultants to assist with three major aspects of management: legal issues, audit, and data management.

Data Management and Analysis

Health planning agencies are required to collect, maintain, and analyze data to develop a health plan. Types of data routinely collected deal with the health status of the population; the status of the health care delivery system; the utilization of that system by the area residents; and the effects of the system, environmental factors, and occupational hazards on the health of the population. Because data are generally collected from a number of different sources, health planning agencies should first seek to form a collaborative relationship with other agencies to obtain data on a routine basis. New data should be collected by health planning agencies themselves only where data are unavailable and will materially benefit the evaluation of key health issues. To ensure expertise in data management, special staff members should be hired to supervise the data management function.

Most health planning agencies keep extensive data files on such health areas as vital statistics, primary care, patient origin, drug abuse, mental health primary care, health status indicators, long-term care, medical facilities inventory, infant mortality, and home health care. They use their data for three basic purposes: review of certificate-of-need proposals, development and updating of their health plans, and development of special studies. A number of agencies are computerizing their data systems. In addition, many agencies hire full- or part-time librarians who obtain books, monographs, magazines, and a wide variety of reference works; run computer searches; and maintain the library. Furthermore, health planning agencies develop agreements with many institutions to exchange data and provide information requested by the public.

Coordination

Health planning agencies should coordinate their "affairs with other entities whose actions are likely to have a significant influence on their plan development and plan implementation activities."[12] Such entities may include institutions engaged in planning, development, monitoring, or evaluation of health resources. Arrangements should be made with other institutions to share data and information, to provide technical assistance to each other, and to coordinate the agency's plan development and implementation tasks. While special emphasis should be placed on coordination with other organizations that have similar functions and purposes, such as Professional Standards Review Organizations (PSROs), agencies, contiguous health planning agencies, state health planning agencies, and the cooperative Health Statistics System, there should also be coordination with other significant agencies, such as medical societies, hospital associations, county governments, mental health agencies, community development agencies, offices on aging, the End-Stage Renal Dialysis Network, and providers of emergency medical services. To maintain continuing relationships with this long list of institutions is a frustrating, time-consuming, and usually nonproductive function, often resulting in maintenance of the status quo rather than any dramatic improvements in care.

In a study of interorganizational relationships of community decision-making organizations such as welfare departments, boards of education, model cities, urban renewal, and health planning agencies, Warren and his coworkers found that what appears to the uninitiated outsider to be chaotic relationships among major and minor organizations in urban communities is in fact a highly regulated, "remarkably stable, patterned, and systematized environment."[13] They go on to state that "much of the coordination that takes place . . . does so through this very process of mutual adaptation at the margins, in processes involving not only cooperation but also contest. . . ."[14] The only changes that take place are those on the periphery of the organization's major functions. Such community decision-making organizations use strategies of preventing, blunting, and repelling to ensure that no one invades their domain. Consequently, they found that only minimal innovations took place with the creation of model cities programs, although the primary incentive was innovative change for urban ghettos. Such initiatives were abortive because the community organizations were satisfied with the methods being used to serve the target population.

It appears, given this brief background, that the health planning agency position resembles that of model cities programs and is further impeded by fewer resources and less authority. The models most likely to accomplish a nonthreatening relationship with the health-related agencies are the partnership and alliance planning models. Minimal change and survival are their innate characteristics, which accommodate and adapt to the amount of change desired by allied health care agencies. Review and planning functions are the logical means by which both coordination and acceptable incremental changes are brought about. As already indicated, the partnership planning model adopts a broad consensus, enabling the diversified participants to collaborate, while the alliance planning model functions in an ad hoc manner, involving passive and active coalitions. The problem of coordination is difficult under the individual action model because of the powerful effect of external influences on the agency's activities. These activities, often arbitrary, are subject to unpredictable forces that render coordinating relationships ineffectual, unless a policy of mutual support is adopted and accepted by the various board members and agency committees. The systems model of planning assumes the health planning agency has good control of its activities so that coordination with other agencies is not required. Reality, however, does not find an agency of the systems style in existence; no health planning agency has the necessary powers for such a model to function. Perhaps the examples closest to this form of planning can be found in New York's Urban Development Corporation and in Boston's Rehabilitation Agency where planning, implementation, and financing are under the control of one agency, and even these agencies are inhibited in the use of their vast authority. Planning and implementation have been deliberately separated in health planning. To date, the health field has seen implementation without planning and coordination without obligation for change.

GOALS OF HEALTH PLANNING AGENCIES

Blum defines goals as "descriptions of aspirations which represent fruition of the ideals established by values . . . their nature may be spiritual as well as practical. It is for this reason in part that they have to be broken down into more tangible subelements, the objectives."[15] Wagner defines a goal as "a long-range, specified state of accomplishment toward which programs are directed. It does not fix a time for its achievement. It may be as idealistic or ambitious as good judgment dictates, but it must be consistent with the mission" of the health agency.[16] Federal guidelines define goals as "statements of desired levels of health status, desired performance of the health system, or desired levels of resources."[17]

All three definitions are future-oriented; they represent ideal states considered necessary for positive health that the society would like to attain. They are also value judgments that the society confirms through its many devices and mechanisms, such as government, legislation, public forums, and mass media. The emphasis may be on body weight or height, ability to induce physical labor, or mental stress. It may be a serenity of mind and body. Whatever the qualities emphasized, these become the values society strives to achieve.

Congress has awarded high value to longevity of life and prevention of illness and disability resulting from such major killers as heart disease, stroke, and cancer. Likewise, it has become cost conscious and places a high value on efficiency in the use of scarce health care resources by emphasizing rational planning through the development of health planning agencies and by screening health facilities' proposals to ensure real need. Such goals generally lack specificity and cannot be measured directly. It is not possible to measure a goal that states people should live a long, useful, and healthy life. Terms "long," "useful," and "healthy" require definition. Is "long" 40 years? 50 years? 100 years? Goals are descriptions of desired end results upon which society has agreed. Thus goals are ends rather than means to those ends. Positive health, long life, robustness of health, freedom from disability are various statements of end states that society hopes to achieve. Thus, goals are indeterminate, represent society's values with respect to health, are too general to be directly measured, and are the end health states society hopes to achieve. Nonetheless, federal guidelines exhort health planning agencies to state their goals wherever possible in quantifiable terms and, if necessary, as a range of minimum and maximum levels of achievement.

Further, goals should be selected based on an examination of

- the concerns of the community
- the present and projected health status
- the needs of the area's population
- the effects of health services delivered
- the National Guidelines for Health Planning and National Priorities
- a study of feasible alternatives[18]

National Priorities and Standards

Unlike PL 89-749, which stated its goal in general terms, PL 93-641 identifies specific national health priorities that focus on measures to produce a more efficient and therefore less costly health system. It encourages the use of multiinstitutional systems, medical group practices, HMOs, and lower cost physician's assistants, as well as a regionalized, integrated health system. It also advocates improving primary care for medically underserved populations, increasing the population's knowledge of personal health care and use of health care services, and preventing disease caused by nutritional or environmental factors. Amendments to PL 93-641 further reenforce the efficiency concerns of Congress by calling for a reduction in the duplication of services, adoption of policies to contain rising health care costs, and competition in the health system. They also focus on improving the care of the mentally ill, especially by providing outpatient community-based mental health services. Obviously, the priorities expressed in PL 93-641 represent a major advance in specifying the health care priorities of the nation.

Congress and the executive branch have gone even further in this specification by setting forth regulations identifying standards of medical care and utilization that health planning agencies are expected to follow in developing their own goals.[19] These are referred to as the National Guidelines for Health Planning. (See Appendix 6-B for a summary of these standards.) These guidelines provide standards on desirable bed/population ratios, occupancy rates and minimum number of births required in an obstetric unit, number of open heart surgery procedures required to justify such a unit, as well as the minimum number of treatments or procedures for cardiac catheterization, radiation treatment, CAT scanners, and end-stage renal dialysis. The standards permit variations based on age of population, geographical area (rural, urban), season (summer/winter resort areas), and levels of treatment. These standards must be taken into account by health planning agencies when they develop their own goals. It can be readily seen that these standards refer primarily to acute care services and the high-cost specialized services offered by short-stay hospitals.

Issues in Standards Development

Development of the National Guidelines was extensive, as shown by Exhibit 6-1. Three volumes of policy papers, numerous meetings with important health groups, and comments on many preliminary drafts by the public at large all slowed the process. From an initial decision to publish 24 goal statements on infant mortality, communicable disease, health education, and health care costs, the Department of Health, Education and Welfare (HEW) decided to limit the first regulations on guidelines to the standards noted previously. The initial response to this publication was some 55,000 comments, mostly from three states with predominantly rural populations who feared the loss of their small community hospitals if the standards on hospital beds and occupancy rates were allowed to become national policy. As a result of this reaction, the proposed guidelines were made more flexible to meet the varying needs of rural and urban populations. The standards were published in their final form as regulations on March 28, 1978, almost three years after the initial formation of a task force to consider them.

Exhibit 6-1 Chronology of Initial Administrative Actions

April 1975	Establishment of Intra-Departmental Committee on Public Law 93-641
May 1975	Establishment of Task Force on the National Guidelines
June 1975	Publication of Notice in the Federal Register
June 1975	Issuance of contracts regarding potential criteria and standards
July 1975	Communications to professional and public organizations and local and State agencies
July 1975	Commissioning of first issue papers
Summer 1975	Three meetings at the Harvard School of Public Health
November 1975	Followup communications to professional and public organizations and local and State agencies
December 1975	Meeting of the first members of the National Council on Health Planning and Development
January 1976	Conference with WHO consultants on health goals and standards
January 1976	Meeting in San Francisco sponsored by University of California School of Public Health
July 1976	Distribution of initial draft of potential guidelines
July 1976	Workshops at American Association of Comprehensive Health Planning meeting in Miami
September 1976	Publication of first volume of "Papers on the National Health Guidelines"
October 1976	Distribution of revised draft of potential guidelines
Fall 1976	National Health Policy Issues Forum, DHEW Region IX
Winter 1976	Local and regional meetings on the draft National Guidelines
January 1977	Publication of second volume of "Papers on the National Health Guidelines"
Spring 1977	Local and regional meetings on the draft National Guidelines
July 1977	Health Resources Administration conference on financial and economic indicators

Exhibit 6-1 Continued

September 1977	Publication of third volume of "Papers on the National Health Guidelines"
September 1977	Publication of notice of proposed rulemaking on initial issuance of the National Guidelines in the Federal Register
September 1977	First full meeting of National Council on Health Planning and Development
November 1977	Five public meetings on the proposed guidelines
December 1977	Meetings of the National Council on Health Planning and Development to make recommendations on proposed guidelines
January 1978	Publication of revised proposal on the initial issuance of the National Guidelines in the Federal Register
March 1978	Publication of final rules on initial issuance of the National Guidelines in the Federal Register
April 1978	Publication of fourth volume of "Papers on the National Health Guidelines"

Source: Daniel I. Zwick, *Initial Development of National Guidelines for Health Planning,* Public Health Reports, Vol. 93, No. 5 (Hyattsville, Md.: HHS, 1978), p. 409.

In April 1980, HHS published draft National Health Planning Goals.[20] These draft goals were produced by the same effort that resulted in the National Guidelines. Because of the experience gained with the guidelines, as well as the increase in knowledge over the intervening three years, the final goal statements are expected to be published in a much shorter time. However, when first published in October, 1979, the comments revealed several issues that would have to be dealt with in revisions as well as in all future guidelines and goal statements. It was clear, for example, that the goals should include those stated in the Surgeon General's report, *Healthy People.* In this document, five goals were proposed for each of five age cohorts, the newborn to the elderly, to be achieved by 1990; health promotion, health protection, and disease prevention were stressed.[21] A second issue involved the special needs of rural areas, including the inadequate medical services available, the lower health status of rural residents, their poverty and inadequate insurance coverage, and the long distances they must travel to obtain medical care. The national goals should be flexible in order to make allowances for the special circumstances of rural populations.

A third issue focused on the level of specificity of the national goals. PL 93-641 requires that all goals be stated in measurable terms where appropriate. Most of the health status goals in the draft national goals were quantified, but only a few of the health promotion and health systems goals were. One group argued that national goals must be viewed as "expressions of desirable aspirations for improving both health status and health care";[22] another group, composed largely of health planning agency officials, felt the need for this quantifiable guidance in the development of their own goals. It was concluded that the tensions generated by efforts to state measurable goals and the diversity of the various regions make it politically inadvisable to state all goals in quantifiable terms. However, health planning agencies were urged to do this, if possible.

A final issue concerned financing the proposed goals. It was pointed out that most of the goals relating to health promotion and education could not be funded under the current reimbursement systems. While acknowledging this, HHS advises health planning agencies to use their influence and ingenuity in advocating changes in the financing system and finding alternate ways of implementing these goals where possible until the present reimbursement systems are changed.

As for the goals themselves, Appendix 6-C provides a summary of the proposed goals. Goals were selected on the basis of six criteria:

1. relevance to the mission of PL 93-641
2. relevance to an important issue
3. consistency with existing federal law or regulations
4. strong possibility of achievement
5. usefulness to health planning agencies
6. timeliness as a national policy statement[23]

An examination of a few goals reveals the nature of national goals being seriously considered:[24]

• Health Status Goals

Reducing the infant mortality rate to less than 11 deaths per 1,000 live births by 1985 and to less than 9 deaths per 1,000 live births by 1990.

The health of adults should be improved and death rates for those aged 25–64 reduced to less than 472 per 100,000 by 1985 and to less than 400 per 100,000 by 1990.

Age-adjusted death rates for heart disease should be reduced to 156 per 100,000 persons and for stroke to 29 per 100,000 persons by 1985. Efforts should be directed toward improvements in survival rates through detection and treatment for all types of cancer.

- Disease Prevention and Health Promotion

  Programs should be undertaken to prevent accidents in the home, during recreation, at work, and on the highway. Particular efforts should be made to reduce accidents involving children.

  People should be informed about what constitutes good nutrition and should be encouraged and aided in obtaining a proper diet.

- Service Delivery

  To the extent that shortages or excesses of primary care personnel or medical specialties exist and are documented, these imbalances should be corrected.

  The integration of mental health services in general health care delivery programs should be increased through in-service mental health training of primary care providers and placement of mental health professionals in primary care programs.

  Providers of health services should be organized into regionalized networks which assure that various types and levels of services are linked together to form comprehensive and efficient systems of care. These networks should work to improve access to health services, eliminate unnecessary duplication of services, and improve quality.

Objectives

If goals represent the general direction in which a society wishes to go, the ways to get there offer the various alternatives. These alternative routes to the stated goals can be called objectives. Wagner's definition of objective "is stated in terms of achieving a measured amount of progress toward a goal, or maintaining a certain measured level of health required by a goal, during a specified interval of time."[25] In different language, but with a similar orientation, Blum calls objectives "the tangible subdivisions of goals toward which specific programs are aimed."[26]

Both of these definitions have in common the characteristics of short-term range, specificity of detail, and measurability. Whereas goals have an indeterminate time orientation and are never fully achieved, objectives have shorter time spans. One thinks in terms of accomplishing an objective in a stated determined period of time, such as one year, 18 months, etc. The objective also states what is to be achieved. To improve on the longevity of a population, alternative objectives to this general goal might be reducing the incidence of the main killers of people, such as heart disease, stroke, and cancer; stressing how people can live a more well-rounded and tension-reduced life; showing people how to prevent through proper diet the occurrence of physiologically induced conditions thought to lead to the development of these diseases; or possibly changing the societal stress on competitiveness as a way of achieving success to one of societal cooperation and helpfulness. It becomes the responsibility of society's decision makers to determine which alternatives to choose or value judgments to make. Some of the alternatives are negative in their approach, such as reducing the conditions that cause high mortality whether through diet or elimination of environmental health hazards. Some are stated in positive terms, such as stressing a more tranquil life style or encouraging the population to lead well-rounded lives that give equal consideration to physical and mental health. Perhaps both approaches are required simultaneously.

Objectives should usually be stated in terms that permit measurement. With respect to the longevity goal, a negative objective might be stated in terms of reducing the number of deaths due to heart disease, stroke, and cancer from 630 per 100,000 population to 500 per 100,000 population by five years from now. If analysis concludes that the take-off point for a rapid increase of deaths due to these conditions is in the 45 to 64 age bracket, then the emphasis would be more specifically defined by age. Likewise, further analysis may indicate that some diseases are more prevalent for one racial group than another, or even that residents of certain geographical areas may be more prone to a certain disease than others. Thus, a combination of value orientation and technical analysis may be able to define ways in which to direct health resources that would reduce causes of disease and thereby increase longevity. With respect to positive objectives, one might be stated in terms of increasing the percentage of children who conform to a certain physical standard with respect to height and weight from 60 percent as currently measured to 80 percent two years from now. Analysis of data may reveal by age categories, geographic location, or ethnicity on which populations to focus.

There may be valid objectives that cannot be measured in a numerical manner. Change in societal mores from competition to cooperation is one such objective that would lead to greater longevity. This may require analytic description and identification of the characteristics of competition and cooperation to determine whether such a shift is taking place. Difficult-to-measure changes such as student emphasis on helping each other or participating in self-help programs rather than competing for grades or athletic awards, or people accepting jobs based on personal satisfaction rather than financial reward are illustrations of changes that would give clues to any shifts taking place in societal norms. While there may be ways to measure such changes, they may well obfuscate what is occurring rather than indicate the trends, and they may offer little or no guidance as to why the changes are occurring.

Actions

Once the objectives are stated, it becomes necessary to outline what specific actions are required to achieve them. It becomes necessary to specify what will be done and by whom, under what circumstances, and in what amounts. These actions are the instruments or means to the ends— the objectives. They are concrete, geographically specific, time-bound, and measurable. In the classic experiment, they are the interventions at time one that test an hypothesis of what is expected to happen at time two. Unlike the inanimate objects of physics and chemistry, which can be tightly controlled, the program interventions used to reach health objectives have people as their subject. It is almost impossible to control all the variables because people are free agents to move and decide for themselves, change their status from unemployed to employed, single to married, residence in one city to another, etc. These factors make it very difficult to measure true change, but within limits change can be crudely measured to determine whether program intervention makes a difference.

As with objectives, there may be many program alternatives that are possible to achieve a single objective. To achieve a reduction in the incidence of heart disease, stroke, and cancer among the 45- to 64-year-olds in urban areas on the East Coast of the United States, an education program aimed at cutting down smoking, a health education program in high schools about these diseases, the guaranteeing of higher education opportunities for the urban poor and working class, or a law requiring annual physical and mental checkups to spot incipient symptoms of these diseases are all possible alternatives. Predictions of the effect each of these alternatives may have on reducing the incidence of the diseases may be made, and selection of the alternative action with the most profound impact can ultimately affect longevity.

When these three aspects of planning are taken together, they are hierarchically linked from the most general to the most specific statement of health. The general is society's symbolic or ideational representation of what it considers important in health matters; the actions are the manifestations of these symbols. Objectives are the intermediary link between the two. Figure 6-1 depicts this linkage.

Figure 6-1 Goal-Objective-Action Relationships

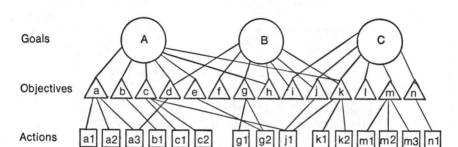

Goals A and B can be partially achieved by five objectives and goal C by four. A few of the objectives in turn can help to achieve more than one goal. Objective "d" is linked to goals A and B while objective "k" is linked to all three goals. Whether it is the most effective objective to achieve any one of the goals or all three is a matter of technical analysis and value judgments by experts and decision makers. More does not mean better or more effective. In turn, the objectives have their own action alternatives. Objectives "a" and "m" each have three action alternatives, while "e," "f," and "h" have no actions identified that will help achieve them. Thus, three major goals expand to 14 objectives and 15 action alternatives. Which to choose and what criteria to use to determine choices become planning decisions requiring the collaboration of planners and decision makers in the health field. This shows how complicated the achievement of a simply stated goal becomes and offers a clue to the reason that health planners and specialists are needed to work with lay decision makers.

Illustration of Goals, Objectives, and Actions

The acute care component from a regional long-range health plan can be used to illustrate the relationships among goals, objectives, and alternative actions. The table of contents (Exhibit 6-2) shows that this plan is divided into four major sections and has 22 health care components. Acute care services are part of Section IV, Health Systems Services, and the subsection dealing with diagnosis and treatment services. It can be readily discerned that this is both a very comprehensive and complex health plan. The first long-range goal of the acute care component states:

> To reduce the excess number of acute hospital beds to a zero level while assuring the required supply of beds, based on current

Exhibit 6-2   1980–1984 Health Systems Plan: Table of Contents

Exhibit 6.2 Continued

and forecasted demographic utilization and related indicators while maintaining a regional bed ratio of no more than 3.3 beds per 1,000 population.

The objectives designed to meet this goal are:

Objective 1:   By 1984, the number of excess beds should be reduced by 50% (current excess range: 368–516 beds).

      Alternative Action 1:   Certificates of need for medical/surgical beds in areas of excess should not be approved.

      Action 2:   The health planning agency and the area hospitals should investigate alternative ways to reduce excess medical/surgical capacity.

      Action 3:   Final plans for the future use of RV Hospital should be implemented.

Objective 2:   By 1984, the number of excess pediatric beds should be reduced by 50% (current excess: 106 beds).

      Action 1:   Certificates of need for pediatric beds in areas of excess should not be approved.

      Action 2:   Pediatric services in M. County should be considered.

Objective 3:   By 1984, the number of excess obstetrical beds should be reduced by 50% (current excess range: 72–104 beds).

      Action 1:   Certificates of need for obstetrical beds in areas of excess capacity should not be approved.

Objective 4:   By 1984, the medical/surgical bed complement should be increased by up to 71 beds in M. County and by up to 103 beds in O. County.

      Action 1:   Hospitals in M. and O. Counties should add up to 71 and 103 medical/surgical beds respectively with emphasis on BC, FA, MM, and PK hospitals.

Objective 5:   By 1984, combined reductions in hospital admissions and average lengths of stay should decrease patient days per 1,000 population by 5%.

Action 1:   All area hospitals should institute same day surgery plus pre-admission testing for 100% of elective admissions.

Action 2:   Inappropriate utilization of acute care facilities by persons requiring lower levels of care should be reduced through the combined efforts of hospitals, long-term care providers, home health providers and appropriate government agencies.

Action 3:   The development of health maintenance organizations should be encouraged by business, industry and providers in the area.

An examination of this goal, its objectives, and actions reveals the following points:

1. Eliminating excess capacity is heavily dependent on the implementation/review function. This strategy will be carried out by denying approvals for certificate-of-need applications where excess beds exist. At the same time, approval of such applications is recommended for two counties with an inadequate supply of beds.
2. Specific numbers of medical/surgical, pediatric, and obstetrical beds are slated for elimination, which should help reduce the overall excess of beds. By specifying the types of bed reductions to be made rather than reducing the number of beds across the board, the health planning agency's board is relying on the planning staff's analysis to make selective cuts. This will have the double effect of increasing efficiency and ensuring the bed needs of the population are being met.
3. Further, reductions in lengths of stay and admissions are also being used to achieve the overall goal.
4. Alternatives to hospitalization, such as same day surgery and greater use of ambulatory services, are viewed as a further means of lowering the occupancy rate.

5. To achieve these objectives, a necessary linkage to other services, including long-term care services, home health care, primary care services with special emphasis on HMOs, pediatricians, obstetricians, and family medicine practitioners would be required.

This illustration shows clearly how a goal to improve the efficiency of the health system through elimination of excessive acute care beds requires a series of five self-limiting objectives and ten alternative actions. An assumption is made that, if the five objectives are achieved, each of which is a partial solution to the problem, the goal of 3.3 beds per 1,000 population will be met. However, to achieve the objectives, the health planning agency will have to overcome the resistance of hospitals to closing or amalgamating beds; at the same time, the agency must encourage hospitals or groups of physicians to develop ambulatory, same day surgery units and must stimulate the regional population's interest in HMOs. None of these strategies is easy to execute, and all require time. Except for decisions on certificate-of-need proposals, decisions are controlled by provider institutions and consumer preferences. It is quite possible that only one or two of the objectives and their actions may be fulfilled. Nonetheless, by stressing alternative strategies, the agency enhances its potential for achieving at least a part of its goal level by 1984.

Relationship of Plan Elements and Planning Models

What type of relationship exists between the four planning models and these three plan elements? The goals-objectives-actions linkages illustrated require the centralization of power in the health planning agency, as is found in the systems planning model. With this health planning agency, however, the implementation of the objectives and actions is dependent on the decision making of a number of provider institutions over whom the agency has limited authority. It cannot force the hospitals in M. and O. Counties to add beds when they are not ready, nor can it dictate that hospitals reduce their admissions by 5 percent. Only a close working relationship and agreement between the health planning agency and the PSRO responsible for monitoring hospital admission and length of stay practices can have any impact on reducing admissions. Likewise, the agency would have to influence state and federal funding sources, as well as private insurance carriers, to reimburse patients for ambulatory care services if it is to have any hope of changing the behavior of consumers. No health planning agency has such authority. Thus, while this health planning agency used a systems concept in developing its plan, it lacks the fiscal power and legal authority to implement its goals without considerable cooperation from the many autonomous actors in the health care system.

With respect to the partnership planning model, agencies are more likely to establish general goals and some measurable objectives, although most are stated in general terms, and to identify general alternative actions. No specific actions are identified because this requires an assignment of power to one group at the expense of another. Individual agencies represented on the health planning agency use established goals and/or general objectives as the basis for promoting the programs in which they have an interest. In this way, the partnership model agency reacts to the initiatives fostered by the individual and autonomous health care services that are promoting their own programs. At present, this is done during review procedures. Even when the decisions on which programs to support are apparently based on objective criteria, it is more likely that a bargaining process is used and that programs are selected on the basis of who promotes them rather than what impact they will have on the achievement of the planned objectives. The last study of certificate-of-need approvals showed that, in 14 of 25 states, the state regulatory agencies continued to approve additional beds in areas where the hospital capacity was in excess of 105 percent of their published need projection for five years.[27] Obviously, bargaining, not objectivity or technical criteria, was used in approving these beds.

The alliance planning model is unlikely to have any goals at all. As a result of studies of health conditions or because of crises calling for a position to be taken by the agency, objectives are developed in an ad hoc and arbitrary manner. Once the objectives are determined, they may be used as a basis for rendering approval to the programs submitted by members of the alliance currently in control. More likely, each committee serves as its own alliance and uses the agency's decision-making approval process to gain a board-approved, rubber-stamped decision. Prior to the passage of PL 93-641 with its statement of procedures and criteria for review of certificate-of-need proposals, health planning agencies were more likely to have their boards rubber-stamp committee review decisions or not review them at all. Under these circumstances, the objectives and approved programs are what the committees say they are, especially when there is neither an accepted plan nor a central coordinating and review board that makes decision in lieu of a plan.

In the individual action model, there is no pretense of an agency setting goals or objectives. Only program proposals submitted by outside groups are approved. The internal decision-making structure of the agency is so fragmented that only the weakest of external organizations has difficulty getting a program approved in the review process. It is unlikely that any health planning agency would be able to operate on this basis for long because of the close monitoring of state and federal agencies.

It appears that the systems model of planning is related to goals-objectives-actions; the partnership planning model to general goals, arbitrary objectives unrelated to the goals, and approval of programs that may or may not be related to the objectives; the alliance planning model, to arbitrarily set objectives and program proposals unrelated to anything except the committee structure; and the individual action planning model, to program proposals initiated from outside the agency, related only to the self-interests of the program initiators. Table 6-5 sums up this relationship.

AUTHORITY OF HEALTH PLANNING AGENCIES

Historically, Congress has been very reluctant to give too much authority to agencies responsible for federally sponsored programs. In the health field, the private sector provides most of the services, although a high percentage of these services are paid for through government-sponsored programs. Congress is consequently very sensitive to the desires, needs, and philosophy of those in the private sector and the professional associations that speak for them. This congressional reluctance is exemplified by the passage of PL 89-749, the Partnership for Health Act, which gave little authority to the planning agencies. Rather, planning depended on the willingness of health provider institutions to work with consumers and government representatives. The AMA even had a clause introduced into the act to prevent the health planning agency from developing any new programs that were not consistent with accepted medical and dental practices.

With the passage of PL 92-603, Section 1122, the federal government gave states that entered into agreements with HEW the authority to review and approve/disapprove capital facilities costing over $100,000. Health care institutions that ignored a state decision to disapprove could be penalized by the loss of that portion of their capital expenditure reimburse-

---

Table 6-5   Relationships of Goals to Types of Planning Model

Planning Model	Goals
Systems	Goals, objectives determine program approval.
Partnership	Arbitrarily set objectives determine some programs; others determined arbitrarily.
Alliance	Programs determined by internal fragmented committee structure; no objectives.
Individual action	Programs determined by external influences on fragmented decision-making structure.

ment for the service funded under Titles V (Maternal and Child Health Act), XVIII (Medicare), and XIX (Medicaid). Regional health planning agencies in whose areas the programs were being proposed were permitted only to comment on these proposals. They were, in effect, recommending what action the state health planning agency should take, but the state agency had authority to make decisions and fiscal power to back up its decisions. Congress gave the states authority they did not previously have to make an impact on the health system.

It is the regional health planning agencies' lack of authority and power that Congress sought to overcome with the passage of PL 93-641. It gave them direct authority to review federally funded programs and make final decisions on such proposals. More importantly, the law demanded that review decisions be based on (a) a minimum set of federal procedures and criteria and (b) the goals, objectives, and priorities of their health plans. Thus, for the first time, planning took precedence over the review function; plans must now be taken seriously by health providers. Proposals they submit now have, as one criterion for evaluating them, their consistency with goal priorities contained in regional and state health plans. Approved health plans thus have a new power, and the regional health planning agencies have a new influence.

At various points in the debate on PL 93-641, consideration was given to granting health planning agencies the authority to be involved in setting rates and correcting problems found in health care institutions during the agencies' appropriateness reviews. However, for the time being, it was decided to permit only demonstrations of alternative rate review systems and publication of institutions' strengths and inadequacies as a strategy to stimulate them to correct problems voluntarily. In short, Congress gave health care providers notice that, unless they voluntarily took steps to improve the efficiency of their institutions, it might well give the planning agencies authority to do it for them.

PL 93-641 also increased the authority and power of health planning agencies by replacing three autonomous health planning agencies with one integrated system in which each was required to collaborate with the other. No longer can the three health planning agencies (Hill-Burton, Comprehensive Health Planning Agency, and Regional Medical Program) ignore each other. They have become part of one health planning system. More importantly, health care providers who formerly ignored one or more of the health planning agencies, or played one against the other, now must work with them. This means greater receptivity on the part of the health care providers to the guidance of the health planning agencies in the system.

While the power and authority of regional health planning agencies have been increased, it is to the state, usually the state health department, that federal legislation has delegated the most authority. As the share of federal health dollars increases, withholding of funds to health care providers results in considerable clout. But Thomas points out that even where this power exists it must be used with discretion.[28] He goes on to make the case that "within a zone of acceptance" planning and action can proceed if "planners check frequently on the program of their plan implementation and make adjustments and readjustments, the steps being small and involving neither great change nor long time periods."[29]

However, the incrementalism described by Thomas is not meant to negate the need for the occasional "giant step" that must be taken periodically. "After a period, perhaps extended, of acquiring information, increasing understanding, and consolidating goals, these factors may also be coalesced, in a giant step, into a new, grand scheme that departs profoundly from past policies to provide more of what society wants from what it has to expand."[30] The passage of the Social Security Act of 1935 and the Hill-Burton Act of 1954, and a national health insurance bill in the future are such giant steps. But, it required a Kerr-Mills and Titles XVIII and XIX of the Social Security Act to pave the way for a national health insurance bill. In short, Thomas asserts that, through incremental steps over a long period of time and demonstrated experience, health planning agencies will be able to accrue the requisite authority to carry out their responsibilities. Thus far, they have had the authority to plan under PL 93-641 and the power to develop comprehensive, long-range systems plans. They have some of the authority needed to implement the goals and priorities of those plans, but not as much as they require to ensure full responsiveness from health care provider institutions. Indeed, one of the questions that confronts all planning agencies is, in a democracy, how much authority and power should be given to a single agency when its decisions can vitally affect the lives of all citizens? That decision can only be answered by elected officials and the decisions they make.

NOTES

1. Health Resources Administration, *Health Systems Agency Performance Standards Guidelines* (Hyattsville, Md.: Bureau of Health Planning, February 1, 1977).

2. Health Resources Administration, *Performance Standards,* p. 3.

3. Michael J. Meshenberg, *Health Planning and the Environment: A Preventive Focus* (Chicago: American Society of Planning Officials, 1974), Chapter 1.

4. Boyd Z. Palmer, *An Advanced Health Planning System* (Springfield, Va.: National Technical Information Service, U.S. Department of Commerce, 1972).

5. *Survey of Selected 314(a) and Area-wide 314(b) CHP Agencies* (Newton, Mass.: Organization for Social and Technical Innovation, 1972), p. 49.

6. Cyril Roseman, "Problems and Prospects of CHP," *American Journal of Public Health,* January 1972, p. 17.

7. David H. Gustafson and Betty Chewning, "Final Evaluation Report: Conference on Health Program Development," mimeographed (Madison, Wisc.: University of Wisconsin, College of Engineering, 1971).

8. See Warren paradigm in Chapter 4, Planning Models.

9. Health Resources Administration, *Performance Standards,* p. 6.

10. Health Resources Administration, *Performance Standards,* p. 3.

11. *Survey of Selected Agencies,* pp. 19–20.

12. Health Resources Administration, *Performance Standards,* p. 6.

13. Roland L. Warren, Stephen M. Rose, and Ann F. Bergunder, *The Structure of Urban Reform* (Lexington, Mass.: Lexington Books, D.C. Heath, 1974).

14. *Ibid.*

15. Henrik L. Blum & Associates, *Notes on Comprehensive Planning for Health* (Berkeley, Calif.: American Public Health Association, 1968), p. 404.

16. Carruth J. Wagner, "A Systems Approach to Health Planning," in *Planning for Health* (Chicago: National Health Forum, 1967), p. 46.

17. Health Resources Administration, *Guidelines for the Development of Health Systems Plans and Annual Implementation Plans* (Hyattsville, Md.: Bureau of Health Planning, February 23, 1979), p. 9.

18. Health Resources Administration, *Guidelines,* p. 9.

19. U.S. Department of Health and Human Services, "Health Planning: National Guidelines," Federal Register, vol 43, no. 60, March 28, 1978, pp. 13040–13050.

20. U.S. Department of Health and Human Services, *National Health Planning Goals: The National Guidelines for Health Planning* (Hyattsville, Md.: Health Resources Administration, April 17, 1980, draft).

21. U.S. DHHS, *National Health Planning Goals,* p. 13.

22. U.S. DHHS, *National Health Planning Goals,* p. 16.

23. Daniel I. Zwick, *Initial Development of National Guidelines for Health Planning,* Public Health Reports, vol. 93, no. 5 (Hyattsville, Md.: HHS, 1978).

24. U.S. DHHS, *National Health Planning Goals,* various sections, pp. 23–29.

25. Wagner, "Systems Approach," p. 46.

26. Blum, *Notes on Planning,* Appendix, p. B.1.

27. Carolyn Harmon, "Efficiency and Effectiveness of Capital Expenditures," *Health Regulation: Certificate of Need and 1122,* ed. Herbert H. Hyman (Rockville, Md.: Aspen Systems Corporation, 1977), p. 42.

28. William Thomas, "Health Planning and Realism," *Hospital Administration* 14 (Fall 1969): 16–34.

29. Thomas, "Planning and Realism," p. 9.

30. Thomas, "Planning and Realism," p. 11.

Appendix 6-A

Checklist for Reviewing HSA Compliance with Performance Standards

A. *AGENCY ORGANIZATION AND MANAGEMENT*

Standard A-1: Organizational and Operational Policies

____The governing body has formally adopted written policies as prescribed in Standard A-1 which satisfy the requirements set forth in:

    ____Standard A-1a (organizational structure)
    ____Standard A-1b (authority, roles, etc., of organizational components)
    ____Standard A-1c (authority, roles, etc., of staff)
    ____Standard A-1d (membership and officers)
    ____Standard A-1e (meetings)
    ____Standard A-1f (other)
    ____Standard A-1g (receipt of funds)

Identify discrepancies: _____

_____

_____

____The agency is organized and operates in accordance with the adopted policies.

Identify discrepancies: _____

_____

_____

____The adopted policies have been reviewed by the governing body (and revised as necessary) at least annually.

Identify discrepancies: _____

_____

_____

Source: Bureau of Health Planning, *Health Systems Agency Performance Standards Guidelines,* February 1, 1977, pp. 30–42.

Standard A-2: Annual Work Program and Budget

____The governing body has formally adopted an annual work program and budget (and any revisions thereto) as prescribed in Standard A-2 which satisfy the requirements set forth in:

____Standard A-2a (work program)
____Standard A-2b (budget)

Identify discrepancies: _____

_____

_____

____The agency conducts its activities and allocates its resources in accordance with the adopted work program and budget.

Identify discrepancies: _____

_____

_____

Standard A-3: Managing and Monitoring Agency Activities

____The agency has developed an internal management reporting system that satisfies the requirements set forth in Standard A-3.

Identify discrepancies: _____

_____

_____

____The management reporting system is utilized to monitor agency progress in accomplishing its work program and the utilization of agency resources, and to identify where corrective action is required in the management of agency resources.

Identify discrepancies: _____

_____

_____

Standard A-4: Financial Administration

____The governing body has formally adopted a system for agency financial administration as prescribed in Standard A-4 which satisfies the requirements set forth in:

____Standard A-4a (fund accounting)
____Standard A-4b (authority and responsibility)
____Standard A-4c (internal control procedures)
____Standard A-4d (procurement and reimbursement policies)
____Standard A-4e (financial statements and reports)
____Standard A-4f (audit)

Identify discrepancies: _____

_____

_____

____The agency administers its financial affairs in accordance with the adopted system for financial administration.

Identify discrepancies: _____

_____

_____

____The agency has made provisions for periodic review of its financial administration system by the governing body and has adhered to those provisions.

Identify discrepancies: _____

_____

_____

Standard A-5: Personnel Administration

____The governing body has formally adopted agency personnel policies and procedures as prescribed in Standard A-5 which satisfy the requirements set forth in:

____Standard A-5a   (staff recruitment, compensation, etc.)
____Standard A-5b   (authority and responsibility for personnel administration)
____Standard A-5c   (staff performance evaluation)
____Standard A-5d   (grievances, disciplinary actions, appeals)
____Standard A-5e   (staff development)
____Standard A-5f   (conditions of employment)
____Standard A-5g   (personnel files and records)
____Standard A-5h   (staffing patterns, etc.)
____Standard A-5i   (staffing patterns, etc.)

Identify discrepancies: _____

_____

_____

____The agency administers its personnel affairs in accordance with the adopted personnel policies and procedures.

Identify discrepancies: _____

_____

_____

____The adopted personnel policies and procedures have been reviewed by the governing body (and revised as necessary) at least annually.

Identify discrepancies: _____

_____

_____

Standard A-6: Orientation and Training of Members and Staff
____The governing body has formally adopted an orientation and training program for members and staff as prescribed in Standard A-6 which:

    ____is based upon an annual assessment of needs as required by Standard A-6a;

    ____provides for a basic orientation program for new members and staff as required by Standard A-6b;

    ____provides for on-going education and training of members and staff as required by Standard A-6c.

Identify discrepancies: _____

_____

_____

____The agency schedules and conducts orientation, education, and training activities as an integral part of its annual work program in accordance with the adopted orientation and training program.

Identify discrepancies: _____

_____

_____

B. *PLAN DEVELOPMENT*

Standard B-1: Health Systems Plan
____The agency has developed and published a health systems plan (HSP) as prescribed in Standard B-1 which has been formally adopted by the governing body, and which:

    ____satisfies the requirements pertaining to the scope of services to be addressed set forth in Standard B-1a;

    ____HSP goals take into account and are consistent with national guidelines as set forth in Standard B-1b;

    ____HSP objectives express desired achievements as set forth in Standard B-1c;

_____includes an assessment of all health services and goals reflecting desired future directions for health systems development within the health service area in terms of their *cost, availability,* and *accessibility* as set forth in Standard B-1d;

_____*includes an assessment of all health services and goals reflecting desired future directions for health systems developed within the health service area in terms of their *continuity, acceptability,* and *quality;* as set forth in Standard B-1d;

_____initially places emphasis upon the area's diagnostic and treatment services as set forth in Standard B-1d.

Identify discrepancies and/or HSP development status: _____

_____

_____

_____The adopted HSP has been reviewed and amended (as necessary) by the governing body on an annual basis.

Identify discrepancies: _____

_____

_____

Standard B-2: Annual Implementation Plan

_____The agency has developed and published an annual implementation plan (AIP) as prescribed in Standard B-2 which has been formally adopted by the governing body, and which:

_____satisfies the requirements pertaining to the scope of services to be addressed referenced in Standard B-2a;

_____AIP's short-range objectives should relate to HSP's high priority objectives and long-range actions as set forth in Standard B-2b.

Identify discrepancies and/or AIP development status: _____

_____

_____

_____The adopted AIP has been reviewed and amended (as necessary) by the governing body on an annual basis.

Identify discrepancies: _____

_____

_____

---

*Not a prerequisite to achieving full designation.

Standard B-3: Specific Plans and Projects

____*The agency has developed, or assisted other appropriate entities to develop specific plans and projects as prescribed in Standard B-3 in accordance with the priorities and recommended actions established in its AIP; such plans and projects have been adopted by the governing body and published.

Standard B-4: Recommendations for the State Medical Facilities Plan

____*The agency has developed and submitted to the SHPDA, on an annual basis, recommendations and priorities for medical facility modernization, construction, and conversion projects within the health service area in accordance with DHEW and SHPDA requirements.

Standard B-5: Planning Process

____The agency has established a planning process for developing (or reviewing and amending) its plans, and a format for presentation of those plans, as prescribed in Standard B-5 which satisfy the requirements set forth in:

____Standard B-5a   (public involvement and participation)
____Standard B-5b   (coordination)
____Standard B-5c   (data acquisition and analysis)
____Standard B-5d   (work program)

Identify discrepancies: _____

_____

____The agency has developed, reviewed, revised, adopted, published, and disseminated its plans in accordance with the established planning process(es) and format(s).

Identify discrepancies: _____

_____

C. PLAN IMPLEMENTATION/REVIEW ACTIVITIES

Standard C-1: Review Procedures and Criteria

____The governing body has formally adopted written procedures for the conduct of agency review activities as prescribed in Standard C-1 which satisfy the requirements set forth in:

_____

*Not a prerequisite to achieving full designation

_____Standard C-1a   (assignment of responsibilities)
_____Standard C-1b   (conflict of interest)
_____Standard C-1c   (coordination)
_____Standard C-1d   (public involvement and participation)
_____Standard C-1e   (technical assistance to applicants)
_____Standard C-1f   (preliminary examination of proposals)
_____Standard C-1g   (monitoring proposals under review)
_____Standard C-1h   (monitoring follow-up activities on approved
                      projects)
_____Standard C-1i   (maintenance of data on proposals)
_____Standard C-1j   (other procedures)

Identify discrepancies: _____

_____

_____

_____ Interested and affected groups or individuals were provided an
opportunity to review and comment upon proposed procedures
(or revisions thereto), and their comments were considered by the
governing body prior to adopting the review procedures.
Identify discrepancies: _____

_____

_____

_____ Interested and affected groups or individuals have been made
aware of, and have been provided an opportunity to obtain copies
of, the adopted procedures.
Identify discrepancies: _____

_____

_____

_____The agency conducts its review activities in accordance with the
adopted review procedures.
Identify discrepancies: _____

_____

_____

_____The adopted procedures have been reviewed by the governing
body (and revised as necessary) at least annually.
Identify discrepancies: _____

_____

_____

____The governing body has formally adopted written criteria for use in carrying out its review responsibilities as prescribed in Standard C-1 which are consistent with, and supportive of, the goals, objectives, priorities, and recommendations contained in the agency's HSP and AIP when developed.

Identify discrepancies: _____

_____

_____

____ Interested and affected groups or individuals were provided an opportunity to review and comment upon proposed criteria (or revisions thereto), and their comments were considered by the governing body prior to adopting the review criteria.

Identify discrepancies: _____

_____

_____

____ Interested and affected groups or individuals have been made aware of, and have been provided an opportunity to obtain copies of, the adopted criteria.

Identify discrepancies: _____

_____

_____

____The agency utilizes the adopted criteria in making its determinations on applications or proposals reviewed by the HSA.

Identify discrepancies: _____

_____

_____

____The adopted criteria have been reviewed by the governing body (and revised as necessary) at least annually.

Identify discrepancies: _____

_____

_____

D. *PLAN IMPLEMENTATION/HEALTH SYSTEM DEVELOPMENT*

Standard D-1: Technical Assistance and Consultation

____* The agency has provided consultation and assistance to appropriate entities as prescribed in Standard D-1 in order to stimulate

_____
*Not a prerequisite to achieving full designation

and encourage health system development activities within the health service area based on identified needs.

Standard D-2: Area Health Services Development Fund

____* The governing body has formally adopted written procedures and criteria for reviewing and awarding grants and contracts through its area health service development fund, and procedures for administering such funds, in accordance with DHEW requirements.

____* The agency reviews proposals and administers its development fund in accordance with the adopted procedures and criteria.

____* The agency has made provisions for periodic review of the procedures and criteria by the governing body and has adhered to those provisions.

Standard D-3: Public Issue Involvement

____* The agency has established a mechanism whereby its members and staff may identify appropriate health related issues upon which the governing body should consider taking public positions as prescribed in Standard D-3.

____* The agency has prepared position statements on such issues that the governing body deems timely and relevant as prescribed in Standard D-3b.

____*All such position statements released by the HSA have been consistent with the adopted plans of the agency, have been approved by the governing body, and have been widely disseminated throughout the health service area.

E. *DATA MANAGEMENT AND ANALYSIS*

____The agency has developed a data management and analysis program and conducts its data activities in a manner which is supportive of its plan development and plan implementation activities, which is coordinated with other appropriate entities and maximizes the use of data maintained by such entities, and which satisfies the requirements set forth in:

____Standard E-1a (status of residents)
____Standard E-1b (status of health care delivery system)
____Standard E-1c (effect of system)
____Standard E-1d (number, type, location, etc.)

---

*Not a prerequisite to achieving full designation

_____Standard E-1e (patterns of utilization)
_____Standard E-1f (environmental & occupational exposure)
_____Standard E-1g (staff responsibilities)
_____Standard E-1h (organizing, storing, retrieving)
Identify discrepancies: _____

_____

_____

F. *COORDINATION*

Standard F-1: Formal Coordination Agreements

_____The agency has established written agreements for coordinating its plan development, plan implementation, and data activities with PSRO, A-95, HSAs, and other appropriate entities as prescribed in Standard F-1 which have been formally adopted by the governing body and which satisfy the requirements set forth in PSRO agreements:

_____Standard F-1a (sharing of data)
_____Standard F-1b (review and comment)
_____Standard F-1c (technical assistance)
_____Standard F-1d (assurance of actions)

A-95 Agreements:

_____Standard F-1a (organizational & procedural arrangements)
_____Standard F-1b (formal arrangements for review)
_____Standard F-1c (technical assistance)
_____Standard F-1d (provision of assurance)
_____Standard F-1e (sharing of data)

HSAs within same SMSA:

_____Standard F-1a (review and comment)
_____Standard F-1b (organizational & procedural requirements)
_____Standard F-1c (sharing of data)

Identify discrepancies: _____

_____

_____

_____The coordination agreements have been implemented and are followed by all involved parties.

Identify discrepancies: _____

_____

_____

Standard F-2: Other Coordination Arrangements

_____The agency has identified other appropriate entities with which coordinative relationships should be established in accordance with Standards F-2a-c and has established formal or informal working agreements with such entities (which at a minimum provide for exchange of information on related activities) as prescribed in Standard F-2.

Identify discrepancies: _____

_____

_____

_____The working agreements are properly observed and adhered to by all involved parties.

Identify discrepancies: _____

_____

_____

G. *PUBLIC INVOLVEMENT AND EDUCATION*

Standard G-1: Public Information

_____The governing body has formally adopted written procedures for providing information to the public as prescribed in Standard G-1 which, at a minimum, include provisions for informing Indian tribes or intertribal organizations located within the health service area (if applicable) of the availability of federal health funds, and which satisfy the following notification and reporting requirements set forth in:

_____Standard G-1a (detailed description)
_____Standard G-1b (notice of time, place, etc.)
_____Standard G-1c (statement of the qualifications)
_____Standard G-1d (summary of comments)

Regular Reports:
_____Standard G-1a (status of each review)
_____Standard G-1b (annual report)

Identify discrepancies: _____

_____

_____

_____The agency conducts its public information activities in accordance with the adopted procedures.

Identify discrepancies: _____

_____

_____

_____The adopted public information procedures have been reviewed by the governing body (and revised as necessary) at least annually.

Identify discrepancies: _____

_____

_____

Standard G-2: Public Access to Agency Records and Data

_____The governing body has formally adopted written procedures for assuring public access to agency plans, review procedures and criteria, reports, records, and data as prescribed in Standard G-2 which, at a minimum, satisfy the requirements set forth in:

_____Standard G-2a (distribution of HSP, AIP, etc.)

_____Standard G-2b (index of agency records and data)

_____Standard G-2c (periodic notices regarding the availability of agency plans and other documentation)

_____Standard G-2d (receiving and processing requests for materials)

Identify discrepancies: _____

_____

_____

_____The agency provides for public access to agency documentation in accordance with the adopted procedures.

Identify discrepancies: _____

_____

_____

_____The adopted procedures have been reviewed by the governing body (and revised as necessary) at least annually.

Identify discrepancies: _____

_____

_____

Standard G-3: Public Input

____The governing body has formally adopted written procedures for public participation and input regarding the organization and operation of the HSA and its planning and implementation activities as prescribed in Standard G-3 which, at a minimum, satisfy the requirements set forth in:

____Standard G-3a ("public" meetings and advance notification)
____Standard G-3b (public input on agency plans)
____Standard G-3c (public input on review procedures and criteria)

Identify discrepancies: _____

_____

_____

____The agency provides opportunities for public participation and input in accordance with the adopted procedures.

Identify discrepancies: _____

_____

_____

____The adopted procedures have been reviewed by the governing body (and revised as necessary) at least annually.

Identify discrepancies: _____

_____

_____

Standard G-4: Public Education

____* The agency has developed and implemented a strategy for promoting educational programs and activities for area residents designed to increase their knowledge and awareness regarding proper personal health care and effective use of available health services, based upon the objectives, priorities, and recommended actions contained in the agency's AIP.

---

*Not a prerequisite to achieving full designation

Appendix 6-B

Summary Statement
of Standards

General Hospitals—121.201 and 121.202
1. No. beds/1,000 (4)
2. Occupancy (80%)

Obstetric Services—121.203
3. No. and percentage of obstetric service facilities with "linkage" (signed agreements) to a regionalized OB network
4. No. births/year for each level II and III facility (1,500 minimum)
5. Occupancy for units with more than 1,500 births/year (75%)

Neonatal Special Care Units—121.204
6. No. and percentage of neonatal service facilities with "linkage" (signed agreements) to a regional OB network (100%)
7. No. neonatal beds/1,000 live births (4)
8. No. beds in each single level II or III neonatal unit (15 minimum)

Pediatric Inpatient Services—121.206
9. No. beds in each urban pediatric unit (20 minimum)
10. Pediatric inpatient occupancy by bed size (20–39: 65%; 40–79: 70%; 80+: 75%)

Open Heart Surgery—121.207
11. No. open heart procedures/year (200 within 3 years in any institution in which open heart surgery is performed for adults; 350 required for approval of additional adult units)
12. No. pediatric heart operations/year (100 within 3 years)
13. No. pediatric open heart operations/year (75 within 3 years and can be included in the required 100 pediatric heart procedures: 130 required for approval of additional pediatric units)

Cardiac Catheterization—121.208
14. No. of cardiac caths/year/adult or unit (300 minimum; 500 required before a new adult cardiac cath unit is opened)

Source: Bureau of Health Planning, *Program Policy Notice: Guidelines for the Development of Health Systems Plans and Annual Implementation Plans,* February 23, 1979, pp. 34–36.

241

15. No. of intracardiac or coronary artery catheterizations/year/adult or unit (200 minimum; must be included in the 300 cardiac caths/year/unit)
16. No. of pediatric cardiac caths/year/pediatric cc unit (at least 150 within 3 years of operation: 250 required before a new pediatric cc unit is opened)
17. No. of units performing cardiac catheterizations which are not performing open heart surgery (0)

Radiation Therapy — 121.209

18. Service area population for each megavoltage radiation therapy unit (300 within 3 years)
19. No. of treatments/year/megavoltage radiation therapy unit (6,000 required before new units are opened)

Computed Tomographic Scanners — 121.210

20. No. CT scanning procedures/year/unit (2,500 within 2 years; 2,500 required before new units are opened)
21. No. and percentage of CT scanning operations that have established data collection and utilization review systems (100%)

End-State Renal Disease (ESRD) — 121.211

These indicators are taken from 20 CFR Part 405, Subpart U.

22. No. transplants/year/Renal Transplant Center (unconditional: 15 or more; conditional 7–14)
23. No. of dialysis/station/week
   For dialysis facilities or centers performing greater than 20% of dialysis on outpatients and located in an SMSA of 500,000 +,
   unconditional: 4.5+/6+ stations/week
   conditional: 4.0–4.5/6+ stations/week, or
                     4.5+/4–5 stations/week
   For renal dialysis centers performing 20% or less of their dialysis on outpatients
   unconditional: 4.0+/3+ stations/week
   conditional: 4.0+/2+ stations/week
24. No. of renal transplants in renal dialysis centers whose hospitals have Medicare provider status.

The remaining ESRD conditions are programmatic in nature and are more appropriately analyzed and applied by the ESRD funding program.

Appendix 6-C
Summary Statement of Goals

PART I: HEALTH STATUS OUTCOMES

1. *Health Status Improvements*

   Health status should be improved in all parts of the country and among all population groups, especially among medically underserved populations.

2. *Infant Health*

   The health of infants should be improved by:

   a. Reducing the incidence of low birth weight infants (prematurely born, or small-for-age infants weighing less than 2,500 grams) for every subgroup of the population (as defined by socioeconomic, ethnic and geographic characteristics) below the lowest reported rate for such a subgroup; and
   b. Reducing the infant mortality rate to less than 11 deaths per 1,000 live births by 1985 and to less than 9 deaths per 1,000 live births by 1990.

3. *Child Health*

   Child health and development should be improved and death rates for those ages 1-14 reduced to less than 39 per 100,000 by 1985 and to less than 34 deaths per 100,000 by 1990.

4. *Preventable Communicable Diseases*

   The incidence of preventable communicable diseases should be reduced, with a mortality rate of less than 22 deaths per 100,000 persons. Diseases and deaths preventable by routine childhood vaccination should approach zero. Measles should be eliminated as an endemic disease in the United States.

5. *Adolescent Health*

   The health of adolescents and young adults should be improved and death rates for those aged 15 to 24 reduced to less than 105 per 100,000 by 1985 and to less than 93 deaths per 100,000 by 1990.

Source: Health Resources Administration, *National Health Planning Goals: The National Guidelines for Health Planning,* April 17, 1980, pp. 23–29.

6. *Adult Health*

The health of adults should be improved and death rates for those aged 25-64 reduced to less than 472 per 100,000 by 1985 and to less than 400 per 100,000 by 1990.

7. *Older Adult Health*

The health and quality of life of older adults should be improved and the average annual number of days of restricted activity due to acute and chronic conditions for those age 65 and older reduced to less than 33 days per year by 1985 and to less than 30 days per year by 1990.

8. *Alcoholism*

The prevalence of alcoholism and related disabilities and deaths should be reduced by at least 5 percent.

9. *Drug Abuse*

Drug abuse should be reduced by (1) interrupting and reversing by at least 15 percent the trend of increased incidence of current marijuana and phencyclidine (PCP) abuse among youth 12-17 years of age; (2) decreasing by at least 20 percent the use of barbiturates and other potentially harmful sedatives used for the treatment of insomnia; and (3) reducing the annual number of amphetamine prescriptions written for the treatment of weight reduction by 20 percent.

10. *Oral Health*

Oral health status should be improved so that (1) for persons 17 years of age, at least 85 percent retain all of their permanent teeth and (2) for persons 55 to 64 years of age, at least 80 percent retain some natural teeth.

11. *Heart Disease, Cancer and Stroke*

Age-adjusted death rates for heart disease should be reduced to 156 per 100,000 persons and for stroke to 29 per 100,000 persons by 1985. Efforts should be directed toward improvements in survival rates through detection and treatment for all types of cancer.

PART II: DISEASE PREVENTION AND HEALTH PROMOTION

1. *Extension of Disease Prevention and Health Promotion* *

Health promotion and disease prevention should be extended through

---

*Goals marked with an asterisk grow out of the National Health Priorities contained in Section 1502 of the Statute [PL 93-641]. They will be identified as such in the text following the goal statements.

both individual and community actions with emphasis on high risk populations, and be an integral component of care provided by health care and other community institutions.

2. *Consumer Information* *

People should be better informed as to how, when, and where to get health care of an appropriate kind and quality at a reasonable cost.

3. *Prenatal Care* *

Programs should be established to assure that all pregnant women receive adequate prenatal care.

4. *Unintended Pregnancy* *

The rate and adverse consequences of unintended pregnancy should be reduced, particularly among teenagers and other high risk groups.

5. *Immunization* *

At least 90 percent of all children under 15 years of age and newborns at the earliest appropriate time, should be immunized against polio, measles, rubella, diphtheria, mumps, pertussis and tetanus.

6. *Environmental and Occupational Health* *

Programs should be undertaken for protection from and reduction of environmental, occupational and product hazards.

7. *Accidents* *

Programs should be undertaken to prevent accidents in the home, during recreation, at work and on the highway. Particular efforts should be made to reduce accidents involving children.

8. *Fluoridation* *

Community water supplies containing insufficient natural fluoride should be fluoridated to optimal levels for the prevention of dental caries.

9. *Nutrition* *

People should be informed about what constitutes good nutrition and should be encouraged and aided in obtaining a proper diet.

10. *Smoking* *

Communities, working through all available institutions and media, should strive to discourage the initiation of the smoking habit among young people, and to break the habit among those who smoke.

---

*Goals marked with an asterisk grow out of the National Health Priorities contained in Section 1502 of the Statute [PL 93-641]. They will be identified as such in the text following the goal statements.

PART III: INSTITUTIONAL AND PERSONNEL RESOURCES AND SYSTEMS OF CARE

A. SERVICE DELIVERY

1. *Access to Care* *

   Every person should have access to the full range of health care services. Equal access to needed health care services for all population subgroups (including racial and ethnic minorities, the elderly, the handicapped, and low income persons) should be fostered through the elimination of financial, physical, geographic, transportational, organizational and other barriers unrelated to the need for care. Planning and review decisions must take into account the specific health care needs of these groups and give priority to projects which seek to address these needs.

2. *Primary Care* *

   a. *Supply*

      The supply of primary care physicians in a health service area should be at least one physician per 2,000 population. Under certain circumstances, services should be enhanced through more effective utilization of other health personnel, including physicians' assistants and nurse practitioners.

   b. *Balance Among Medical Specialties*

      To the extent that shortages or excesses of primary care personnel or medical specialties exist and are documented, these imbalances should be corrected.

   c. *Integration of Mental Health*

      The integration of mental health services in general health care delivery programs should be increased through in-service mental health training of primary care providers and placement of mental health professionals in primary care programs.

3. *Mental Health* *

   An increasing proportion of mentally ill persons should be restored to productive living by:

   a. developing community-based services for unserved, underserved, or inappropriately served populations, especially children and youth, the aged, the chronically mentally ill, racial or ethnic minorities, poor persons, and persons in rural areas,

---

*Goals marked with an asterisk grow out of the National Health Priorities contained in Section 1502 of the Statute [PL 93-641]. They will be identified as such in the text following the goal statements.

b. minimizing unnecessary or inappropriate institutionalization and ensuring that persons requiring long-term residential care due to mental illness or disability receive such care in the least restrictive settings which assure high quality care and services appropriate to the patient's needs, and

c. providing economical and high quality health facilities for chronic mental patients who require prolonged periods of care.

4. *Child Mental Health* *

Services should be available to improve the level of social and cognitive functioning for children identified as "most in need' of mental health services.

5. *Alcoholism and Drug Abuse* *

Alcoholism and drug abuse services should be organized in ways that further the development of comprehensive community-based prevention and treatment services, and which are integrated into the mainstream of health care.

6. *Dental Services*

Dental services should be available and reasonably accessible to all persons in need of dental care.

B. *SYSTEMS OF CARE*

1. *Regionalization* *

Providers of health services should be organized into regionalized networks which assure that various types and levels of services are linked together to form comprehensive and efficient systems of care. These networks should work to improve access to health services, eliminate unnecessary duplication of services, and improve quality.

2. *Multi-Institutional Systems and Shared Services* *

Efficiency and productivity of health care institutions should be furthered through the development of multi-institutional arrangements for the sharing of clinical, administrative and support services.

---

*Goals marked with an asterisk grow out of the National Health Priorities contained in Section 1502 of the Statute [PL 93-641]. They will be identified as such in the text following the goal statements.

3. *Emergency Medical Systems*

Networks of emergency medical services systems should be developed and improved in order to effectively coordinate the delivery of emergency medical care to all who require it.

4. *Options for Care**

Every resident within the health service area should have available the widest possible range of options for health care services with respect to both the organizational model for delivery and financing mechanisms.

  a. The option of joining a federally qualified or similarly constituted group practice health maintenance organization or other prepaid system of health care, such as a qualified independent practice association, should be available to every resident without reimbursement sanctions.
  b. The number of group practice arrangements for the delivery of medical care should be substantially increased.

5. *Quality of Health Services**

Health planning and review decisions should take into account the results of quality assessment and utilization reviews to support efforts to improve the quality of health services.

6. *Management Procedures**

Efficiency and productivity of health care institutions should be furthered through the adoption of uniform cost reporting, equitable reimbursement arrangements, utilization reporting systems and improved management reporting procedures.

7. *New Technology**

When found safe and effective, the introduction of new procedures and equipment should take place in ways that enhance economy, equity and quality. Reimbursement policies should foster the appropriate use of all technology.

8. *Energy Conservation**

Efforts should be made to promote an effective energy conservation and fuel conservation program for health service institutions to reduce the rate of growth of demand for energy.

---

*Goals marked with an asterisk grow out of the National Health Priorities contained in Section 1502 of the Statute [PL 93-641]. They will be identified as such in the text following the goal statements.
* Not a prerequisite to achieving full designation

C. *COORDINATING COMMUNITY RESOURCES*

1. *Access to Support Services for the Chronically Ill and Handicapped*

A full array of support services should be accessible to those with chronic or prolonged illnesses and/or physical or mental handicaps.

2. *Services Coordination and Case Management*

There should be close coordination among the various medical, social, rehabilitative and other human services which those with chronic or prolonged disabilities often require. Case management should be available to the chronically ill and handicapped to direct them to needed medical and support services.

Chapter 7

Implementation of Health Systems Plans: Reactive Approach

Since the inception of comprehensive health planning in 1965, health planning agencies have focused primarily on the planning function. When the passage of Section 1122 of the Social Security Act in the early 1970s gave them review responsibilities for capital expenditure projects, the project review function assumed major importance for planning agencies. Some agencies even equated comprehensive health planning with decisions on capital expenditure facility and service projects. With the passage of PL 93-641, the different orientations of these two functions, planning and project review, have been clearly delineated. Congress emphasized that it was as much concerned with the implementation of plans as it has been with this development.

Except for those planners intimately involved in Regional Medical Program (RMP) projects, health planners have had very little experience with implementation. It will take professionals in the health planning agencies some time to develop the credibility that comes from experience with plan implementation. Planners must learn to deal with two opposite models of implementation: the reactive and the proactive. Reactive implementation refers to the regulatory functions of certificate-of-need and 1122 reviews, appropriateness review, and reviews of proposed uses of federal funds. For many health planning agencies, it also involves rate review at the state level. This form of implementation involves approving changes in existing and new services, facilities, and programs, as well as new fiscal arrangements. Services and facilities are added, eliminated, modernized, or converted in order to improve availability, accessibility, or quality of programs to the public. This model of implementation is reactive because proposed projects and changes are initiated largely by health care providers; health planning agencies react to proposals presented to them. This situation may also produce an adversary relationship between the providers and planning agencies. As a price for approval providers must meet certain schedules, provide specific information, and prove the program is needed. The burden of proof is placed squarely on the shoulders of the providers to show the significance of their proposal. The benefit for complying with the regulatory process and substantive criteria is usually acceptance and approval by health planning decision makers.

Even with respect to appropriateness review, where the health planning agencies take the initiative in evaluating medical facilities and services in their regions, it is still the health care providers who determine what changes to make from the recommendations contained in the evaluations. Thus, implementation takes place only when the providers perceive the need and take the necessary steps. While a cooperative relationship is desired by the health planners, they are often confronted by providers who feel distrust, consternation at having to modify what are to them perfectly reasonable proposals, and frustration at the length of time it takes to obtain approvals. Providers may even show outright hostility should the proposal be disapproved or should they be forced to add conditions odious to them. The forces at work and the behavior of both planners and providers can create barriers to the very cooperation that both sides desire.

Proactive implementation requires a very different set of conditions, circumstances, and skills. In this model of implementing the goals and objectives of the health plans, health planning agencies must depend on the voluntary cooperation and collaboration of many actors at both the regional and state levels to achieve changes in the health care system. Proactive implementation is, in essence, an extension of what should have been a deeply involved relationship among planners, health care providers, and consumers in the development of the health plans, particularly its goals and high-priority objectives. An atmosphere of good will generated at this stage is readily carried over into plan implementation.

The real issues of this model revolve around technical, legal, and fiscal matters, such as changing reimbursement patterns, adding a health maintenance organization (HMO) in one part of the health service area while eliminating a little used outpatient clinic in the same area. Proactive implementation requires political, organizational, fiscal, and managerial skills. It depends on using influence in an appropriate manner, knowing when to fight or to collaborate, and timing decisions and actions. Unlike reactive implementation, this concept is flexible and dynamic; it is based on the best values and instincts of professional interrelationships among planners, medical care providers, consumers, legislators, budgeting personnel, and a host of significant others.

When the same health planning agency has the responsibility for both types of implementation, the way in which reactive implementation is carried out will have a profound effect on the agency's capacity to engage in proactive implementation. A hospital administrator whose proposal has been disapproved or saddled with difficult and costly conditions may not be willing to cooperate with the same agency (even if the planners come from a different division within it) in developing health services to meet the high-priority goals of the health plan. That hospital administrator may still cooperate in implementing the plan's high-priority objectives, however, because of competition with a nearby hospital, need to upgrade and maintain a high level of services, or the influence of a hospital trustee. Thus, while decisions made by the health planning agency in carrying out its reactive implementation function may affect its capacity to work in a proactive milieu, there is no way to predict what the effect of mixing these two types of implementation in the same agency will be on its capacity to achieve its goals and objectives.

CERTIFICATE-OF-NEED/1122 REVIEWS

The certificate-of-need requirement was originally based on state law. New York passed the first certificate-of-need law in 1964, the Metcalf-McCloskey Act. From that time to the passage of Section 1122 of the Social Security Act in 1972, another 18 states passed certificate-of-need legislation. Section 1122 was enacted because many states resisted any form of regulation dealing with health facilities and services. While Section 1122 involved a voluntary agreement between the state and the federal government, it was passed with an implied threat of mandatory federal regulation if the states did not follow up with some form of health facilities regulation. As of 1975,[1] the year in which PL 93-641 was enacted, all states except one had either passed a certificate-of-need law (29 states) and/or had made a Section 1122 agreement (39 states) with the Department of Health, Education, and Welfare (HEW). While there are differences between the two laws, Section 1523 of PL 93-641 and Section 1122 of the Social Security Act, they have generally the same intent. The major goal of the laws is to reduce expenditures for medical facilities and services that are not needed in the health service areas. Section 1523 requires a state health planning agency or another agency designated by it to administer a state certificate of need program which applies to new institutional health services proposed to be offered or developed within the state and which is satisfactory to the Secretary of the Department of Health and Human Services (HHS). It further requires that no service should be started before the state agency has made a determination of its need. All states were required to pass a certificate-of-need law by a designated date.

While the regulations spell out minimum requirements, states can pass laws that are more stringent. The minimum requirements were developed to ensure that a common denominator would be adhered to by all states. Prior to federal involvement, there had been considerable variation among states with respect to which health institutions were reviewed, the financial threshold at which a review must take place (ranging from $25,000 in one state to $300,000 in another), and the review process itself.

The facilities covered are defined by Section 1531 of PL 93-641 as "health services which (A) are provided through private and public hospitals, rehabilitation facilities, nursing homes, and other health care facilities . . . and (B) entail annual operating costs of at least" $75,000. Other covered health care facilities include psychiatric hospitals, tuberculosis hospitals, kidney disease treatment centers, and HMOs, where applicable. Not covered by the federal regulations are home health services, ambulatory care facilities, and physicians' offices.

Threshold for Certificate of Need

A review of any proposed service is required if any one of the following conditions are present. These are known as the thresholds that trigger certificate-of-need review:

1. any capital expenditure that exceeds $150,000 for a new health facility.
2. a change in bed capacity that increases, decreases, or relocates the number of a facility's beds by ten beds or ten percent, whichever is less.
3. the acquisition of major medical equipment costing more than $150,000 to be used on a regular basis for inpatients, regardless of where the equipment is located, i.e., in the hospital itself or in a nearby physician's office or a clinic. Any office-based physician, failing to file notice of purchase of major medical equipment 30 days before it is to be purchased, will require a certificate-of-need review.
4. the addition of any health service not offered in the previous 12 months and having operating expenses of a minimum of $75,000 annually.
5. a change in the services listed in an approved certificate of need within one year of its approval.[2]

Because states may make these thresholds more restrictive, they can increase or decrease the number and type of health facilities and services to be reviewed. Thus, a state may set the threshold for review of major medical equipment purchases at $25,000 instead of $150,000, or it may require home health services to be reviewed, even though federal regulations do not require it. HMOs are exempt from certificate-of-need review if they (a) enroll 50,000 persons, (b) the facility is readily accessible to enrollees, and (c) 75 percent of the persons served by the facility are enrollees.

Procedures

All state certificate-of-need laws must adopt a minimum set of procedures outlined in Section 1532 of PL 93-641. These are to ensure fairness and objectivity in the reviews. The health care provider must give the planning agency reasonable notice of intent to file a certificate-of-need proposal, and the planning agency must notify the health provider of any additional information needed and the date of the beginning of the review. Recommendations or decisions made by planning agencies must be in writing. The public shall have access to all information contained in the applications, except those covered by the Privacy Act. Further, any person or institution affected by the application may request a hearing and must be permitted to speak or submit written evidence concerning the proposal. Providers are to be given timely notice of the status of their proposals as they move through the review process. Contacts between parties to the application, both for and against, and those state officials responsible for reviewing and evaluating the proposal are prohibited. Finally, all similar proposals must be reviewed together, no less than twice each year. This last procedure is known as "batching" and is an exception to the general rule that the agency must complete its review within 60 days following the notification of the applicant of the beginning of the review. While there are exceptions to these procedures, these minimum requirements govern all reviews undertaken by health planning agencies, including reviews of proposed uses of federal funds and appropriateness reviews.

Figure 7-1 shows the steps in the review process. The review is initiated by the health provider, who generally submits an application to the regional and state health planning agencies. Each reviews the applications from different perspectives. Within the regional health agency, a minimum of two bodies review the proposals: a project review committee and an executive committee or governing body. Additional reviews may be undertaken by subarea councils, or county or borough councils. Regardless of the number of review bodies, most reviews, unless "batched," are completed within the 60-day review period permitted to regional planning agencies. At the state level, a review committee and its overall general council examine certificate-of-need/1122 proposals. In Figure 7-1, the State Hospital Council, its review subcommittee, and the decision maker, the State Health Commissioner in this instance, are all involved in the

Figure 7-1 Certificate-of-Need Review Process

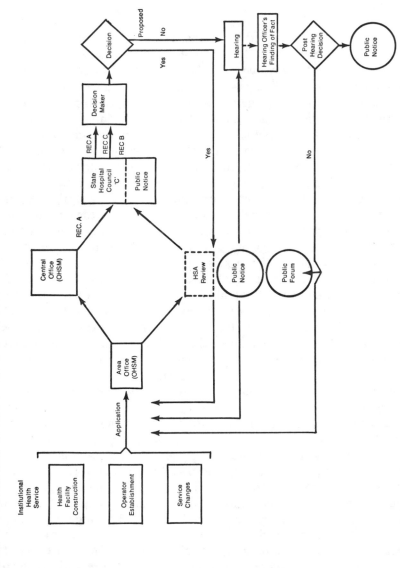

Source: New York State Office of Health Systems Management

process. The state usually has 90 days to render its decision, beginning with notification of the applicant at the regional planning level. Thus, it is possible that four to eight groups may be involved in an application review. If adverse decisions are appealed, then added to these procedures are an administrative hearing and, possibly, a judicial decision. Regional planning agencies make recommendations to the state agency, which has final decision-making authority, barring appeals. The great majority of regional health planning agency recommendations are supported at the state level.

Substantive Criteria

Whereas review procedures are mainly concerned with fairness, substantive criteria focus on whether the proposed project is really needed and feasible. These criteria indicate whether the proposal is consistent with the health planning agencies' plans and the health care provider's own health plan. The proposal must meet the needs of the population to be served and increase access to low-income persons, racial and ethnic minorities, women, handicapped persons, and other underserved populations. Further, the proposal must show how it is competitive with existing services as well as why the alternatives are not as efficient or effective. The applicant's past experiences in providing access to the medically underserved are also considered. For example, agencies examine the degree to which applicants provided "free" medical services to those unable to pay under their Hill-Burton commitment and the degree to which physicians admitted Medicare and Medicaid patients to facilities in which they have admitting privileges.

Generally, the burden of proof is on the applicant to establish the need for the proposed service or facility. Nonetheless, there are ways for applicants to predict an agency's receptivity to proposals. One procedure calls for presubmission consultation with the planning agency. During these meetings, the applicant is in a position to gauge the attitude of the agency toward the proposal. Second, an applicant patterning a proposal after one of the regional health plan's high-priority goals can be fairly confident that it will be approved, barring competition.

Outcome

There are only fragmented and inconclusive data that show the outcome of certificate-of-need regulations. Lewin's study, completed in 1975, showed that 93 percent of all projects were approved as well as 91 percent of the dollar values.[3] Of 1,943 projects, 1,806 were approved; of $3.8 billion, $3.4 billion were approved. Approval of major medical technology, including EMI Scanners, radiological x-ray, renal dialysis, cardiac catheters, and others was approved at an even higher rate—almost 96 percent. Lewin further found that "nearly 75% of the sample states and areas (30 of 41) approved hospital beds in excess of 105% of their published need projection . . . . Fourteen of these began the period overbedded and approved additional beds; five others became overbedded during the period studied as a result of the projects they approved."[4]

Bice and Salkever studied investment, costs, and utilization data of nonfederal, short-term general hospitals in the entire United States for the 1968–1972 period.[5] During this period, certificate-of-need laws were just beginning to be passed by a number of states, and Section 1122 had not yet been enacted. They found that the certificate-of-need requirement had the desired effect of reducing bed expansion, but there was nonetheless an increase in overall capital expenditures because hospitals were increasing their purchases of major medical equipment and modernizing their facilities. Further, they stated that "the overall effect of CON [certificate-of-need] regulation on the volume of inpatient services was to reduce utilization."[6] Inpatient days were reduced by 2.15 to 8.30 percent; admissions per capita, by 4.92 to 8.30 percent. It was concluded that "the pattern observed across several indicators of costs clearly provides no support for the widely held presumption that these controls have reduced costs."[7]

Both of these studies were made before the implementation of PL 93-641. The American Health Planning Association (AHPA), commissioned to study the effects of certificate-of-need/1122 reviews for the period 1976–1978, sent survey questionnaires to 204 health planning agencies; 166 responded.[8] The report makes a distinction between "official" and "unofficial" decisions. Official decisions involve proposals duly submitted and acted upon by the health planning agencies. Unofficial decisions concern presubmission actions taken by the applicants, usually as a result of conferring with agency planners; such actions include not submitting the application, modifying the proposal, or deferring submission. During this three-year period, the agencies reviewed certificate-of-need proposals with a value of $12 billion, including $10.6 billion that were officially reviewed. Of the official reviews, proposals in the amount of $2.3 billion were disapproved (22 percent). Of the $1.4 billion proposals unofficially reviewed, $1.1 billion, or 79 percent, would probably have been disapproved had they been officially submitted. Of the 11,500 official new hospital bed requests made, 3,700 were disapproved (32 percent), while 24 percent of the 85,000 officially submitted requests for nursing home beds were denied. Adding the unofficially disapproved hospital beds (4,200) and nursing beds (29,000), the study concludes that more than $10 billion in operative costs would be saved in the 1980s by these agency decisions.[9] Even allowing for admitted limitations in the data, these findings show a far greater impact of certificate-of-need reviews on capital expenditures than had been revealed by the previous studies. This may be an indication that health planning agencies are beginning to mature; they have been most successful in developing their health plans with measurable goals and objectives precisely in those areas where most certificate-of-need requests are made: acute care beds, nursing home beds, and major medical equipment. National guidelines and standards have assisted health planning agencies in making their recommendations and decisions. Thus, it is possible that the agencies' use of certificate-of-need/ 1122 regulations is beginning to retard the expansion of capital expenditures.

Yet, an unpublished draft of a 1978 report by Rubel and Troyer-Merkel suggests that certificate-of-need regulations may not be having the large impact inferred by the AHPA's study.[10] That report expected $7 billion in capital spending in 1979, of which $1.6 billion was for new beds. They stated that "if there is no change in current policy (and that includes CON [certificate-of-need]/1122 regulations), capital spending in 1982 is expected to range from $9.2 billion to $11.6 billion, with at least 56,000 net new beds added to the system."[11] This will add to the operating costs of those additional units. In 1979, the $7 billion was expected to increase hospital operating costs by 4 percent. Thus, the optimistic picture of one report is countered by the pessimistic forecasts of a second.

A review by this writer of the data available from 12 northeastern health planning agencies' work programs shows that for 1979, 637 projects were reviewed. Of these, 563, or 88 percent, were approved, 7 percent were still pending, and only 5 percent were disapproved. These data are consistent with the Lewin findings as well as those suggested by the Rubel and Bice studies. These projects were valued at $252 million with $217.2 million (86 percent) approved, only $10.7 million disapproved or withdrawn (4 percent), and $24.5 million still pending.

In the most recent study of data still in the refinement stage, a 50 percent sample of certificate-of-need/1122 review decisions made in the United States for the period July, 1979–June, 1980 was made by the Certification Programs Branch of the Bureau of Health Planning. These data reveal that

- 63 percent of the proposed 7,270 hospital beds were approved.
- 84 percent of the proposed 23,053 nursing home beds were approved.
- 92 percent of the proposed $2.9 billion worth of hospital beds were approved.
- 95 percent of the proposed $1.5 billion of nursing home beds were approved.

While health planning agencies denied an increasing number of hospital and nursing bed proposals, there was an overwhelming tendency for them to approve the larger, more costly projects and reject the smaller, less expensive ones. When all proposals are considered (e.g., equipment, HMOs, and ambulatory services) planning agencies approved 93 percent of the 3,246 submitted.

Several points must be made about these data. First, 85 percent of the disapproved hospital beds are accounted for by only five states (Arizona, Florida, Nevada, Tennessee, and Texas). Second, six states (Florida, Indiana, Louisiana, Pennsylvania, Tennessee, and Virginia) accounted for 54 percent of the disapproved nursing home beds. This would indicate that the overwhelming majority of health planning agencies tend to approve most of the bed proposals submitted. Thus, while these data support the AHPA and Bice findings with respect to reduced bed expansion, they also support the findings of Rubel and this author that there continues to be a high rate of approvals.

Other data from this study reveal that regional and state health planning agencies agree in their decisions 96.5 percent of the time. It is also shown that 6.7 percent of the proposals were revised. It is not clear, however, whether revisions occurred in the presubmission phase or were withdrawn after submission and revised. One of the findings of the Lewin study, which is supported by the AHPA study, is that health planning agencies do, in fact, influence health providers during the presubmission phase to revise, withdraw, or recast their applications. If this occurs on a larger scale than noted by the Bureau of Health Planning's data, then the process may be working better than is indicated; many more proposals may have been withdrawn or scaled down than would have occurred otherwise. Since the bureau's information is still tentative, it is hoped that future findings will show trends of whether certificate-of-need/1122 reviews truly result in cost containment and where in the process the planning agencies have the most impact: in the presubmission phase, during the course of the review, or in the appeal/litigation stage. In spite of the increasingly rich data on certificate of need, it is still not possible to form a consensus of the true impact of these regulations as a strategy for containing the rise of medical costs.

Issues Involved

There are a number of issues involved in certificate-of-need/1122 strategy, e.g., methodology, determination of need, data base, and linkage to health plans.

Methodology

No methodology has as yet been fully accepted by all researchers studying certificate-of-need/1122 data. Whether new data are developed, as in the AHPA and Lewin surveys, or whether pooled multiple regression analyses are made of previously collected data, as by Bice and Salkever, there is little uniformity in the type of data collected, the period of time for which they are collected, and the manner of statistical manipulation. This makes it very difficult to compare results, establish trends, or determine the significance of findings. Whether health economists should be optimistic over the findings of the AHPA study or pessimistic over the research done by Bice and Salkever cannot truly be determined. Agreement must be reached on methodology to be employed in carrying out future research.

Determination of Need

An important part of cost containment strategy rests primarily on the judgments of health planning agencies about whether particular proposals meet some health need in the region or state. Up to this date, no quantified standards have been fully agreed upon respecting the need for medical facilities or services. Even the 11 standards promulgated in the *National Health Guidelines* on the need for acute care hospital beds and use of specialized medical technology such as computerized axial tomography (CAT) scanners and renal dialysis units are issued as guidance statements only. Most state Hill-Burton plans had previously used some variation of the four beds per 1,000 population as a standard, but the Lewin study clearly documents how that standard was often disregarded. Exceptions were continually made to circumvent state plan standards. It will be much more difficult to set standards for other services and medical procedures where there is less consensus and acceptance of a standard. Is an input measure such as bed capacity or number of CAT scan procedures a better measure of need than an output measure such as mortality, reduced morbidity, length of stay, or duration of a patient's illness? What standards should be set for the care of those afflicted with behavioral problems, such as mental illness or alcoholism? With increasing emphasis on positive health, how can this ambiguous and undefined concept be measured? by the number of miles or laps persons run or swim each week? by their capacity to carry out their basic functions in life? or by some measure of their satisfaction with life? In short, while crude measures of need are used in making judgments about important certificate-of-need/1122 proposals, no one should be deluded that these seemingly scientific and technical measures really offer the guidance review committees need. It is not surprising that these committees put so much faith in their collective, subjective judgments in making certificate-of-need decisions.

Data Base

It is also difficult to obtain valid and reliable data on which to base judgments. Only 166 of the 204 health planning agencies responded to the AHPA survey. Were these self-selected? Were the data submitted by the agencies based on a similar statistical format? For example, the AHPA study stated that

> another source of confusion in the . . . reporting is the categorization of projects reported—into a "hospital beds" proposal, or a "hospital renovation" proposal. . . . Many projects actually involved more than one type of proposal, but where the types and costs were not separable, they were coded into only one category. Hence the figures showing the *results by category* . . . are rough.[12] (Emphasis added.)

All studies are faced with the limitations of the data available, coding consistency, and reliability. Researchers, aware of these data problems, usually identify the limitations of their study's findings or the conditions under which the data and the findings ought to be interpreted. Although planners involved in certificate-of-need evaluations are in reality action-oriented researchers, they usually lack the knowledge or capacity to interpret the data properly, and they may have a tendency to accept the validity and reliability of the data too easily. This, of course, may well influence review committee members who rely upon professional staff for technical guidance and may result in their unwittingly making poor decisions.

Linkage of Review Decisions to Health Plans

One reason that the development of health plans is so important is that planning agencies must use high-priority goals and objectives as one major basis for making review decisions. Through research, analysis, and a democratic decision-making process involved in plan development, it was hoped that there would be sound factual and technical bases, in addition to community values, on which to determine the need for a proposed service. However, because so many of the goals and objectives are couched in general terms, tend to have limited measurability, or do not pertain to the proposal, the agency's review committee often cannot use the health plan as a basis for review decisions. Further, the difference in orientation and thinking between planners and regulators often produces an antagonistic environment that inhibits coordination and dilutes the strength of each. Further, health planning agencies tend to lodge planning and review activities in separate divisions, each with its own director.

This structural separation creates a situation in which each can readily ignore the other's activities. Thus, while linkage between planning and regulation is considered essential, it is the unusual agency that can actually forge this linkage into a cooperative relationship between the professionals and their lay committees when considering certificate-of-need/1122 decisions.

PROPOSED USES OF FEDERAL FUNDS

A variant of the certificate-of-need/1122 strategy, proposed uses of federal funds (PUFF) are to be reviewed by regional health planning agencies "for the development, expansion, or support of health resources" and "shall be consistent with and will help to implement the plans" of the planning agencies.[13] Funds are provided as grants, contracts, loans, or loan guarantees under the Public Health Service Act, the Community Mental Health Centers Act, and the Comprehensive Alcohol Abuse and Alcoholism Prevention, Treatment, and Rehabilitation Act of 1970. Such funds are also made available from allotments to states, which in turn give grants to develop, expand, and support regional health services. Most of the discussion about certificates of need also applies to PUFF; however, there are a few major differences.

Coordination of Reviews

Since proposals funded under PUFF may also require a certificate of need, the health planning agency's review procedures and criteria should be similar enough to those for a certificate of need that both reviews can be made simultaneously. This is an important consideration because applicants for PUFF funds are usually under strict federal deadlines. Planning agencies have 60 days to review a PUFF proposal unless they require a longer time, and the provider agrees to the extension. In most cases, the provider agrees to give the agency more time so that the 60-day limit may not be held as often as the regulations had intended. If a certificate of need is required and the PUFF funds result in competing proposals, they are batched so that similar applications are reviewed together within a six-month schedule. In New York State, six or more months are needed to complete reviews of batched applications. Consequently, it becomes important that this consideration be taken into account when simultaneous certificate-of-need and PUFF reviews are mandated by regulation.

Involvement of More Than One Health Planning Agency

Some proposals may involve one or more health service areas, such as migrant health grants, the National Health Service Corps program, crippled children's services, or specialized medical facility programs. When more than one planning agency's service area is involved, then one agency becomes the lead, or coordinating, agency and the others submit their recommendations to it. This responsibility falls on the planning agency in the area from which a health provider will administer the program. If a majority of the services are to be provided in a health service area other than the one from which the program is administered, however, then that planning agency may be assigned coordinating responsibility. When a planning agency disapproves a program for its service area, that portion of the funds designated for the program in its area will not be used. The secretary of HHS, upon request of the applicant, will decide how to allocate those funds.

Programs Subject to Review

The secretary of HHS is periodically required to list those federal programs subject to review. However, the listing of a program does not necessarily mean that all parts of it must be reviewed, nor does the fact that a program is not listed mean that it is not subject to review. The list is to guide health planning agencies. Federal funding agencies are expected to inform health planning agencies which of their programs are subject to review. Also, the planning agencies can request such information from the federal agencies. As a general rule, three criteria guide the health planning agencies in determining which federal programs are subject to review:

a) Whether the proposed use falls under one of the four Acts.
b) Whether it is a grant, contract, loan or loan guarantee or a proposed use made available from allotment funds through grant or contract.
c) Whether it would develop, expand, or support health resources as defined in these regulations.[14]

A large number of PUFF applications are for noncompeting continuation grants. To reduce the workload of planning agencies, such applications are subject to review under only four conditions:

1. The health planning agency asks to review the application.
2. The proposal has a 20 percent or more change in its funding level.

3. There will be a major change in the service program, as determined by the applicant or the federal funding agency.
4. It has been five years since the last review.

Over 40 programs that may require either a regional or state level health planning agency review have been listed. Examples of federal programs subject to regional review are

- drug abuse community service programs
- mental health—children's services
- alcoholism demonstration program
- community mental health centers—service support
- medical facilities construction—project grants
- family planning projects
- emergency medical services
- home health services program
- maternal and infant projects
- urban rat control project grants
- venereal disease control grants
- HMO development

PUFF grants subject to state review are

- crippled children's services (state plan and application for allotment grant)
- state medical facilities plan and application for allotment grant
- comprehensive public health services health incentive formula grants (state plan and application)
- state plan required by Section 237, Community Mental Health Centers Act
- alcohol formula grants (state plan and application for allotment grants)

The state agency reviews only the state plan and application based on allotments to which it is entitled. However, since most of the service programs involve regions within the state, any requests to use allotment funds for regional services require a PUFF review. This means that two reviews are required, one for the state plan and a second for the individual projects funded under the allotments.

Written Notification of Beginning of a Review

PUFF review procedures are stricter in requiring that the applicant be given notice of the beginning of a review than are certificate-of-need review procedures. Under the latter, a planning agency may delay the beginning of a review until it has sufficient information to make an evaluation. Under PUFF procedures, written notification cannot be delayed. Should the planning agency determine that it does not have sufficient information to make a review, the agency may disapprove the application. On the other hand, should the planning agency fail to make a decision on a PUFF application by the end of the 60-day period, the federal agency may make its own decision without regard to the planning agency. This more rigid schedule is necessitated by the federal agency's own tight review schedule. Federal review committees or panels almost always have experts from all over the United States who come together for brief two- or three-day periods to review PUFF proposals. Since they meet only two or three times per year, they must make decisions based on applications before them.

Submission of Information to the Planning Agency

Federal agencies and regional planning agencies generally require different types of information from applicants. Federal agencies are interested mainly in the technical merits of the proposal and the capacity of the applicant to carry it out as proposed. Planning agencies are more concerned with whether the proposal is consistent with planning goals and objectives, how it meets the needs of the populations it serves, the cost-benefit of the service compared to alternatives, and the impact on the costs of health services. To ensure that both types of information are provided, the planning agency may also request the information required by the federal agency, provided it informs the applicant in advance of the information needed. By giving the applicant advance notice, the planning agency may be able to reduce the number of times it is forced to disapprove an application because it lacks the complete data needed for review.

Approval/Disapproval of Applications

Unlike certificate-of-need reviews where conditions may be placed on proposals, a planning agency must approve or disapprove a PUFF proposal with no conditions. If an applicant asks for a review of a disapproved proposal within 15 days of notification, then the secretary of HHS is required to make a review and asks the state health planning agency for its comments. The applicant, in asking for the secretary's review, must provide justification for approval by answering in detail the written reasons for disapproval offered by the regional planning agency. The secretary's decision is final and is generally based on four criteria:

1. whether the planning agency adhered to its own review procedures and thus showed fairness to the applicant.
2. whether the agency's decision was consistent with its established review criteria. Since these have been previously approved and widely circulated, the agency cannot change its criteria for a specific application. This, again, is to ensure consistency and fairness in the review.
3. whether the disapproval harms the health status of the residents of the health service area(s). This is to ensure that bias or prejudice does not interfere with the provision of health services to needy and/ or underserved populations within the region.
4. whether the proposal meets a national or regional need that cannot be provided elsewhere. For example, some end-stage renal dialysis networks cover more than one state, especially in sparsely settled populations of the West. Disapproval of such a service may adversely affect those persons with this potentially fatal disease unless service is guaranteed.

It should be noted that when Congress gave the secretary of HHS the authority to override a PUFF disapproval, it did so with the intent that this authority would be used infrequently. Congress intended that planning agencies retain the authority to determine the health services needed by the residents of their service areas.

PUFF Review Process

PUFF applications, unlike certificates of need, are generally reviewed at the regional level. The state becomes involved in two circumstances. If a regional planning agency disapproves a PUFF application, the state planning agency provides comments for the secretary's consideration in making a final decision. However, where a regional planning agency disapproves a grant request for approved state allotment funds, it is the governor and not the secretary who makes the final decision, after receiving advice and comments from the state health planning agency. Figure 7-2 illustrates a typical review process.

PUFF Review Issues

In addition to issues discussed under certificate-of-need/1122 strategy, there are a few other issues peculiar to PUFF reviews.

Figure 7-2 Decision Sequence for Reviews Involving Multiple Health Systems Agencies (HSAs)

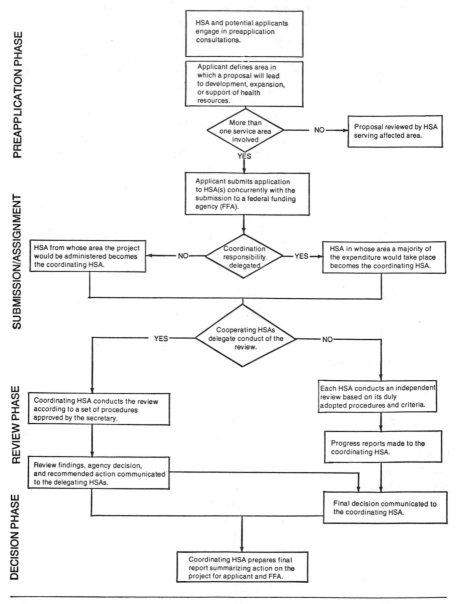

Source: Bureau of Health Planning, HHS. Prepared by the Institute for Health Planning, April 1980, p. 16.

Approval/Disapproval

The fact that no conditions can be placed on PUFF applications necessitates much greater preapplication discussion between the two parties to ensure that the proposal meets regional as well as federal intent and that the application is complete. A very good application with one or more minor deficiencies that could readily be resolved during the implementation of the program is more likely to be disapproved under PUFF than under certificate-of-need reviews. Because there is heavy competition for federal funds, an applicant whose proposal was disapproved may not get a second chance to apply for these funds. On the other hand, if a planning agency approves an application with obvious deficiencies, then it will not usually have an opportunity to influence applicants to correct their programs' shortcomings at a later date. Thus, both sides have a problem that is not readily resolved under an either/or decision mechanism, except by appeal to a higher authority, the secretary of HHS or the governor. However, except for the most important reasons, even they will not normally override an agency's disapproval. This calls therefore for a close agency-applicant relationship in the development of PUFF proposals.

Technical versus Need Review Criteria

Closely related to the approval/disapproval issue is the problem of the distinction between technical and need criteria. Under PL 93-641 (Sec. 1532), health planning agencies are required to consider technical criteria, such as whether less costly alternative services have been considered or whether a proposal fits in with the existing health services, in rendering their decisions. Yet, the regulations call for health planning agencies to limit their reviews to a proposal's conformity with regional health plans and not the technical and scientific merits of the proposal. It is obvious that there is a gray area concerning what a technical criterion is. The more the planning agencies encroach on what the federal agencies consider their domain of expertise, the greater the potential for conflict between the agencies. It would seem that this issue can be resolved only on a case-by-case basis and over a lengthy period of time. The difficulty of resolving such issues is evidenced by the fact that, more than five years after the passage of PL 93-641, no decision has been made to define when research or training programs, especially those funded by the National Institutes of Health, significantly change the health delivery services of a region and are thus subject to review. Although there is general agreement that the goal of PUFF applications is to improve and expand regional health services, this end may be tangled in the means to achieve it when different autonomous agencies, health planning agencies and federal funding agencies, attempt to control how that goal will be met.

APPROPRIATENESS REVIEW

The third regulatory function bestowed on health planning agencies is appropriateness review. It is the newest, the most threatening, and the most challenging. No one really knows what it is, whether it will work, or its true impact on the health care system. It is based on two brief paragraphs of PL 93-641. Section 1513(g) states:

> . . . each health planning agency shall review on a periodic basis (but at least every five years) all institutional health services offered in the health service area of the agency and shall make recommendations to the State health planning . . . agency . . . respecting the appropriateness in the area of such services.

The first review must be completed within three years, and the state is required to make its findings public within one year of the completion of the review by the regional health planning agencies. Essentially, appropriateness review is to *existing* health services what certificate-of-need review is to *new* institutional health services. Since the services already exist, the planning agency cannot ask the politically explosive question, Are such services needed? Rather, it asks whether they are appropriate.

Definition of Appropriateness

Never given an explicit definition of its own, appropriateness review is defined by what it does. "A finding of 'appropriateness' means a finding that a service meets the needs of a population, in accordance with the criteria development. . . ."[15] This makes the definition of criteria, i.e., availability, accessibility, quality, acceptability, continuity, and cost, basic to the meaning of appropriateness. In other words, appropriateness cannot be more explicitly defined until these important characteristics of the health care system are defined. Then, a reviewer might ask whether a specific health service was available, accessible, etc. Since these questions must be asked of *all* existing institutional health services, it can be readily perceived that the state of the art is simply too crude to provide standards regarding, for example, the acceptability of a community mental health center service or home health care. It is because of the immense complexity of appropriateness review that the term has been deliberately left vague at this stage of planning development.

Goal of Appropriateness Review

Appropriateness review can be either a planning tool or a regulatory tool. As a planning tool, it can be used to uncover deficiencies in the health care system with respect to the six characteristics noted previously. If appropriateness review showed a lack of primary care services in the health service area, the health plan would normally be modified to take this finding into account. On the other hand, appropriateness review can be used as a tool to identify inadequacies of specific hospitals, rehabilitation facilities, or nursing homes and the services provided by them. Although the findings are intended to be recommendations to the state health planning agency, their publication threatens institutions. As one critic of appropriateness review states, "AR [appropriateness review] will be a costly enterprise, but the largest costs may not be in dollars, but in prestige and influence" to the health institutions.[16] The Bureau of Health Planning gives no clear-cut picture of appropriateness review, describing it as "an extension of the health planning process"[17] in which the health plan is improved by the findings, which in turn serve as important aids in rendering regulatory certificate-of-need/1122 decisions and improving the health care system. However, since there are twin goals in the everyday utilization of appropriateness review, there is strong institutional concern that federal officials, more concerned with cost than with quality of care, may opt to emphasize the regulatory goal of cost containment as a way of reducing duplication and eliminating inefficient, obsolete, or underutilized institutional services. Only experience can determine whether the goals will complement each other or be in conflict.

Process of Appropriateness Review

Basically, the state health planning agency, with the cooperation of the regional agencies, will take the lead to

- establish the definitions of services to be reviewed
- determine the priorities among the services
- set the schedule for the reviews

The first round of reviews must be completed within three years; subsequent reviews must be made at least every five years. The services to be reviewed are those in private and public hospitals, rehabilitation facilities, and nursing homes. Services in other institutions, such as HMOs, kidney dialysis centers, and ambulatory surgery facilities, may be reviewed on an optional basis. If the state agency fails to begin appropriateness reviews within the required six-month period, then the regional agencies may come together to develop their own work program and schedule of activities.

The state agency takes the further responsibility of notifying the institutions to be reviewed of the type and kind of data needed for the review. Within six months from the time the institutions have been notified of the beginning of the review, the review must be completed and recommendations submitted by the regional agencies to the state. Reviews must be areawide rather than institution-specific, i.e., all the services of the same type located in a health service area must be reviewed together. For example, are there enough intermediate nursing care beds? Are they accessible to all segments of the population? Can everyone afford them? Are they acceptable to the residents who use them? Do they guarantee continuity of care so that patients can obtain other types of medical care as needed? Although deficiencies must be cited for the service as a whole, regional planning agencies have the option of also making institution-specific findings. When published, the findings are accompanied by a series of recommendations for dealing with the deficiencies. The procedures and criteria used for undertaking appropriateness reviews are the same as those that apply to certificate-of-need and PUFF reviews, with some minor exceptions.

Issues

Impact on Provider Institutions

There is a major concern that appropriateness review is really a weak form of decertification of health facilities. Because of the opposition of the American Hospital Association (AHA) to the initial bill, which included "decertification of excess hospital capacity," this was watered down from a mandatory decertification to a voluntary action by the institution.[18] Nonetheless, because the watered down version requires publication of findings, the AHA views this as a form of coercion. Since a positive and cooperative relationship between provider institutions and health planning agencies is essential, it is feared that conflict over appropriateness findings may develop into an antagonistic relationship that will disrupt or retard the work of the planning agencies. On the other hand, federal officials view appropriateness review "as an excellent opportunity for providers and planning agencies to assess cooperatively the current health care system and to make changes which can benefit the community."[19] Thus, each side views appropriateness review from its own perspective: health providers from their concern at what might happen to their own institutions (self-interest) and federal officials and planning agencies from their concern for what might happen to the community (public interest). This difference can be resolved only after several years of actual practice.

Capacity of Planning Agencies to Carry Out Appropriateness Review

There is general concern expressed by the numerous comments submitted in response to the notice of the proposed federal regulations that the planning agencies do not have the personnel, expertise, and experience to carry out such a complex and vast undertaking as appropriateness review in the short period of three years. Federal funding for health planning is being challenged by opponents to PL 93-641. They are trying to curtail the size of the planning budgets. Because of their political influence, professional associations may succeed in holding down or reducing funds for planning. Should this occur, it will be increasingly difficult for the already overburdened agencies to carry out their PUFF functions and certificate-of-need reviews, and to implement their plans at the same time. Proponents agree that more funds are needed to carry out appropriateness reviews, but feel that it is necessary to "conduct [only] a selected number of reviews annually" because there "has to be the planned elimination of existent excess capacity" and this will "not be accomplished without actual or threatened outside intervention."[20] They believe appropriateness review should focus on high-priority areas contained in the health plans and that it should be institution-specific rather than areawide. However, the federal regulations make it explicit that, whether the agencies are ready or not, they are obligated to carry out an appropriateness review for *all* designated institutions within a three-year period. The attitude expressed in the regulations is that, as the agencies gain experience in this first review cycle, future cycles will be completed more efficiently, with greater sensitivity to both the public and private interests.

Obtaining the Necessary Data

Appropriateness review depends on provider institutions to submit data needed to develop criteria and standards for the various system characteristics of availability, accessibility, and cost. However, many states do not have legislation that will compel institutions to supply data if they refuse. At the same time, in order to avoid duplication, planning agencies are explicitly forbidden to develop their own data without HHS approval. Without these data, agencies will be forced either to make reviews on limited, unreliable, and fragmented data or to forego making the reviews at all. While it is too early to know how the provider institutions will respond to planning agencies' requests for data, the nature of that response will indicate how cooperative they plan to be in the appropriateness review process. Because the appropriateness review process is just getting under way, it is too soon to anticipate the impact of the reviews on the health system as a whole or on the specific institutions that comprise it.

PROFESSIONAL STANDARDS REVIEW ORGANIZATION

Another element in the effort to implement changes in the health care system is the Professional Standards Review Organization (PSRO). Its twin emphases are on improving the efficiency and increasing the quality of care. PL 93-603, passed in 1972 as Title XI of the Social Security Act, was enacted because of congressional dissatisfaction with the existing medical utilization reviews set up by hospitals to ensure that care provided to Medicaid and Medicare patients was both necessary and of good quality. Rather than relying on hospitals to police themselves, the PSRO legislation created autonomous, outside organizations to monitor the quality of care in an objective manner.

PSROs pass through three stages: (1) a planning stage, in which the focus is on the development of the structure and organization of the PSRO; (2) the conditional stage, in which PSROs have up to four years to prove their capacity to operate in an efficient and effective manner in carrying out the mandate of the law; and (3) the fully designated stage, in which they have demonstrated their ability to meet the requirements of the law. Within two years after being fully designated, a PSRO must begin to review ambulatory services.

The board of the PSRO is composed almost exclusively of physicians. Where three or more PSROs are active and established in a state, a statewide PSRO council is formed.

Goals

The two goals of PSROs (cost containment and improved quality) created a conflict from the very beginning because of the difference in the emphasis given them by the two main bodies involved in implementation of the program. Physicians, who were to comprise the dominant constituency of the board of directors of the local PSROs, conceived the program as a means of raising the quality of care while HEW and the president's Office of Management and Budget (OMB) focused on cost containment. While in theory these two goals complement each other, in practice they tend to clash. Raising the quality of care usually results in increased costs. Reducing the number of days of unneeded hospitalization; using less expensive, but equally effective, medical procedures; and providing a lower level, appropriate service, such as outpatient care, are fostered by HEW and OMB as ways of reducing costs without jeopardizing quality. Section 1151, Title XI of the Social Security Act spells out the mandate of the law.

> . . . that payment for such services will be made—(1) only when, and to the extent, medically necessary, as determined in the exercise of reasonable limits of professional discretion; and (2) in the case of services provided by a hospital or other health care facility on an inpatient basis, only when and for such period as such services, cannot, consistent with professionally recognized health care standards, effectively be provided on an outpatient basis or more economically in an inpatient health care facility of a different type, as determined in the exercise of reasonable limits of professional discretion.

PSRO Process:

To carry out this mandate, three review components were established:

1. concurrent review. In this review, eligibility for admission is determined by comparing the patient's diagnosis to established criteria of the medical need for hospitalization. If admitted, the patient is permitted to stay a certified period of time, according to the diagnosis and specific norms of care. Extensions beyond that time require approval by the PSRO. Failure to comply results in nonpayment by Medicaid, Medicare, or Maternal and Child Health Programs for all days not certified and authorized.
2. retrospective review. Also known as medical care evaluation (MCE), retrospective review is used to assess whether previously determined criteria for medical need and accepted standards of care were met. Failure of physicians or hospital units to meet such standards usually calls for educational remediation to assist in their future compliance.
3. profile analysis. Statistical analysis is applied to aggregate data collected on patient care. Patterns of utilization by specific diagnostic categories, mortality rates, and morbidity rates are examined and compared with area norms. Sharp deviations call for analysis of the causes and eventual resolution.

PSROs have put the most emphasis on concurrent review and the least on profile analysis at this stage of their development.

PSROs either delegate the responsibility to a hospital to carry out the three review components or, if the hospital refuses or is judged unable to assume the responsibility, the PSRO will do the reviews itself. About 80 percent of the review responsibility is delegated to hospitals.[21] Where the review function is delegated, PSROs take on a largely monitoring, evaluative, and educational role. As of 1979, of the 195 areas designated for a PSRO, 186 PSROs held conditional status, 3 were in a planning state, and 6 were still unfunded. Of the 5,524 short-stay hospitals with patients paid out of federal funds, 82 percent were covered by PSRO reviews.[22]

Sanctions

Three kinds of sanctions are used to ensure compliance with PSRO standards. (1) PSROs can disapprove health services and thereby deny federal payment; (2) individual hospitals or physicians who fail to comply with PSRO mandates can be suspended or excluded from the program, or they can be forced to return excess payment they have already received for services; or (3) HHS can terminate its contract with a PSRO for failing to carry out its agreement. When this occurs, the state PSRO council will attempt to find a substitute organization to assume the PSRO responsibilities.[23]

PSRO Issues

PSROs have been embroiled in controversy since their inception. As one writer has stated, "For reasons that are not entirely clear, the PSRO program has been subjected to a greater evaluation effort than any other federal program in history."[24]

Quality of Care versus Cost Containment

It has been noted that two potentially incompatible goals were mandated in the PSRO legislation. Blumstein points out that there is a subtle, but important, distinction between Congress' concern with "waste" of health care services and cost containment. He points out that PSROs may reduce waste (by reducing the length of stay, by denying inappropriate admissions, or by raising questions about the use of certain ineffective medical procedures) but at the same time PSROs may foster the use of high-cost technology that may have only a minor impact on the patient's condition and thereby raise the cost of care.[25] Physicians, not necessarily motivated to reduce waste, would resist any effort to lower the quality of care they offer, as measured by their use of the latest medical technology. This would directly threaten their status, prestige, and income. The OMB has seen few cost reductions resulting from the PSRO program; at one point, the OMB recommended the program's elimination from the 1979 budget, but lost out on the HHS secretary's direct appeal to the president.[26] Because the program appears to have more antagonists than proponents, its future will continue to be clouded until it shows conclusive evidence that both its cost and quality goals can be reached.

Development of Standards

It is important that clear-cut, measurable standards be developed so that decisions can be consistent with professional usage. There are three types of measures:

1. norms, defined as typical professional practices, or what is.
2. criteria, defined as guidelines against which every day practice is measured, or what ought to be.
3. standards, defined as professionally developed measures that fall within a zone of acceptance based on a norm or criterion, or how much professional practice can deviate from a standard and still be considered acceptable.[27]

The real issue is who defines the criteria and standards. The norms are self-defined because they are based on actual practice. Originally, HHS and its PSRO national council were to be responsible for developing the criteria and standards. However, under pressure of physicians and the American Medical Association (AMA), it was decided to let each local PSRO set its own. This, of course, makes it difficult to compare one PSRO region with another, since there are no common criteria or standards. On the other hand, there may be valid reasons for different regions of the United States to have varying standards. Temperature differences, cultural traditions in the use of medical services, income, availability of physician services, and physician practices all have a bearing on who uses medical services and how these services are used. Thus, the PSRO program is caught between national criteria and standards that are questionable, and local criteria and standards that are valid and reliable but not amenable to interregional comparison.

Expectations of Cost Containment

It may be that too much is expected of PSROs in reducing cost. A Health Care Financing Administration (HCFA) evaluation of PSROs clearly shows that 65 percent of hospital cost increases from 1970 to 1978 were due to inflation; 29 percent, to greater service intensity, i.e., more costly medical technology and associated personnel costs. Only 6 percent was due to population growth.[28] Since quality of care is generally related to the more intense use of medical technology, it is not likely that PSROs can have much impact on that area of cost increase. In fact, their push would be in the opposite direction. By denying unnecessary care to some of the 6 percent population increase, PSROs may have a small impact on that component of cost increase. However, even a major impact on this element would show only a marginal change in the overall escalation of medical costs. The PSRO program was designed to affect hospital utilization, not how hospitals use medical technology. Whether these impacts are of sufficient importance for Congress to retain the program is a value judgment, not a technical issue. Congress must determine whether the small decrease in "wasted" resources is sufficient to offset the increased costs of higher quality of care in order to continue the program. The program should be judged by what it can reasonably be expected to accomplish, not by some inflated notion that exaggerates its potential.

Status Quo versus Innovations

PSROs are designed to maintain the status quo in medicine. Criteria and standards are generally set close to the actual practice of physicians. "Normal" measures cannot be expected to change significantly as a result of PSRO activity. Further, PSROs do not make choices between one mode of care and another. For example, their emphasis is on diagnosis and treatment services; they do not involve themselves with health promotion or prevention services that may have a greater impact on the diseases under study. By limiting themselves to diagnosis and treatment "after the fact," they also limit their impact on mortality or morbidity rates for specified diseases. The innovations they can foster are circumscribed by the medical care system. They may encourage greater use of HMOs, home health care services, ambulatory surgery, supervised physician's assistants in place of higher cost and potentially less appropriate medical care. Within their boundaries, the PSROs can opt for medical innovations, but they cannot make the political decisions on cost and quality goals that can better be met by some nonmedical intervention.

Outcome

Although it is too early to determine the effectiveness of the program, annual evaluations have been carried out to assess the program.[29] Most of the data in this section are based on HCFA's 1979 assessment report. Measures used to reveal changes in the program are average length of stay and total days of care by diagnosis. The HCFA study compared active and inactive PSROs of aged Medicare beneficiaries by region:

The results of the regional analysis show that PSRO areas in the Northeast and North Central regions have a statistically significant impact in reducing the Medicare days of care rate. The PSRO impact in the West region is in the direction of reducing days of care but does not attain statistical significance. In the South region . . . PSRO activity apparently contributes to a significant increase in the days of care rate.[30]

In regard to Medicare days of hospital care, 948,430 days, or 1.7 percent, were saved in 1978. Over 950,000 days in the Northeast and 325,000 days in the North Central regions were saved, but these were offset by an increase of 450,000 days in the South. The West showed a small decrease of 115,000 days saved.

In a study of four surgical procedures (hysterectomy, cataract surgery, cholecystectomy, and breast cancer surgery) and one diagnosis (acute myocardial infarction) for the period 1973–1977, it was concluded that active PSROs had a lower utilization rate than inactive PSROs; these rates were statistically significant for four of the five instances. There was a decline in the utilization rate for all conditions except hysterectomy, which showed no significant difference. The results of these findings must be accepted with caution, as the study may contain sampling errors and coding inaccuracies. At best, the findings can be accepted as a beginning trend.[31]

Finally, with respect to cost-benefits, the report shows an estimated saving of $21 million in Medicare expenditures over the cost of operating the PSRO program.[32] While this figure is encouraging, most of the data are preliminary and thus subject to change. Chassin's review of the literature on a number of small area utilization studies shows that the "impact of UR on hospital utilization and costs are . . . inconclusive. Some studies suggest that this technique may reduce hospitalization; others suggest it has no effect. None is sufficiently valid to enable any firm conclusions to be drawn."[33] This review involved studies completed before the passage of PSRO legislation and during the early years of the program. The consistency of these findings with the 1978 PSRO findings leads to the conclusion that it is still too early to determine the effectiveness of the program.

RATE SETTING

Based on the assumption that hospitals lack incentives to curb costs if they are allowed rates sufficient to cover their previous year's expenditures (retrospective rate setting), Congress and various state governments developed a new system of reimbursement. This form of payment, known as prospective rate setting, is defined as "any means for determining the financial remuneration of hospitals whereby the amounts to be paid for specified units of service are established by some external authority *prior* to the period in which the services are to be given."[34] (Emphasis added.) The strategy is based on the notion that, if hospitals are given incentives to do so, they will become more efficient in the use of resources and thus operate at lower costs than they would have without these incentives. Planners envision transferring funds saved by more efficient hospital operation to the development of other high-priority programs. In this way, they foresee a link between cost containment in one sector of the medical system and the creation of quality programs in other sectors.

Forces Pressing for Rate-Setting Mechanisms

For a variety of different reasons, a number of primary actors have supported rate setting. Legislators, concerned with out-of-control rises in Medicaid payments, have pressed for a mechanism that could help them forecast the future year's cost of hospital services. Blue Cross programs, fearful that the rapidly rising costs of hospital care would bankrupt them, have favored such mechanisms. State insurance commissions have also been concerned with the potential insolvencies they foresee with the rapid rise of hospital costs. Consumers, especially middle-class families, have been concerned about rising tax rates and have supported any strategy that controls the costs of any tax-supported program, including those that involve hospitals. Hospitals themselves have supported rate-setting commissions. Their professional association has claimed that hospitals have been made the scapegoat of rising medical costs and that these costs are really outside hospitals' capacity to control. It believes independent, rate-setting commissions would relieve the pressure placed on hospitals. Such a commission could also be a third party to support hospital's efforts in rejecting suggestions by physicians for medical technology that they either do not need or cannot support. Thus, a strong constituency has developed to support the rate-setting experiments Congress authorized in PL 93-641.

Methods for Setting the Rates

Rate setting can be based on a per diem, per admission, or per specific service basis. While hospitals will closely monitor changes in any of these rates, they may offset lower per diem rates by increasing the number of patient days. Some states, such as Maryland and Washington, set total allowable revenues per hospital. This requires the rate-setting commission to specify what the marginal (or variable) cost of a unit of service is. As Abernethy and Pearson point out, "if a hospital gains (or loses) only the marginal costs associated with an increase (or decrease) in volume, there is a smaller incentive toward volume increases, and a positive incentive toward volume decreases. This occurs because the revenue per admission will increase as volume decreases, as only the marginal cost of reduction is subtracted from total revenue."[35]

While these are the basic units for evaluating an individual hospital, rate-setting commissions have used one of three methods for determining the prospective budgets for hospitals.[36]

1. cost-budget reviews. These are line-item reviews of each hospital's budget for additions to personnel, facilities, and services, as well as cost trends by departments. Through negotiation with each hospital, a final budget for the coming year is determined. Hospital administrators are free to shift funds as long as the bottom line amount remains the same. This scrutiny tends to make hospitals more cost conscious.
2. interhospital comparisons. Hospitals are grouped into categories based on size, type, and other such characteristics. Analyses of each hospital's service, department, or cost center are made in order to find a measure of central tendency, such as mean or median, for each hospital group. Budgets are then set at some specified point in the range of hospitals in the group. Those beyond the set cut-off point usually have their rates adjusted downward to the predetermined ceiling.
3. limitation of rate increases to the rate of inflation. In this method, an index or set of economic indicators is developed to measure changes in the general economy of the region. At quarterly or semiannual periods, adjustments are made in the hospital budgets to take into account these economic changes. New York, Massachusetts, and Western Pennsylvania use this method.

Rate-Setting Issues

There are a number of issues associated with prospective rate setting.

Noninvolvement of Physicians

Probably the most important issue is that physicians, heavily involved in PSROs, are not asked to participate in prospective rate setting. This is unfortunate, since physicians generate most of the costs in hospital care. The main targets for hospital cost control are management; hospital staff, facilities, and equipment; underutilized beds; and inefficiencies in supportive services.[37] None of these involve physicians. It may be that physicians already view themselves as heavily involved in quality and utilization review and feel they do not have time for other aspects of operating the hospital. If that is the case, then it becomes essential for the two programs to be more closely coordinated.

Incentives for Controlling Costs

Although most rate-setting programs have incentives for hospitals to reduce costs by allowing them to keep a part of the savings, in reality it pays for them to spend to the ceiling of their total budgets and a little beyond, if they can manage to do so legitimately through appeals or any other means. This is because, as Bauer points out, an "institution's future rates are calculated primarily on the base of its historical and current year spending; to reduce this spending base would, therefore, run completely counter to its long-run interests."[38] Since a hospital will get a bigger budget based on its previous year's spending habits, the pressure is to spend rather than save money during the year, particularly if its state commission has a history of rejecting appeals.

Rate Setting and Innovation

Setting rates based on the previous year's experience tends to discourage innovations. A number of states, such as New York, do not allow start-up costs for innovations in the first year. If innovations fail to generate sufficient income to cover initial costs, hospitals will be forced to use funds from other cost centers to make up losses in the new programs. Thus, if there is some doubt that innovations, such as hospital-based home health care, ambulatory surgery, or renal dialysis centers, will pay for themselves in a relatively brief period of time, then hospitals with limited or no reserves may not be willing to risk the operation of their more successful divisions. This, of course, may become a negative factor in health planning agencies' efforts to influence hospitals to expand their services in accordance with some of the high-priority goals of the regional health plans.

Setting Hospital Rates

One of the real problems is setting hospital rates at a level that will encourage efficiency in service and still permit hospitals to function properly within their budget ceilings. If the rate is set too low, the hospital will either have to cut low-volume, but necessary services or reduce the quality of efficient services. Appeals can be made to change the rate, but if the appeal is denied, the hospital may go bankrupt. This has already happened to many marginal hospitals. In many cases, these beds represent an overall surplus for the region, however, and rate setting is merely one strategy used by the state to force them to close, convert, or integrate with stronger hospitals.

Hospitals that have a higher ceiling than is really needed will, in effect, be overpaid. This sometimes happens because a hospital may have a less complex case mix than comparison hospitals, the case mix becomes less complex over time, or the hospital becomes more efficient in its operation.[39] The nature of the rate-setting process is such that this type of change is not readily detected nor sought in the analysis of hospital budgets, and hospitals are not likely to call attention to such changes that work in their favor.

Outcomes of Rate Setting

A number of studies have been completed regarding the effects of rate setting on cost savings. Different studies come to different conclusions, however. Bauer concludes that "experience during the 1970s indicates that in and of itself, hospital rate setting is by no means the way to salvation."[40] The development of rate setting is still too primitive and there are too many unknowns to know what impact rate setting has on containing costs. When Chassin examined studies of different states, he found that a Blue Cross of Western Pennsylvania study showed that the control hospitals had average annual cost increases of 13 percent to 11 percent for the prospectively reimbursed hospitals for the period of 1970–1974.[41] After examining an early 1970 study of New Jersey hospitals, he concluded that "prospective reimbursement did not work in New Jersey."[42] New York State's rate-setting strategy worked much better than those in Ohio and New England. The reason cited is that New York State has a much stricter rate-setting commission, as shown by the fact that New York hospitals experienced deficits in every year of the 1970–1974 period of the study; this was not true of Ohio and New England. However, Bulgaro and Webb point out that hospital debt declined from 6.7 percent in 1969 to 3 percent in 1977 in spite of tightening rate review regulations in New York.[43] Finally, Abernethy and Pearson state that preliminary results of studies of Connecticut, Washington, Maryland, and Massachusetts showed that all four had cost increases less than the 1977 national average of 14.2 percent.[44] Thus, while there is no certainty, prospective rate setting appears to be helpful in cost containment.

In addition to these potentially quantitative gains, there are other positive results from rate setting. It has generally forced hospitals to become more cost conscious and efficient in their operations. The initial high expectations from rate setting are giving way to a more realistic understanding of the gains that are possible in containing hospital costs. It is being recognized that rate setting must be coordinated with health planning and certificate-of-need strategies to promote a synergistic impact on costs. Finally, the methodologies of rate setting are improving and better information on which to base decisions is forthcoming. However, at this point, no authority can conclusively state there is one best method of rate setting applicable for most states.

IMPLICATIONS FOR REACTIVE IMPLEMENTATION

Each of the regulatory strategies has its own goal(s). The findings noted in the previous sections have shown that, at this stage of development, none of the regulatory strategies has conclusively achieved its goals. However, health planning agencies depend on one or more of these regulatory strategies to achieve their plans' goals. Reduction in bed expansion heavily depends on certificate-of-need/1122 decisions. Regionalization of high-cost medical technology procedures depends on certificate-of-need/1122, PSRO, and appropriateness reviews. Certificate-of-need review determines whether the equipment is needed; appropriateness review determines if it is used appropriately; and PSRO, whether the procedures are overused. Implementation of the 11 medical practice standards contained in the *National Guidelines* depends on one or more of these strategies, but planning agencies that use them to contain unnecessary medical costs and improve quality and availability of care may run the risk of putting too much emphasis on an unproved line of activity. Regulators will be looking to regional and state health plans for guidance in making decisions. While these plans provide some direction, they have many gaps that prevent them from being used as a comprehensive tool to understand the full range of medical issues that come before regulatory bodies. Furthermore, hospitals, researchers, and physicians have the ingenuity to counter regulatory techniques in order to gain favorable decisions for their interests. Yet, in spite of these limitations, these strategies can potentially be of major assistance to health planning agencies in achieving their high-priority goals.

Reactive Strategies as Conservative Strategies

By themselves, the effects of the regulatory strategies are conservative. They aim primarily at improving what is or making it work more efficiently. All of these strategies accept established forms of medical diagnosis and treatment. Their aim is to ensure that all institutions provide care at some minimum level of quality by using these established procedures. It is the overuse and underuse of accepted medical practices that lead to waste, duplication, and higher costs of poorer quality medicine and concern the regulators. They are not in a position to state whether another alternative is superior or to suggest an innovative form of care. Their task is to react to what is presented to them and make a judgment as to whether it meets some accepted standard of practice. The only exception to this is PUFF; many federal grants encourage innovative demonstrations of new techniques, forms of treatment, or alternative structures in which to render services.

On the other hand, when a regional health plan is used as one of the standards for rendering decisions, then innovative elements of the plan may well encourage regulators to give favorable consideration to unusual or experimental programs, proposals, or organizational models of medical practice. These could include acceptance of biofeedback techniques, mental health services operated by nonprofessional ethnic faith healers, or use of emergency medical service equipment by nonmedical personnel such as teachers, scout leaders, or stockbrokers dealing with worried investors. While health plans are being developed with a greater degree of quantitative specificity, they are still fairly crude to be used as more than a general guide to regulators who must make decisions on innovative practices, however. Because of potential challenges in courts of law by dissatisfied medical providers, regulators need a greater degree of certainty and specificity than is generally found in present plans. Lacking the type of formal standards they require, they either develop their own or fall back on traditional practice, both of which usually result in conservative standards.

Defensive Posture of Providers

The nature of regulatory review is to develop an adversarial atmosphere between medical providers and regulators. Unless the regulators have been "captured" by the regulated, the cooperative spirit called for in the appropriateness review Public Policy Notice of the Bureau of Health Planning is likely to be observed only when the ideas of health providers are accepted with a minimum of difficulty. This is generally the case with certificate-of-need/1122 decisions, which have an approval rate of 80 to 95 percent; however, the approval rate on PUFF proposals is only 20 to 50 percent.

If the regulators are strict in applying their criteria and standards, an adversarial relationship is likely to develop; if they are lenient, a more open and cooperative relationship is possible. When new regulations are first issued, regulators tend to interpret and apply them in a strict fashion; their performance and decisions are being closely scrutinized by legislators, federal officials, public interest groups, and evaluators. Once a basic pattern of decision making has been accepted and become routine, providers may ask for and receive greater leniency with respect to their proposals, grants, or operational practices. A cooperative relationship develops under these circumstances so that it is not always clear whether regulatory decisions are serving a public or private interest. Fortunately for the health care field, most of the regulations are so new that they are still subject to close legislative scrutiny and the public interest is still very much in the minds of the regulators as they make their decisions. They may be influenced by hospitals and their professional staffs, medical researchers and others, but that influence is not at this time the controlling factor in regulatory decisions. Because PL 93-641 calls for early discussion between applicants and regulatory staff of the planning agencies, it is impossible to judge what a high approval rate of these applications means. Have the poor proposals been weeded out in the preliminary stage so that only the best have gone forward to more certain approval, or have the regulators approved a high rate of applications on a more indiscriminate basis?

Regulation is relatively new to the medical field and its impact on hospitals and physicians has not yet been determined. The defensive posture readily apparent in most of the professional journals attests to the growing tension between regulators and providers, however. The problem is intensified by the fact that, under PL 93-641, both regulators and planners are sometimes found in the same agency. Certificate-of-need/1122, PUFF, and appropriateness reviews are all mandated functions of health planning agencies. PSRO reviews are carried out in a separate, autonomous agency. Rate review, as a state function, may be part of a larger comprehensive health department or an independent commission or council. When these functions are carried out in the agency that is also responsible for planning, it can be expected that the hostile relationship developed in the reactive implementation strategy will adversely affect the efforts of the proactive plan implementors to involve these same medical providers. While this atmosphere may abate over time, during the initial stages of implementing new regulatory programs, a tense, noncooperative environment is more likely to be the rule.

Minimal Role of Physicians

Except for PSRO reviews, which are effectively controlled by physicians as mandated by law, none of the other regulatory strategies make a strong effort to involve physicians. Bauer considers this a major tactical error regarding rate review, because she notes that they control about 75 percent of the hospital expenditures. Their assistance and cooperation are needed if hospital rates are to be contained. Wennberg, Gittelsohn, and Shapiro are more emphatic with respect to certificate-of-need decisions:

> . . . experience in Vermont suggests that population-based data can help distinguish between "need" based on overutilization and need as defined by a consensus of regional experts. The key role of a regional management committee comprised principally of physicians in making the determination of need emphasizes the importance of including a properly constituted panel of physicians in the decision process established under certificate of need program.[45]

Health planning agencies are beginning to understand the importance of using physician experience and knowledge. More physicians are being used as consultants to explain complex medical procedures, use of medical technology, or interpretation of utilization and personnel data. While some physicians sit on review bodies, by law the majority of the members of these bodies are consumers. Other providers on these committees may include medical administrators and hospital trustees who, while knowledgeable, do not possess the same depth of medical information as do the physicians. Furthermore, since physicians are usually apt to benefit or suffer as a result of programmatic changes, they are the ones who will fight to limit or nullify their losses while maximizing their gains. It is only with their direct involvement that changes can be made, accepted, and implemented as intended.

Synergistic Impact of Regulation Strategies

It has already been noted how the various regulatory strategies by themselves have had either limited or no impact in achieving their goals. It has also been inferred that, when these strategies act in concert, they can produce a positive impact greater than that of their individual effects. Lewin found this in his certificate-of-need/1122 study. In five of the six states that were consistently ranked the highest in controlling hospital beds and assets, prospective reimbursement systems were in place. "Officials in these states expressed the view that, by placing provider institutions at risk with respect to future revenues, rate controls force these institutions to more carefully weigh the economic and financial feasibility of capital projects."[46] Under prospective rate review, losses resulting from a new program, for example, are not usually accepted by rate review commissions as a reason for justifying a higher rate.

Remarking on the experiences of the cooperative relationship between planners and rate reviewers in Rhode Island, Bauer found that rate reviewers approved expenditures of *new* programs "in strict conformance with written listings of priorities of statewide community need established by the planning agency."[47] She felt similar links between PSRO and rate review bodies were equally essential if the cost effectiveness of hospitals was to be improved. As the guardians of quality in medical practice, PSROs are in an excellent position to signal certificate-of-need review, rate review, and planning bodies about their findings in the region as a whole or in a specific hospital. Inefficient, low-quality institutions may well be penalized by rate reviewers, while planners may propose marriages between weak and strong medical institutions to improve the overall quality of care of the weaker one. The question is whether these organizations, especially the planning agency and other regulatory bodies, can work together.

Planners' Orientation versus Regulators' Orientation

Health planners are primarily concerned with improving the availability, accessibility, quality, and acceptability of health care services, whereas regulators are mainly concerned with reducing the inefficiencies that raise the operating costs of medical institutions. Nonetheless, one of the mandates of planners, under PL 93-641, is to contain costs while raising the quality of care. Since cost containment was not initially one of their high priorities, health planners are guided by a different orientation and set of techniques than regulators. At times, they disagree on how proposals should be handled, since each perceives the proposals from a different perspective. For example, planners concerned with providing hospital beds or primary care services in underserved areas of their region may find their interests conflict with those of regulators concerned with the fact that in the region as a whole there are too many beds and too many primary care physicians. The regulators may conclude that the problem is one of inappropriate allocation of services, and it is not their responsibility to shift resources from overserved areas to underserved areas. That is a planning problem to be solved by a proactive implementation strategy.

Planners are constantly being urged to consider innovative ways of solving old problems, while regulators look to the traditionally accepted practices for providing medical care. Innovations may require the introduction of new standards and a search for new ways to make decisions. Regulators are more cautious when faced with innovative proposals. Their standards and criteria cannot adequately evaluate them, and unfairly or not, such projects may be disapproved.

Planners seek to meet the needs of specific populations—senior citizens, low-income families, single parent families—even if this means violating prescribed standards. Regulators use standards based on demand, irrespective of what segment of the population uses the service, and make decisions based on those standards. One of the major criticisms of the initial set of *National Guidelines* was the apparent rigidity of standards. These were made more flexible as a result of the outcry and were issued as guidelines to regional and state health planning agencies rather than as mandated standards. This difference in how planners and regulators make decisions is a constant source of tension between them.

Finally, planners use political trade-offs to develop their goals and priorities. This permits negotiation and compromise. In contrast, decisions are made in a legally, formalistic manner by regulators. For example, PUFF regulations require that a proposal be approved or disapproved. There is no room for compromise, for conditions of approval to be set. Either the proposal meets the criteria, or it does not.

In spite of the potentials for conflict along these dimensions, planners and regulators must work together, as called for in various federal laws, and this requires that they learn to understand and find some way to compromise with each other. Bauer and Altman, fully aware of these differences and bureaucratic rivalries, believe that effective relationships can take place provided there is

—Agreement on common policy objectives;
—A common overall strategy for working towards these
  objectives;
—Clear legal authority that spells out the respective
  functions of the parties;
—Sufficient funding and staff to carry out the common purpose;
—Shared information on which to base decisions;
—An administratively feasible process to link activities.[48]

Needless to say, this is a formidable array of conditions. Although mandated by PL 93-641 to share information, PSROs sometimes put up barriers to sharing data with health planning agencies. They expressed concern that the confidentiality of patients would be violated. While this was obviously an important issue, they may have tried to prevent the exposure of other inefficiencies such as a poorly operated department within a hospital or a hospital with low quality care and/or extended lengths of stay. Only after much bickering and the passage of several years has an understanding been developed around the sharing of information, as well as technical assistance. This example illustrates the major difficulty planning agencies can expect to encounter in meeting the conditions delineated by Bauer and Altman for a fruitful and cooperative relationship.

If implementation depended only on a reactive strategy, then it would appear health planning agencies would have a most difficult time achieving their goals. There are simply too many barriers to overcome, too high a potential for disagreement that dissolves into acrimony. More than that, most of the newly developed regulatory strategies have not yet had time to do what they are mandated to accomplish. The little that is known shows that regulatory agencies are likely to accomplish more and be more effective if they learn to work together. This may be more difficult for regulators, who have an innate tendency toward formalistic behavior, than for health planners, who have learned to negotiate compromises among competing or conflicting parties. When regulatory agencies work together, the reactive implementation strategy can be a very potent tool for achieving change in medical care. When each works alone, there will be a few successes, some "no changes," and many failures, if the early studies are any indication of future impact in achieving regulatory goals.

SUCCESS STORIES

Illustrations of successful cooperation and coordination among health providers, health planners, and health regulators are difficult to find. The following two, taken from a recent Bureau of Health Planning document,[49] show the synergistic impact in two health service regions when health planners, certificate-of-need regulators, and rate review professionals work closely together to implement health planning goals for the benefit of the community.

Consolidating Two Hospitals into a New Facility

On March 23, 1978, the Board of Trustees of the Health Planning and Resources Development Association of the Central Ohio River Valley (CORVA) gave unanimous approval to a proposal for construction of the new 240-bed St. Francis-St. George Hospital in the Western Hills neighborhood of Cincinnati. This action not only brings a new hospital to this working class community but also ends months of controversy and confrontation over the best way to consolidate two inappropriate hospitals and to reduce excess bed capacity. The struggle towards compromise was one that entangled business and religious leaders, politicians and legislators, citizens of Cincinnati's west side neighborhoods, and leaders of the health care community.

This case study summarizes the struggle and highlights the role of CORVA, the HSA which serves the Greater Cincinnati metropolitan area. The HSA negotiated the compromise proposal that consolidated the two hospitals into one new hospital with 74 fewer beds, representing savings of approximately $18.5 million in capital and long-term interest costs and $53 million in operating expenses over a ten-year period over the hospital's original proposal.

The 232-bed St. Francis Hospital is a 93-year-old facility that has been remodeled and renovated so often that its departments are no longer functionally integrated. As long as seven years ago St. Francis noted in its 1971-72 Long Range Plan that the population in its immediate area was declining and that future occupancy levels could be expected to dwindle, especially in the face of the obsolete physical plant.

St. George Hospital, which opened in 1968, is an 82-bed acute care hospital located only about 15 minutes away from St. Francis and serving the same area. Although it originally was designed and funded as a chronic care facility, as it reached the final design stages, it was redesigned, and it subsequently opened its doors as an acute care hospital. During its first five years of operation, St. George experienced a consistent 90 percent occupancy rate, with nursing units and emergency room operating at near capacity. However, the hospital had one major drawback: it was too small to provide the Western Hills community with the sophisticated services it needed, and its patients frequently had to be transferred elsewhere for care.

In 1972, CORVA's predecessor CHP agency, recognizing that St. Francis was physically outdated and operationally inefficient, while St. George needed more beds to remain an economically viable institution, recommended that the two hospitals begin planning for eventual consolidation. The officials of the two hospitals were amenable to CORVA's idea of a single Western Hills hospital, and, in September 1974, after two years of joint planning, representatives of the hospitals and the Archdiocese of Cincinnati signed articles of incorporation creating the St. Francis-St. George Hospital Corporation.

During the next two years, the Corporation worked on plans for the joint venture, and in December 1976, it announced that it was planning to build a 320-bed hospital on a 22-acre lot roughly equidistant from the two existing hospitals at a cost of $36 million.

Shortly thereafter, Corporation officials, concerned about losing the option to buy the new lot, asked CORVA for preliminary approval of this plan. The CORVA Board of Trustees, however, agreed to endorse only the concept of merging the hospitals, not the proposed plan itself. CORVA's review boards were concerned that the plan called for building six more beds than already existed at the two hospitals when the area already had a projected 1980 surplus of 77 beds—a figure later revised upwards to 224 surplus beds when a projected 5 percent reduction in medical/surgical bed utilization was applied to the estimated 1980 population data. CORVA officials also questioned how the building of an entirely new hospital could be less expensive than expanding the 10-year-old St. George facility. They had problems with the total costs of the project, the future uses of the two existing hospitals, and the new site. In the end, CORVA told the St. Francis-St. George Corporation to "significantly reduce" the size of its project.

In August 1977 Corporation officials submitted their proposal. The number of beds had been reduced from 320 to 300. Costs also were slightly down—from $36 million to $34.1 million. However, the plan still called for construction of a totally new facility.

Battle lines were quickly drawn. In an unprecedented move, leaders of other area hospitals came out in opposition to the proposal because it would add unneeded beds to the County. The local Blue Cross plan took the unusual step of buying newspaper space to explain why the proposal was "a serious mistake." As CORVA's staff analysis proceeded, it became apparent that the proposal was headed for trouble, and relations between the Corporation and the HSA became increasingly strained.

On December 2, 1977, the CORVA staff released a negative report that surprised no one. It recommended that the CORVA Board of Trustees should urge Corporation officials to withdraw their application and to continue to plan, with emphasis on expanding the St. George facility into a 200-bed hospital. The staff's recommendation reflected three major concerns about the Corporation's proposal: (1) that the proposed use of public taxable bonds, as opposed to tax-exempt revenue bonds, would mean higher long-term interest expenses of up to $6.7 million; (2) that construction of a new hospital did not foster cost containment since it appeared to be more costly than expansion of the St. George facility; and (3) that the proposal was inconsistent with the CORVA Health Systems Plan.

The Corporation's board secretary, Eugene P. Ruehlmann, swiftly announced that he was "outraged" by the CORVA staff review. Accusing CORVA of discriminating against the west side of town and fabricating the 224-bed surplus, Ruehlmann insisted that there would be no change in the proposal and the Hospital sponsors would be going forward with their proposal. (Ironically, it had been Ruehlmann who, as Cincinnati's Mayor, had chosen in 1966 to bypass traditional political and medical powers and to ask businessmen familiar with the health care field to take the initiative in creating CORVA.)

At this point, the Hospital's sponsors embarked on an intense lobbying campaign aimed at gaining endorsements for their proposal from key political leaders. Petitions supporting the proposal were circulated in the Western Hills community. When the Subarea Advisory Council for the Western Hills area met to review the proposal, buses were chartered to bring several hundred supporters to the meeting. Waving placards and supported by the endorsements of the Cincinnati City Council, the County Commissioner, Cincinnati Archbishop Joseph L. Bernardin and other key political, medical, and civic leaders, the proponents attempted to win approval of their proposed new hospital. Although Corporation officials agreed to revise the long-term financing method from taxable to tax-exempt revenue bonds, the SAC Board, basing its decision on its study of community need, voted 12-3 to recommend disapproval of the project.

A month later, the proponents suffered another setback when the proposal was rejected by CORVA's Proposal Review Committee. This set the stage for a confrontation before the CORVA Board of Trustees. However, a mid-winter blizzard forced postponement of the trustees' meeting for a week, giving participants extra time to work out a compromise. When the Trustees finally convened on February 1, the Corporation Board asked them for a sixty-day postponement to allow it time to study its proposal further and to arrive at a "mutually acceptable" position with CORVA. This decision to request a delay came out of a last minute private meeting between the Archbishop, Corporation board members, CORVA staff and a Procter & Gamble group vice president (a former CORVA president) who had been persuaded to act as a mediator by local business leaders.

During the next six weeks, a task force comprising the Corporation Board and CORVA's staff and Board met weekly to hammer out a compromise. Finally, on March 23, 1978, an amended proposal for a 240-bed hospital was submitted to CORVA for approval. In a memorandum to the CORVA Board, CORVA director James F. Sandmann outlined several reasons for recommending approval:

(1) That the revision in the financing method represented a savings of approximately $5.4 to $6.7 million;
(2) That the number of beds had been reduced from 300 to 240 and that this was expected to produce savings of $9.0 million in capital costs and $9.5 million in long-term interests costs. What is even more significant, the reduction in beds was expected to produce savings of more than $53 million in operating expenses over a ten-year period, and
(3) That the move to a new site was necessary because services at the St. George facility would be seriously disrupted while the facility was being remodeled, and the program plan, as redeveloped, could not be implemented in a remodeled facility.

Further, the new site provided excellent traffic accessibiilty. The amended proposal received the unanimous approval of the CORVA Board of Trustees.

This decision will have a decided impact on future health care projects in Cincinnati. CORVA has shown that it is a planning body that must be "reckoned with" and that in these days of cost containment, shared services and reduction of excess system capacity, no hospital can plan alone or expect to get everything it wants.

Developing a Regionalized Hospital System*

The Finger Lakes Health Systems Agency (FLHSA) serves a nine-county area in the western part of New York State. Although

*This case was adapted from a case study prepared by the Alpha Center for Health Planning, Syracuse, New York, January 1979.

this area encompasses the city of Rochester, it is primarily rural, with many dairy and apple farms and small vineyards.

Its four-county (Ontario, Seneca, Wayne and Yates) Central Area is the home of eight hospitals, clustered in a Y-shaped area 35-miles long and 26-miles wide. While the bed/population ratio of 3.7 bed per 1,000 population is nearly 18 percent below the national average and is 7½ percent below the level called for in the National Guidelines, there is a serious maldistribution of beds, with some underutilization, and shortage of long-term and ambulatory care services.

This case describes how the Finger Lakes HSA and its Central Subarea Advisory Council, spurred by New York State health planning authorities, have begun to shape a regionalized hospital system by promoting cooperative hospital planning, decertification of underutilized beds and conversion of beds to new uses.

In April 1974 the F.F. Thompson Hospital, a recently rebuilt, 101-bed acute care facility located in the Ontario County town of Canandaigua, filed an application to build 40 new medical-surgical beds at an estimated cost of $25 million. To explain the need for the additional beds, Thompson cited such factors as (1) a doubling of utilization in the past five years; (2) an overall occupancy rate of 92-95 percent; (3) a projected population increase in the area of more than 25 percent by 1980, and (4) the fact that its capacity had been cut from 125 to 101 beds when it was rebuilt three years earlier.

Soon after the application was submitted, Thompson and FLHSA's predecessor CHP Agency were informed that the application probably would not be acted upon until a cooperative planning study, begun a year earlier at the State's request, had been completed. This study of acute care services in the Central/ Finger Lakes Area was being conducted by the Finger Lakes Hospital Planning Group, a four-county organization composed of representatives of each of the eight area hospitals, including Thompson, and of consumer groups. This organization was an advisory body to the local health planning agency.

The acute care services study was completed in the fall of 1974. It reported excess capacity of 59 to 60 beds, due primarily to maldistribution, and stated that there was "no apparent need demonstrated for additional beds in the four-county area at this time." It further recommended a one-year moratorium on approvals of new beds in the area.

Despite this study, Thompson's application, along with an application for 50 new medical-surgical beds filed by the Geneva General Hospital, a 130-bed acute care facility located just two towns away from Thompson in Ontario County, were approved by the Ontario County subarea council in the summer of 1975. Shortly thereafter, however, the applications were disapproved by the HSA review and full boards.

As a result, in November 1975, Thompson submitted a scaled-down version of its application, requesting only 20 new beds. This application was approved by the HSA Board despite the strong opposition of SHA staff and forwarded to the State Hospital Review and Planning Council in January 1976. The State subsequently disapproved the application, and the Hospital requested a hearing.

Ten months later, the State still had not acted on the hearing. Central/Finger Lakes Subarea Advisory Council Chairman Robert W. Purple, inquiring about the reason for the delay, learned that the State did not intend to recommend approval of this or any other application from the area until a plan reviewing the acute care bed situation and recommending "which underutilized beds in Ontario County (or the surrounding area) should be decertified," had been completed.

Subsequent discussions with the State confirmed that a recommendation for approval of 20 beds at F.F. Thompson Hospital would have to be accompanied by "a recommendation for decertification of a number of beds in the surrounding area which would result in a net shrinkage" and "a net actual cost reduction."

As a result, on December 1, 1976, the Central/Finger Lakes Subarea Council adopted a resolution directing its Chairman to appoint a small task force to develop an acute care plan.

This Acute Facilities Task Force, composed of representatives of the HSA Executive Committee and Board, the Subarea Council, the Regional Hospital Council and the Central/Finger Lakes Hospital Council, began meeting in February 1977 and, during the next six months, gathered data on beds and utilization and consulted with representatives of each of the hospitals in the area. Operating on the premise that closing whole hospitals or hospital units, rather than converting beds on a piecemeal basis, was the most effective way to achieve cost savings, the Task Force saw its charge as one of producing a plan of action which would recommend bed decertifications, service consolidations or hospital mergers.

After six months of study, the Task Force released an initial report. This report so enraged the administrators, boards and medical staffs of the local hospitals that for the first time, the eight hospitals in the Central/Finger Lakes Subarea joined together in a Hospital Cooperative (COOP) to undertake a formal joint planning venture. This was a development that had been urged by the HSA for a number of years.

During the next six months, the Task Force held hearings on its report, and the COOP spent its time attacking the report and developing its own counter-report.

In November 1977, the COOP released its report. Although the number of overall bed reductions proposed in this report was close to the number recommended by the Task Force, major differences existed in regard to where the beds should come from and whether medical-surgical or pediatric and obstetric beds should be decertified.

A month later, the Task Force released its final report, and in January 1978, both reports were forwarded to the Central Subarea Council for its consideration.

The Council met on January 4, and after listening to lengthy testimony from the administrators of each of the affected hospitals, decided to table any action and review all of the recommendations in detail at the following meeting.

When it reconvened on February 1, a motion was put forward to approve the Task Force's report as it stood. This opened up a new round of debate over the assumptions utilized in preparing the report, and the motion was defeated.

A counter-motion for approval of the COOP plan was then put forward by a representative from Canandaigua who was anxious to see the recommendations for Thompson Hospital approved. After a number of floor amendments were offered, the Subarea Council adopted the bed changes offered by the COOP with two amendments. Although these changes amounted to a net decrease of more than 30 acute care beds, they resulted in a net increase of four medical-surgical beds and no cost savings, with the possible exception of savings that might accrue as a result of obstetric bed consolidations approved in 1974.

The FLHSA Executive Committee met on February 28 and spent four hours reviewing the Subarea Council's recommendations. After an initial motion to accept the Council's recommendations failed, a procedural resolution to consider each hospital and the related recommendations individually was adopted. Then, the Executive Committee approved the following recommendations by roll-call vote:

1. F.F. Thompson Hospital—approve pending 20 medical-surgical bed application; convert 13 pediatric beds to medical-surgical use.
2. Newark-Wayne Hospital—decertify 13 obstetric beds and at least 17 medical-surgical beds.
3. Seneca Falls Hospital—decertify 2 medical-surgical beds.
4. Taylor Brown Hospital—decertify 14-bed obstetric unit per 1975 obstetric plan.
5. Seneca Falls-Taylor Brown Memorial Hospitals—corporate merger within 36 months, if legally possible.
6. Clifton Springs Hospital—decertify 8-bed obstetric unit as adopted in 1975 obstetric plan.
7. Myers Community Hospital—decertify 4 pediatric and 2 obstetric beds.
8. Finger Lakes Health Services Cooperative—continue its cooperative planning efforts with the Subarea Council.

Postscript

The above recommendations were forwarded to the State Office of Health Systems Management in March 1978. Two months later, the State informed FLHSA Executive Director Anthony T. Mott of its willingness to proceed with a favorable Thompson Hospital review pending receipt of decertification requests from the affected hospitals. As of September 1978, all but one of the requests had been received. State action on both decertification and approval of Thompson is likely to go through as negotiated, and the Central/Finger Lakes area of New York State will have a more rational, efficient and responsive health care delivery system.

NOTES

1. Samuel V. Stiles and Katherine A. Johnson, *Regulatory and Review Functions of Agencies Created by the Act,* Public Health Reports 91, no. 1 (Hyattsville, Md.: HHS, 1976), pp. 25–28.

2. Michael Runner, *Certificate of Need Regulations Proposed by HEW-Comments Needed by May 27, 1980* (Santa Monica, Calif.: National Health Law Program, April 25, 1980 Memo), pp. 1–2. See also *Developing Complying Review Programs under P.L. 93-641: IV. Certificate of Need/Section 1122 Review* (Madison, Wis.: Midwest Center for Health Planning, undated, but around 1978).

3. Lewin and Associates, *Evaluation of the Efficiency and Effectiveness of the Section 1122 Review Process-Part III: Executive Summary* (Washington, D.C.: September, 1975), Table 6, p. 6.

4. *Ibid.*, p. 13.

5. Thomas W. Bice and David S. Salkever, "Certificate-of-Need Legislation and Hospital Costs" in *Hospital Cost Containment*, eds. Michael Zubkoff, Ira Raskin, and Ruth Hanft (New York: Prodist, 1978), pp. 429–460.

6. *Ibid.*, p. 450.

7. *Ibid.*, p. 451.

8. American Health Planning Association (AHPA), *Second Report on 1978 Survey of Health Planning Agencies* (Washington, D.C.: February, 1979).

9. *Ibid.*, p. 1 of Executive Summary.

10. Eugene Rubel and Marian Troyer-Merkel, *Reducing Excess Institutional Capacity.* A draft memo, presumably to Health Care Financing Administration (Washington, D.C.: June 13, 1978).

11. *Ibid.*, p. 2.

12. AHPA, *Second Report*, p. 7.

13. "Health Systems Agency Reviews of Certain Proposed Uses of Federal Health Funds," *Federal Register* 44, no. 156 (August 10, 1979): 47064–47091.

14. *An Analysis of the Final Rules: Federal Register (44:156) August 10, 1979.* (Madison, Wis.: The Institute for Health Planning, August 16, 1979), p. 7. Other parts of the discussion on PUFF are based on this and other analyses undertaken by the institute and the House Subcommittee on Health and the Environment, 96th Congress, on the amendments to PL 93–641, October 1979. In addition, Technical Assistance Memorandum No. 20, published by Alpha Center for Health Planning, Bethesda, Maryland (March 3, 1980) describes and analyzes the relationship between use of mental health, alcoholism, and drug abuse funds and health planning agency reviews.

15. "Health Systems Agency and State Agency Reviews of the Appropriateness of Existing Institutional Health Services: Final Regulations," *Federal Register*, 44, no. 239 (December 11, 1979): 71769.

16. Wood McCue, Charles F. Pierce, Jr., and Anthony T. Mott, "Appropriateness Review: Which Road to Take?" *American Journal of Health Planning* 3, no. 4 (October 1978): 10–16.

17. "Appropriateness of Existing Services," p. 71755.

18. McCue, Pierce, and Mott, "Which Road to Take?" p. 10.

19. U.S. DHHS, *Final Regulations for Reviews of the Appropriateness of Existing Institutional Health Services,* Program Policy Notice 80-03 (Hyattsville, Md.: Health Resources Administration, January 16, 1980), p. 1.

20. Social Security Act, Title XI, Section 1151.

21. Health Care Financing Administration (HCFA), *Professional Standards Review Organization 1979 Program Evaluation* (Washington, D.C.: Office of Research, Demonstrations and Statistics, May, 1980), p. 3.

22. *Ibid.*, p. 13.

23. James F. Blumstein, "The Role of PSROs in Hospital Cost Containment," in Zubkoff, Raskin, and Hanft, *Hospital Cost Containment,* p. 466.

24. Ruth M. Covell, "The Impact of Regulation on Health Care Quality," in *Regulating Health Care,* ed. Arthur Levin (New York: The Academy of Political Science, 1980) p. 120.

25. Blumstein, "Role of PSROs," p. 470.

26. David S. Abernethy and David A. Pearson, *Regulating Hospital Costs* (Ann Arbor, Mich.: AUPHA Press, 1979), p. 67.

27. Blumstein, "Role of PSROs," p. 467.

28. HCFA, *Professional Standards,* p. 3.

29. *Ibid.*

30. *Ibid.,* p. 8.

31. *Ibid.,* pp. 44–58.

32. *Ibid.,* p. 14.

33. Mark R. Chassin, "The Containment of Hospital Costs: A Strategic Assessment," *Medical Care* 16, no. 10 (October 1978): Supplement.

34. Katharine G. Bauer, "Hospital Rate Setting—This Way to Salvation?" in Zubkoff, Raskin, and Hanft, *Hospital Cost Containment,* p. 325.

35. Abernethy and Pearson, *Regulating Costs,* p. 60.

36. Bauer, "This Way to Salvation?" pp. 345–350.

37. *Ibid.,* p. 344.

38. *Ibid.,* p. 359.

39. *Ibid.,* p. 358.

40. *Ibid.,* p. 362.

41. Chassin, "Containment of Hospital Costs," p. 42.

42. *Ibid.,* p. 43.

43. Patrick J. Bulgaro and Arthur Y. Webb, "Federal-State Conflicts in Cost Control," in Levin, *Regulating Health Care,* p. 109.

44. Abernethy and Pearson, *Regulating Costs,* p. 61.

45. John E. Wennberg, Alan Gittelsohn, and Nancy Shapiro, "Health Care Delivery in Maine III: Evaluating the Level of Hospital Performance," *The Journal of the Maine Medical Association* 66, no. 11 (November 1975): 306.

46. Lewin and Associates, Inc., *Evaluation of the Efficiency and Effectiveness of the Section 1122 Review Process* (Washington, D.C.: September, 1975), p. I–14.

47. Bauer, "This Way to Salvation?" p. 364.

48. Katharine G. Bauer and Drew Altman, *Linking Planning and Rate Setting Controls to Contain Hospital Costs* (New York, N.Y.: Public Health Service, Region II, Division of Resource Development, October 24, 1975), p. 12.

49. U.S. DHHS, *Health Planning in Action: Achieving Equal Access to Quality Health Care at a Reasonable Cost,* HRP-0150101 (Hyattsville, Md.: Bureau of Health Planning, Health Resources Administration, Public Health Services, October, 1979).

Chapter 8

Proactive Implementation

Implementation is defined by this writer as the application of resources and the use of appropriate strategies and legal/legislative forces as needed to convert symbolic goals and objectives into real products (facilities and services) to improve the health of a region's population. Unlike reactive implementation, in which planners respond to provider initiatives, proactive implementation requires planners to take the initiative in seeking resources and using the regulatory or legislative processes to promote their high-priority health goals and objectives. This is the essential difference between the two processes, and it leads to a variety of different strategies and techniques. Whereas in reactive implementation providers must prove that they have the resources to implement their proposed services, in proactive implementation planners must discover the resources and learn to tap them. Whereas in reactive implementation providers are required to go through a formalistic process to gain approval for their proposals, in proactive implementation coalitions of community actors must be built to promote each priority goal and objective. Whereas in reactive implementation providers know beforehand the process and criteria they must meet to gain approval, in proactive implementation new strategies and techniques must be devised in a dynamic and ad hoc manner for each situation as it arises. Proactive implementors must be opportunistic, flexible, sensitive to organizational needs, adroit at organizing relevant community health and nonhealth factors, knowledgeable about the use of strategies, and capable of providing guidance to secure desired goals. Thus, while the general definition of implementation applies to both orientations, reactive and proactive implementation processes are quite different.

THEORIES OF CHANGE

There are three basic theories of change. One focuses on ways of maintaining the viability of a given social or health system. A second is concerned with making adaptations in an organization or system to overcome its dysfunctional manner of operation. A third involves changing the structure of a system and its mode of operation to make it more effective in meeting people's needs. The first, the interaction process of change, is based on community organization theory and the principles fostered by Ross.[1] The second, the therapeutic process of change, is based on Lewinian[2] principles; the third, called intervention process, is based on Morris and Binstock's concepts of change.[3]

Interaction Process

The focus of the interaction concept is on maintaining the sensitive and tenuous balance that exists in the system by reducing tensions or structural stresses. This means that a hospital would fight to keep its pediatric ward department open, for example, even if the regional and state goal mandated its closing. In a recent case in New Jersey, one hospital with 400 fewer births than the minimum of 1500 required by federal guidelines and state regulations was able to get a positive vote from the regional health planning agency when it secured 12,000 signatures on petitions to keep its pediatric department open. Faced with a serious threat to its obstetric services (a basic part of its structure), the hospital fought back with its full resources to counter the threat and maintain its equilibrium.

Maintenance of the status quo requires much effort and good will among the institutions that comprise the health system. Through coordinative and collaborative strategies, these institutions find ways to resolve differences and bring about orderly and nonthreatening changes. In various consortia and federative bodies, medical institutions have developed forums for discussing potential sources of tension and dealing with them in a positive way. In addition, these forums are able to promote needed changes that meet community health needs without disrupting the basic relationships developed over time among the medical institutions.

Health planning agencies are striving to become accepted as the change agent for the health system. Since most planning agencies in the United States have developed along the lines of the partnership model, their values and attitudes are relatively consistent with those of the health system components of the medical system. Planning agencies play the roles of guide by helping the medical system and the health care consumers of the community to establish goals that are achievable; of enabler by working with the health care institutions to achieve those parts of the planned goals in which they have a vital interest; of expert by providing the technical knowledge and data needed to determine the suitable priority, timing, and location of medical services and facilities; and of social ther-

apist by assisting troubled and/or failing units of the system to heal themselves in order to provide the services required by the population. All of
these roles are played by health planning agencies to ensure the integration,
coordination, and wholeness of the medical system. No attempt is made
to transform the system into some other form, preservation and maintenance are its major concerns. All of these roles and strategies involve the
formal and informal interaction of the health system's leadership with the
community's lay leadership. This cooperative interaction is essential if the
collaborative techniques of education and persuasion are to produce the
positive results intended.[4]

Therapeutic Process

Like the interaction model, the therapeutic model accepts the assumption that a health system exists; however, in the therapeutic model, the
system is not considered static. Rather, the components within the system
are believed to be constantly in a process of changing: adapting, adjusting,
and reorganizing themselves to maintain their place in the system and their
own stability. Each unit grows and develops in its own way, partly in
response to the other units of the system and partly as a result of its own
internal goals. To illustrate, as the number of elderly with chronic conditions increases, hospitals must learn to help them cope with their problems;
a new specialty of medicine—geriatrics—develops. Nursing homes
develop into specialized units that differentiate the services provided the
elderly according to their capacity to cope: home health services for those
able to live at home; apartments for those able to care for their basic needs
but unable to cook or run errands; intermediate care nursing facilities for
those needing closer medical attention, but able to move around without
too much help; and skilled nursing facilities for those in need of total
supervision. Thus, both hospitals and nursing facilities expand, adapt, and
develop to meet the varied and complex needs of senior citizens.

Should the nursing homes in the community not recognize the increasing
numbers of elderly who require their services, or should they not respond
to the phenomenal growth of knowledge about the elderly, their needs,
and capabilities, then these institutions are said to be "frozen" in a dysfunctional mode of operation that is not providing sufficient services to all
those who need their services. Pressures then build on the nursing home
industry to change its ways.

Change agents, in the form of outside consultants or health planners,
are asked to intervene either by health planning agencies or by the nursing
homes themselves in an effort to "unfreeze" their system from an out-
moded form of organization and operation. The change agent plays a

particularly active role in diagnosing what is wrong and making recommendations for developing a new equilibrium that will more readily meet the existing needs of the elderly. It may require the nursing home industry to increase in size; to develop distinct, but coordinated, specialized functions; or to redistribute the location of individual institutions for greater accessibility to the elderly population. Eventually, a new "frozen" stability occurs that enables the nursing homes to function well within the changing larger system. Inevitably, however, the new frozen position will again become dysfunctional and be required to change once more to meet other needs of the population. Thus, the system and its components are in a constant state of development that requires continuing self-diagnosis and treatment to ensure its continued health.

The role of health planning agencies is to ensure the system's efficiency and effectiveness. Data analysis enables the planning agencies to call attention to potential and actual problem areas that require attention. Agencies can also serve as active catalysts by locating the specialists who can assist the health institutions to resolve problems. They stop short of providing the treatment themselves. Thus, like the planning agencies in the interaction model, they play largely catalytic, technical, and quiet advocacy roles. They call attention to a problem, but do not force health institutions to make changes. To a greater degree than change agents in the interaction model, they play an active role in helping to develop and maintain the growth of the system at higher levels of stability.[5]

Intervention Process

The intervention model is based on the assumption that change takes place to meet some glaring unmet need of a whole or of a segment of a population. Through analysis, it may be concluded that the existing medical system or its components are dysfunctional and incapable of meeting those needs. Therefore, an outside change agent finds it necessary to intervene because of the system's tendency to resist change and maintain its equilibrium, even if it is in a state of tension. Thus, unlike the other models of change, an interventionist takes direct action to bring about changes in the system, forcibly if necessary, or to eliminate it or its failing parts to ensure that the needs of the population are served. Emphasis is thus not necessarily on improving the existing system, even if its components are functioning in a coordinated, integrated manner. That system may still not be meeting some basic needs of the population. As an example, a smoothly operating emergency medical service, appropriately integrated with specialized acute care hospitals to treat patients with heart attacks, victims of automobile accidents, or severe burns may not be able to reduce appreciably the morbidity or mortality rates of these conditions. Reductions in these rates require a different type of approach, such as an improvement in the way highways are built, in the way people live, or in the availability of better jobs and housing for the poor and other marginal segments of the population. However, to achieve these goals may require a shrinkage of the medical diagnostic-treatment system or the elimination of inefficient or redundant components of that system. Interventionists would not hesitate to do what is necessary to achieve those ends.

While interventionists prefer the use of collaboration to achieve their ends, there are a number of arguments in favor of the use of conflict.[6] It tends to accelerate the pace of social change. Any change forced on a health institution usually results from a conflict tactic. Rejecting a certif- icate-of-need request, lowering an institution's reimbursement rate, taking away its license, striking, or demonstrating are examples of conflict tactics.

Conflict also sharpens the issues so that the general public can clearly see the difference between the competing or conflicting forces. Differences between conservatives and liberals in Congress over the form comprehen- sive health care should take have been revealed in the various bills intro- duced on national health insurance legislation. The scope of services, the method of payment, the administration of the insurance plan, and those who should be included among the beneficiaries are some of the major areas of contention between the two sides. In addition, a third group, smaller but vocal, has pressed for a national health service that is even more sharply at variance with national health insurance programs that have been advocated.

Conflict is often a creative force. Any major innovation in society that displaces an existing and once accepted service usually comes about only after conflict. Medicare was finally enacted over the strong opposition over a 30-year period of the American Medical Association (AMA). The first health maintenance organizations (HMOs) in the United States were established over the opposition of physicians. Hospitals were initially as strongly opposed to certificate-of-need regulation as physicians were opposed to Professional Standards Review Organizations (PSROs). All of these innovations threatened one influential medical institution or another. Once these new programs were instituted, opponents not only came to terms with the innovations, but often benefited greatly by their successful operation.

Conflict "is useful in overcoming the blight of institutionalism. Most institutions . . . tend to become conservative as they grow older."[7] It has long been said that today's innovators are tomorrow's conservatives. Conflict forces a rethinking of goals. The hold of the AMA on the younger physicians is weakening, as seen by the growing unionization of interns and residents, the development of a black national medical organization, and the fact that less than 50 percent of physicians are now members of the organization. These forces have forced the AMA to rethink its traditional goals in order to recapture some of the influence it has lost to emerging forces, such as the American Hospital Association and the American Nurses Association. Local chapters of the AMA, although they had ignored the planning efforts of the Comprehensive Health Planning Agencies in the 1960s, became much more involved in the new Health Systems Agencies (HSAs) in the 1970s and thereby recognized the presence and potential influence of these agencies.

Finally, conflict often results in the emergence of new forces and a shift in the distribution of power. With the passage of Medicaid and Medicare, HMO legislation, health planning laws, and health personnel acts, the federal government has entered what was once an exclusive, privately operated medical system to influence the type of medical practitioners educated, the fees hospitals and private physicians may charge tax-supported patients and facilities, and the facilities and services developed and their location. Because they pay for an increasingly large share of medical costs, the federal and state governments are taking more initiative in setting policy, and are being begrudgingly accepted by professional associations as partners. Also, the emergence of hospitals as the most important medical institution in the community has resulted in its leaders' claiming more power in determining what services are needed and who should use them. The AMA is no longer the monolithic influence in the field of medicine it once was. Now it must share its power with hospital officials, government officials, and a growing force of consumers. None of these changes and shifts in power came without conflict.

The organization and structure of most health planning agencies are generally not conducive to an intervention model of change. The fact that a very wide representation of the medical and lay leadership composes health planning agency boards, each representing special concerns that sometimes compete with those of other board representatives, makes it very difficult for boards to take on aggressive battles to achieve their goals. Consensus is not likely to be reached on specific objectives, but rather on the more general, broad goals on which all can agree on ends, if not on means. Highly explosive or crisis issues can sometimes produce a consensus, but that would be the exception to the rule.[8] Only if an agency is organized around the systems or individual action models (see Chapter 4) can the intervention model of change be successfully implemented.

Implications for Planned Change

Roles of Health Planning Agencies

A variety of roles are available to health planning agencies. However, depending on the organizational structure and composition of the particular agency's board, some may be functional and some may be dysfunctional. Most agencies can carry out the roles of guide, enabler, and technical advisor. In fewer instances can they play the role of ardent activist, in which an agency imposes its point of view of the health system.

Use of Strategies

Collaborationist techniques are more likely to be used by the interaction and therapeutic models of change; contest techniques, by the interventionist model. The values and beliefs held by board members affect the type of strategies they can use in bringing about planned change. Board members must agree almost unanimously on their objectives in order to use collaboration techniques. For example, board members of a mental health agency are likely to hold common values, which permits the board to act aggressively in dealing with its own problems. However, if the desired changes affect other parts of the medical system or need the approval of a partnership planning agency, then those changes must be consistent with what the planning agency board members are able to accept. This tends to restrain the mental health agency's board from promoting radical changes or using conflict techniques in resolving its problems. Finally, the intervention model assumes that board members hold similar values and therefore more activist contest techniques can be used to resolve problems or promote objectives. It is almost a truism that the use of conflict techniques by a board with similar values draws the members closer together.

Goals of the Models

Interaction and therapeutic models seek to resolve tensions by making adjustments within the system. The aim is to maintain and stabilize the existing system. For interventionists, where the functioning system meets the needs of the population, the goal is also to repair it. However, where it fails to do this, the goal is to change the structure or to replace the system outright with a new one. It is for this reason that interventionists are said to be task-oriented while the others are more maintenance-oriented. One works to achieve a tangible, substantive goal (more primary physicians, a better home health care system), while the others work to

achieve stability and a higher level of integration among the system components (improvements in the referral system; reallocation of services;
less costly, appropriate care).

Values of System Members

The similarity or variance of values held by system members determines
to a great extent the type of change model best used by them. If a system
is composed of generally like-minded components, such as home health
care agency representatives, it can use the more activist intervention
model of change because there is agreement on goals and the values they
hold about home health care are similar. If nursing homes are added to the
system, however, their representatives view home health care services as
a direct threat to their viability—the more comprehensive and available
home health care services, the fewer persons referred to nursing homes
for care. Thus, their differing values and goals require a change model that
is sensitive to these differences. Seeking goals that bring greater benefits
to one component at the expense of the other produces great inner tension
within the system and may lead to its breakdown. If acute care hospitals
are added to the system, it becomes even more difficult to set specific task
goals. Maintenance of the system becomes more important than achieving
task goals, which may favor one part of the system over another. Most
existing health planning agencies find the interaction or therapeutic implementation models more effective for achieving changes and these changes
are focused primarily on maintaining stability and greater efficiency within
the existing system.

Table 8-1 shows the relationship between selected characteristics of
change such as source of change, goal of intervention, and roles of change
agents and the planning models.

IMPLEMENTATION PROCESS

Basically, implementation involves answering a series of questions:[9]

- What is to be implemented?
- For whom is it to be implemented?
- In what priority should the goals be implemented?
- When should the implementation begin?
- Who should be involved or neutralized in the implementation process?
- What actions should be taken to foster the implementation?
- What resources are available?
- How successful was the implementation?

Table 8-1   Planning Models by Planned Change Concepts and Selected Characteristics

Selected Characteristics	Planning Models			
	Systems	*Partnership*	*Alliance*	*Individual Action*
Change concept	Intervention	Interaction	Therapeutic or interaction	Intervention
General goal	Substantive change	Maintenance of system	Maintenance of system	Substantive change
Source of change	Rational planning selected goals	Tension in system	Tension or dysfunctional goals of system subunit	Subjectively perceived tension or dysfunction in a systems subunit
Goal of intervention	Improvement of system or one of its subunits	Adjustment, adaptation	Adjustment, adaptation, or removal of blockages	Improvement of a systems subunit
Roles of change agent	Technician, active advocate of change	Guide, enabler, technician	Guide, technician, moderately active advocate of change	Active advocate of change

These questions form a logical implementation cycle (Figure 8-1). Basically, the cycle implies that implementation involves a combination of technical and political activities.

What Is To Be Implemented

All health planning agencies have developed implementation plans based on their long-range health plans. A series of one- to two-year high-priority objectives has been selected as a beginning effort to achieve high-priority

---

Figure 8-1   The Implementation Cycle

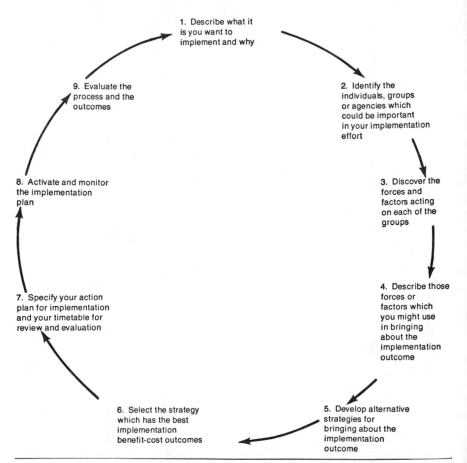

1. Describe what it is you want to implement and why

2. Identify the individuals, groups or agencies which could be important in your implementation effort

3. Discover the forces and factors acting on each of the groups

4. Describe those forces or factors which you might use in bringing about the implementation outcome

5. Develop alternative strategies for bringing about the implementation outcome

6. Select the strategy which has the best implementation benefit-cost outcomes

7. Specify your action plan for implementation and your timetable for review and evaluation

8. Activate and monitor the implementation plan

9. Evaluate the process and the outcomes

Source: Health Resources Administration, *A Course on Resource Development and Implementation* (Hyattsville, Md.: U.S. DHHS, undated), p. C-15.

long-range objectives. The following examples of these one-year objectives have been selected from a variety of health planning agencies:

- There should be no additional obstetrical beds added to areas of excess capacity until the State Perinatal Designation process is initiated. (Central New Jersey)
- By September 1981, all school districts in health service area VII will be in compliance with a ninety percent (90%) required immunization level as mandated by the newly amended school code. (Suburban Cook County-Dupage County, Illinois)
- To have an ordinance adopted which permits the fluoridation of community water supplies in at least one Region II city with a population greater than 5,000 by 1981. (North Central Florida)
- By December 1980, two additional family planning programs shall be operating specialized teen clinics. (Currently, 3 out of 8 programs offer specialized teen clinics.) (Mid-South Medical Center Council, Memphis, Tennessee)
- By 1979 there will be a net increase of at least four new primary care physicians in the Grays Harbor/Pacific subarea. (Southwest Washington)

A plan implementation committee or some similar body is asked to rank these short-range objectives. Exhibit 8-1 shows the successive steps required. In step 1, each person ranks the objectives based on the two criteria noted or on other criteria determined by the committee. In step 2, those objectives that were rated high on both "importance to the region" and "agency's ability to impact" are placed in the upper left-hand box. Others are placed accordingly. Those that fall into one of the three boxes labeled high-high, high-medium, or medium-high (step 3) are candidates for implementation. These objectives could be labeled high-priority objectives; the vertically lined boxes, medium-priority objectives; and the blank boxes, low-priority objectives.

Generally, this can be considered a technical step, with the rankings based on the democratic selection process of the committee members. However, if inadequate knowledge or biased voting was involved, modifications can be made in the final rankings to take these value factors into account.

Who Is To Be Involved

Once it has been determined what is to be implemented, the actors who can assist in implementation must be identified. An implementation strategy worksheet (Exhibit 8-2) may be used to determine who should be

Exhibit 8-1   Implementation Portfolio

1. For each major implementation activity or program rank the importance to the region and the agency's ability to impact.

Implementation Activity	Importance to the Region (High, Medium, Low)	Agency's Ability to Impact (High, Medium, Low)
1.		
2.		
3.		
4.		
5.		
6.		
7.		
8.		
9.		
10.		
11.		

2. Using the ratings on the previous page enter the implementation activity in the appropriate box.

Agency's Ability to Impact

	High	Medium	Low
High			
Medium			
Low			

3. The relative agency emphasis (measured by allocation of Agency resources) should be in tune with the position of the implementation activity in the diagram.

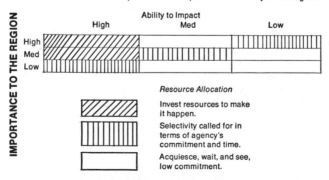

IMPORTANCE TO THE REGION

Ability to Impact

	High	Med	Low

Resource Allocation

Invest resources to make it happen.

Selectivity called for in terms of agency's commitment and time.

Acquiesce, wait, and see, low commitment.

Source: State Plan Implementation Workshop, Alpha Center for Health Planning, October 10/11, 1979.

involved. With respect to the five examples of short-range objectives noted earlier, some of the actors identified by these planning agencies were county health departments, Planned Parenthood, neighborhood health centers, city council, department of aging, parent-teacher associations (PTAs), school district officials, local hospitals, and district planning councils. In Exhibit 8-2, actors include the director of ambulatory services,

Exhibit 8-2 Worksheet for Implementation Strategy

Activity:	Develop a county detection and treatment center
Constraints:	Residents of the county have to be stimulated to come in and to undertake follow-up. Deadline 1/1 of next year.

Implementation Strategy:

(who does what)	(when)
1. Director of Ambulatory Services develops proposal for detection/treatment center	1/1
2. County Board funds proposal	3/1
3. County renovates facilities	6/1
4. Director hires staff, including administrator and medical director	6/15
5. Administrator and medical director develop protocols and procedures, including special effort to motivate residents to participate and to follow up	8/15
6. Administrator acquires equipment and supplies	8/15
7. Data specialist develops patient record forms	9/15
8. Health educator develops education materials	9/15
9. Staff and volunteers are trained by medical director, health educator and head nurse	10/1
10. Administrator tests methods and materials with county residents	10/15
11. Staff begins detection and treatment services to county residents	11/15
12. Administrator evaluates detection and treatment services	11/15

Source: National Heart, Lung, and Blood Institute, *Handbook for Improving High Blood Pressure Control in the Community* (Washington, D.C.: U.S. Government Printing Office, 1977), p. 37.

county boards, medical administrator, data specialist, health educator, and volunteers. Responsibilities, time schedules, and decision points are assigned to each of the actors. For example Exhibit 8-2 reveals that the data specialist and health educator have to develop patient record forms and education materials by September 15.

Forces and Factors Acting on Each Actor

Three groups can be identified by an analysis of the forces and factors acting upon the various actors: (1) allies, who are willing to assist in the achievement of the objective; (2) opponents, who can be expected to take a strong stand against the objective; and (3) neutrals, who will do nothing to assist or obstruct achievement of the objective. A health planning agency can use the techniques of scanning, focusing, and mapping to identify actors who might be involved in the achievement of specific objectives.[10] For example, scanning to identify all those actors who might conceivably be concerned with water fluoridation in a North Central Florida community of at least 5,000 population might show:

- Dentists
- Middle-class families
- Environmentalists
- School officials
- Social agencies
- Welfare rights groups
- Pharmacists
- Health insurors
- Lay groups fearful of harmful effects
- Some PTAs
- Some religious groups as Jehovah's Witnesses
- Some unions
- City council members
- Hospital officials
- Businesses
- Commercial, factory owners
- Chamber of Commerce

The next step is to focus on each group and predict, based on research, past actions regarding the same or similar objectives, and personal contacts, what position each group is likely to take. In focusing, it is necessary to state why the group takes its position. Some positions can be altered through persuasion or education; others are impossible to change. For example, a chart might be drawn that shows

1. Pro

- dentists: Prevention of tooth decay is one of their major concerns.
- middle-class families: Health conscious, interested in prevention of tooth decay.
- environmentalist: Water fluoridation is viewed as a positive example in the use of the environment.
- school officials: Healthy body and mind are considered aids to promote learning and reduce absenteeism due to illness.
- welfare rights group: Fluoridation is considered a cost-efficient way to reduce dental bills that they cannot normally afford.
- health insurors: Fluoridation is seen as a way to hold down cost of health insurance and avoid confrontations with consumers and state officials over requests for rate increases.

2. Con

- lay groups: Many consumers are fearful of potential dangers to their own and their children's health due to accidents or toxicity of fluoridation.
- some PTAs: Groups strongly opposed to fluoridation can use PTAs to oppose it.
- religious groups: Groups such as Jehovah's Witnesses oppose anything that interferes with nature's way.

3. Neutrals

- city council members: Although individual members may take a stand for and against, the council will generally stay neutral until a consensus forms, pro or con.
- hospital officials: Usually not concerned about prevention issues, these officials will be indifferent to the situation.
- Chamber of Commerce: As long as it does not affect business profits, the Chamber of Commerce will not take sides.

Through analysis of each of the actors and their likely positions, the health planning agency can determine whom they can involve to support its fluoridation objective and who the opposition might be.

Based on this analysis, the agency will map the interaction of the forces uncovered with respect to fluoridation. Mapping involves looking "intensively at individual key factors in order to deal with critical linkages and interactions.[11] It cannot be taken for granted that either individual dentists or the local dental association will automatically become an ally to support this objective. They may have other priorities; one influential leader might be opposed to fluoridation and prevent the overwhelming majority of dentists from taking an active stand; or in this particular community, the overabundance of dentists may cause dentists to oppose fluoridation because it will further reduce their incomes. Health insurors may support fluoridation as a cost-free form of health insurance. They view it as a means of opposing future dental association efforts to raise dental fees. Thus, while both may be in favor of fluoridation, they may support it for divergent reasons. This may well lead to tensions within the support group, unless their motivations are kept at a low profile.

Through this type of analysis, a map should be made that shows how all the forces interact with each other and the potential motivations for their positions. Mapping further permits the health planning agency to assess the influence each actor has and can bring to bear on the issue. Groups have various types of influence: money, social status, control over votes, access to mass media, knowledge, political status, energy to work hard, and capacity to legitimize an action. Dentists would normally be expected to have at least social status, some economic status, knowledge, and an informal capacity to legitimize the positive effect of fluoridation. Ardent opponents would usually possess a great deal of energy; some control over votes, depending on the size of the group; some access to media; and knowledge of the issue. The planning implementor assesses the potential resources for influence of those taking each position.[12]

It is not enough to know the sources of influence available. It is important to evaluate how this influence can be used effectively. Banfield defines influence as the "ability to get others to act, think, or feel as one intends;"[13] it is essential to know the various avenues or pathways on which influence can be exerted. Among these avenues are (a) using good relationships or friendship; (b) selling a position to persons open to persuasion; (c) calling in an obligation, possibly owed for a past favor; (d) inducing one to do as you wish because of power you may hold over him, e.g., you assisted in his getting his position; or (e) engaging in outright conflict through the use of votes, demonstrations, or other contest means.

It is entirely possible that there may be no appropriate pathway to use the resources possessed by a coalition of actors. For example, dentists may possess extensive knowledge about the impact of fluoridation, but city council members, in order to maintain a neutral position, are not interested in hearing or being persuaded by it. The knowledge of the opponents may be just as persuasive. Rather than take a position, they close this pathway to both sides. A health insuror may possess money and economic status, but the Chamber of Commerce and city council cannot be reached by this pathway because it is not relevant to their political or business needs. On the other hand, a member of a civic association may be a close social friend of the mayor. The avenue of friendship can be used to persuade the mayor to support fluoridation. An anti-fluoridationist, however, may be able to induce two council members to oppose the objective because the anti-fluoridationists command sufficient votes to defeat them in the next election. In such a case, these two council votes may well neutralize the influence of the mayor.

Because of the cross patterns and multiple sources of influence and pathways to key persons, it is important to map these relationships in order to assess the feasibility of achieving the objective. Banfield states that, when there are a number of autonomous actors and each has some influence over the outcome of the objective sought, it is necessary to centralize control over all of these actors to ensure success. As he states,

> Control over an actor may be secured by an exercise of power.
> . . . No actor . . . ever gives a requisite action unless control
> over him has first been established by an exercise of power.[14]

Resources of influence are the power elements of which Banfield is speaking. Thus, mapping should end with a chart that demonstrates the actions needed for success and the means for controlling the actors. While technical analysis is an important aspect of assessing the forces at work, political values and actions determine the final result.

As Getson has stated with respect to implementation at the state level in Massachusetts, however, the key actors who will later be responsible for decision making should be involved *early in the planning stage.*[15] Waiting until the plan is completed simply complicates matters and makes the capacity of the agency to involve those decision makers more doubtful. In addition, with early involvement a network for planning becomes a network for implementation. Getson points out that it took two years of education and the involvement of five major state agencies and a health insurance organization to develop HMO regulations that were acceptable to a skeptical legislative body. Its members were fearful that too stringent regulation would create difficulties too great for HMOs to overcome and that too loose regulation could be abused by the HMOs themselves. Through this two-year period of working together and involving key legislators, acceptable HMO regulations were approved.

When a single provider is needed to meet an objective such as an expansion of ambulatory care services to underserved areas, the planning agency may have less of a political problem and more of a technical and evaluative one. Some points that should be kept in mind in selecting the proper health care provider are

- The provider should already have experience in the delivery of the services required.
- The provider should be capable of delivering the services without overextending the provision of its current services, since such an overextension could result in their future curtailment.
- The planning agency should cater to those providers who seek and are capable of supporting new or expanding services.
- The planning agency may use a trade-off strategy whereby the provider is encouraged to add a new and needed service in exchange for eliminating a duplicative and/or inefficient service the planning agency would like to see eliminated.[16]

If the provider selected had been involved in the development of the plan, then the agency's analysis of the provider's ability to implement a selected objective would be that much easier. Likewise the cooperation of the provider could be more readily anticipated.

Forces or Factors for Achieving Objectives

In addition to examining the actors involved, it is also necessary to analyze the forces or factors that facilitate or obstruct achievement of the objective. In this analysis, attention should be paid to four basic sets of influences: (1) legal/structural, (2) technoeconomic, (3) sociocultural beliefs and values, and (4) health status and health policy.[17] With respect to the objective sought, certain questions must be asked:

1. Does the objective require legal action, such as a certificate of need?
2. Is the project technically and economically feasible given the reimbursement patterns?
3. Will the services be provided in a way that the target population will feel comfortable using them?
4. Will the service improve the health status of the target population in the manner expected?

Health planning agencies have placed their greatest stress on modifying the hospital industry, e.g., closing down unnecessary and inefficient hospitals, reducing the number of beds, combining the units of two different hospital pediatric or obstetric units into one, fostering reduced usage of certain types of expensive medical technology such as computerized axial tomography (CAT) scanners and open heart surgical units, and expanding existing services to underserved populations.

A number of trends occurring in the hospital industry may enable planning agencies to orient hospitals to the agencies' objectives with respect to hospital care. The following are among these trends:

- The system is shrinking.
- The growth rate of expenditures is leveling off.
- Small hospitals are disappearing.
- Inpatient activity is stable.
- The mix of hospitals is changing.[18]

These trends are threatening to hospitals. Added to these are four other factors that place further tensions on hospitals: (1) the threat of new entrants, (2) the rising bargaining power of consumers, (3) the bargaining power of suppliers, and (4) the threat of substitute services. Most of these factors have intensified since the advent of health planning in the mid-1960s, and they have reached alarming proportions for hospitals in the 1970s. Many hospitals are thus potentially susceptible to health planning agencies' offers of assistance in reducing the impact of certificate-of-need requirements and the development of HMOs, or in finding sources of funds for the high capital costs of new services. By trading on these trends and factors, planning agencies are in a position to participate in reshaping the acute care system so that it is consistent with their goals and objectives.

In working with hospitals, planning agencies must ask a number of important questions:

- Should planning agency activities be focused on a few objectives or be more comprehensive?
- Should the agency be more concerned with the process (maintenance goal) or the outcome (task goal)?
- Does the planning agency see the hospital as an adversary or a supporter?
- Does the agency spend resources to make the weak hospitals stronger or ignore them in favor of the strong ones?
- Should the agency bring about change in hospital behavior by punishment (disapproving hospital certificate-of-need proposals, lowering reimbursement rates) or by reward (providing technical assistance, encouraging their expansion or modernization plans)?[19]

In their eagerness to achieve change, planning agencies must be aware that far-reaching change is time-consuming and involves providers and consumers in a constant, ongoing dialogue. Given the composition of the planning agency's board and its need for hospitals' support to foster the changes it seeks, the emphasis should be on building a cooperative process rather than on ramming through changes to achieve the plan's objectives, regardless of the negative impact on the institutions.

The planning agency must be aware of the forces at work in the environment and make an evaluation of how they can be used to achieve its goals and objectives. The way in which it makes this assessment will affect its image in the community, volunteers' commitment to agency activities, the community's perception of its technical and professional competence, its capacity to gather political support, and its ability to involve other institutions in a cooperative manner. Thus, the stakes involved in the agency's implementation of its objectives are high, for its future acceptance may depend on it.[20]

Alternative Implementation Strategies

Federal health planning guidelines require that "recommended actions" be developed for each short-range objective.

> ... the descriptions of recommended actions specify: (1) the population or geographic area affected, (2) the type of health service affected, (3) the type of facility affected, and (4) the organization, agency, or individuals responsible for the actions.[21]

Actions are directly related to short-range objectives. Their alternative or collective results should be the achievement of the one-year objective. Only by identifying the specific alternative actions sought is the planning agency in a position to select the best alternatives.

Actions are selected after determining whether resources are available, whether a health care provider is willing to take the lead in promoting it, whether the impact of the target population is beneficial, and what the impact on other components of the health system will be. Most agency recommended actions are stated in general terms. An examination of some of the actions linked to the objectives described previously illustrates their specificity and permits an analysis of whether they individually or collectively will achieve the one-year objective.

Objective: Moratorium on new obstetrical beds until state Perinatal Designation Process is initiated.

Recommended
   actions: 1. All agencies in area IV to be notified of the schedule and procedures for implementing the Perinatal Designation Process.

2. Update the long-range plan dealing with obstetrics and maternal and infant health with latest data, taking state recommendations into account.

The planning agency takes on the responsibility of notifying the agencies and updating its plan. Both actions are necessary to keep the plan current and offer guidance to health facilities in the region. There is no need to name specific health institutions or cite specific target populations at this stage. The actions as stated will meet the one-year objective. However, although two actions are mentioned, they are not alternatives, but rather different elements of the same action, both of which are necessary to achieve the objective.

Objective: All schools in service area VII to be in 90 percent compliance in immunization of their school children.

Recommended
  actions: 1. Establish a program to monitor the compliance of schools with the immunizations requirements.

2. Enforcement agency develops a mechanism to enforce compliance.

The actions are specific in naming the population to be affected, all school children in area VII. The PTAs, school district officials, and the state's office of education will monitor the voluntary compliance, and the Department of Public Health is to enforce it for those not in compliance. Again, the actions are not offered as alternatives, but as two levels of achieving compliance, voluntary and mandatory means.

Objective: Add two teen clinics in existing family planning programs.

Recommended
  actions: 1. Obtain information on the extent and type of teen services offered by Planned Parenthood, County Health Department, and the Health Center.

2. Encourage five existing family planning programs to add teen clinics with priority to those able to reach the largest number of teens.

A population is named as the recipient of special services in the recommended action. Also, the actions cite the names of agencies that should provide such services. These are positive and accepted ways of describing the recommended actions. Once again, however, the actions are not alternatives, but rather two different types of activities: seeking information and encouraging providers to become involved.

All of the action statements in the three examples cited can be considered correct as far as they go. Furthermore, two of the three objectives can be reached by the actions (development of a regional perinatal system and 90 percent immunization of school children). In the third, no measurable objective has been stated for the first year, although the long-range goal calls for births to teen-agers to be below the 190 per 1,000 live birth national rate. The effect of opening two additional teen clinics is not stated. Even so, what has been done can be considered positive in these three sets of recommended actions.

The main problem with these recommended actions is whether in fact true alternatives have been offered. For example, reducing teen-age childbirths could be accomplished by establishing teen-age peer discussion groups in schools, increasing the amount and broadening the range of sex education taught in schools or at home, or having churches and teen-age athletic programs take a larger role in sex education. By citing such alternatives, it may then be possible to determine which are the best for achieving the objective.

Likewise, with respect to obtaining compliance for immunization of school children, no true alternatives are offered. Since the law mandates compliance, voluntary action is no real alternative because legal recourse is always available in recalcitrant cases. Since the objective is 90 percent immunization of school children, the real focus is on the method for achieving that rate. This is where alternatives could have been offered, e.g., public health announcements, loss of state-allotted education funds, or personal persuasion by local caretakers, such as family physicians and pharmacists. The true objective is to attain a high rate of voluntary compliance by use of alternative strategies, not to resort to mandatory, legally expensive, and tension-raising means.

If true alternatives are adopted by health planning agencies, then it may be possible to consider techniques for determining which are the best. Cost-benefit analysis has been suggested by federal guidelines as one technique to use in selecting among alternative actions. It was noted in an earlier chapter that detailed data generally do not exist to carry out the type of analysis necessary to make a definitive decision. Rather, "what is needed is enough qualitative and quantitative information to show whether one alternative is likely to be *more* costly or provide *less* benefits than another alternative. Something more than personal judgment is needed, but an elaborate, strictly quantitative analysis should not be expected or needed."[22] Types of benefits that should be examined are

- improvement of health status
- improvement of the health system (e.g., availability, accessibility, or quality of services)

- greater efficiency in the use of high-cost personnel or equipment
- achievement of national and state standards of performance

On the other hand, costs must also be taken into account. Factors that should be considered are

- costs of improving medical services
- likelihood of achieving the desired objective
- the possibility the situation will deteriorate if nothing is done

By analyzing such factors, it may be possible to make a choice among alternative actions based on more than personal opinion, even though a full-fledged, quantitative assessment cannot be made.

A second way of choosing alternatives is to subject each alternative action to a series of questions. Exhibit 8-3 is a checklist of questions that

Exhibit 8-3 Checklist Questions for Assessing Change Strategy Impacts

---

a. What Consequences Does Each Choice Have on the Following?

  1) The HSA's point of view
  2) The community's point of view
  3) The focal organization's point of view
  4) The priority perspectives of:
    The plan
    The board of directors
    The executive director
    The AIP
  5) Short time-frame for implementation

b. What Consequence Does Each Choice Have on the Following Functions?

  1) Agency organization and management
  2) Plan development
  3) Plan implementation/review activities
  4) Plan implementation/health systems development
  5) Data management and analysis
  6) Coordination
  7) Public involvement and education

c. What Consequences Does Each Choice Have on the Following?

  1) Increasing the agency's overall image in the community
  2) Increasing the volunteer's commitment to participation in the agency

Exhibit 8-3   Continued

  3) Increasing the professional competence of the agency in the community
  4) Increasing the agency's image of technical competence in the community
  5) Increasing the image of the agency as an organization which initiates change
  6) Increasing the political support for the agency
  7) Increasing the legal mandate of the agency
  8) Increasing the cooperation of other organizations with the agency
  9) Increasing the collaboration of other organizations with the agency
 10) Increasing the support of other institutions for the agency
 11) Increasing the potential for voluntary compliance with the agency's goals and objectives

d. What Consequences Does Each Choice Have on the Following?

  1) The agency's ability to increase inputs of:
       Additional financial resources
       Staff resources
       Consumer support
       Provider support
  2) The agency's ability to increase the availability of:
       Information
       The HSA's image or status as a
       key community resource
  3) The project's feasibility in terms of:
       Physical and fiscal resources
       Technical resources
       Staff resources
       Volunteer resources
  4) The project's promotion of outputs which relate to:
       A general acceptance of the strategies used by the HSA
       System changes
       Improvement in health status
  5) The project's ability to develop spinoffs which will help the agency implement more of its plan in the future.

Source: Health Resources Administration, *A Course on Resource Development and Implementation* (Hyattsville, Md.: U.S. DHHS), p. C-42.

can be used to examine the consequences of each action from a number of points of view, e.g., that of the health planning agencies and that of the community. Committee members consider the questions by asking whether the action enhances, diminishes, or has no effect on the achievement of the objective and consequences for the community actors involved. If necessary, the questions could be weighted by giving higher numerical values to some than to others. The sum of the answers are then totaled and averaged to determine which alternatives to select for each action. The total range of recommended actions for all objectives could be ranked in this way, or they could be ranked within the functional area under discussion such as mental health, hospital services, or disease prevention.

Implementation Work Program

Having determined the objectives to pursue through a combination of analyses, the planning agency must now incorporate these objectives into a viable work program. Several forms are used in this process to encourage creative thinking and informed judgment and to help the agency manage the implementation process. One such form is a scheduling work sheet (Exhibit 8-4). After the planning agency has decided on its objectives and the functional or core areas (mental health, acute care, primary care, etc.), a staff person should be assigned to coordinate the work for each objective. Through discussion among staff, providers already involved in the functional area of the objective and implementation committee members, the series of tasks that are required to achieve the objective should be cited. For example, suppose the objective is to encourage two health agencies to add teen family planning clinics. The resources needed have already been determined and are potentially available. Discussion reveals that at least the following tasks are required:

- development of a committee of providers, consumers, and teens to determine policy for the teen program
- identification of target schools and neighborhoods for services
- development of an outreach program
- a public information campaign
- hiring of staff to operate the program
- contact with directors of several family planning programs to elicit their interest and commitment to establishing such teen clinics.
- development of assessment measures of success

Each of these activities could be labeled milestones in the development of the clinics, because they represent completions of significant tasks. Each

Exhibit 8-4 Objectives/Tasks/Milestone - Scheduling Work Sheet

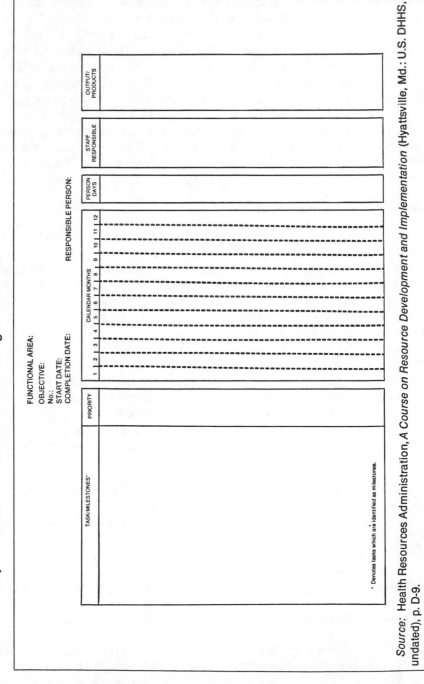

FUNCTIONAL AREA:

OBJECTIVE:
No.:
START DATE:
COMPLETION DATE:

RESPONSIBLE PERSON:

TASK/MILESTONES*	PRIORITY	CALENDAR MONTHS 1 2 3 4 5 6 7 8 9 10 11 12	PERSON DAYS	STAFF RESPONSIBLE	OUTPUT/ PRODUCTS

* Denotes tasks which are identified as milestones.

Source: Health Resources Administration, *A Course on Resource Development and Implementation* (Hyattsville, Md.: U.S. DHHS, undated), p. D-9.

milestone is made up of a series of specific tasks related to it. For example, developing a committee requires

- soliciting names for the committee among providers, consumers, and teens
- evaluating their background, their interest in the objective, their capacity to work with others, availability of time to work on committee and assume responsibility, etc.
- determining the role each might play in the committee (leader, follower, liaison with community or other providers, schools)

A milestone could be a product (e.g., bylaws or a health education program), an event (e.g., a health fair or a ceremony to open the clinic), or the formation of an important relationship (e.g., a hospital's agreement to become a backup facility for the teen clinic). The tasks and milestones should be placed in logical, sequential order in the left hand column of the scheduling work sheet (see Exhibit 8-4). The approximate time it requires to complete the tasks and the various milestones should be placed in the "calendar months" section. Some tasks may be performed simultaneously; for example, outreach and public information programs can be developed at the same time. The time periods for each task should be set so that, when the end date for completing the implementing tasks arrives the teen clinic can be opened and operated in an efficient manner.

Total person days to achieve each milestone should be estimated. Person days involve planning agency staff, volunteers, and staff from coordinating agencies. It is necessary to estimate the person days required so that the planning agency can determine whether it has sufficient personnel to carry out all of its high-priority objectives. Having too few personnel not only overburdens those who are available, but also leads to inefficiencies, as competing program objectives vie for personnel. Having too many personnel wastes precious staff and volunteer time. As it is quite likely that more than one staff will be involved, it is essential to state who has what responsibility, particularly if volunteers are involved. The agency's director may ask other agency directors or their representatives to serve on the committee, while a staff associate seeks out the volunteer and teen members.

Finally, the output involves such things as completing the organization of the committee, naming schools to participate, or producing an outreach manual. All of these tasks and milestones complete the planning agency's implementation phase. The actual operation of the teen family planning clinic is an administrative function and the responsibility of another health service agency.

Network scheduling techniques are important. One such technique, known as PERT (Performance Evaluation and Review Technique) and CPM (Critical Path Methods), is a graphic method for illustrating how long each task takes. It also identifies the series of tasks from the beginning of the project to the end that requires the longest time to perform. This is known as the *critical path* because it indicates the limits within which all other tasks must be completed if the activities are to be completed on time. PERT has the virtue of linking all the tasks into an integrated whole. Exhibit 8-5 is an illustration of PERT applied to developing an open heart surgery unit. Note that the milestones are the completion of planning, renovation of the unit, training of the team, and the installation of the equipment. The last three milestones are to be carried out in parallel. The critical path, shown in dotted lines, is the longest period of time required to complete the surgical unit, some 25 weeks from the equipment order to its installation in the surgical unit. Under ideal circumstances, the equipment portion might be completed in as little as 15 weeks. It can be seen from the best to the worst estimates of time needed that a range of 10 weeks is allowed as slack time.

The PERT technique can be used to uncover potential problems in the network of activities, such as failure of one activity to connect with at least one other activity (known as a "dangle"), or the completion of a milestone in such a way that it does not parallel completion of a second milestone or the end of the project (known as a "loop" problem). If the surgical team were trained but could not practice because the equipment never arrived or the renovation of the surgical unit was incomplete, this would be a loop problem.

If the PERT network were imposed on a time chart, such as is shown in Exhibit 8-4, this would be known as the Gantt technique, a way of depicting tasks on a time line. By reviewing the tasks involved in the action(s), it is possible to reschedule tasks, start activities at different times, or link different groups of tasks with others. It permits the simulation of reality. If alternative actions are required to achieve a short-range objective, the development of PERT and Gantt charts can become quite complex.

Monitoring the Implementation Plan

To ensure that tasks are being carried out consistent with the actions desired, it is necessary to develop a monitoring or tracking system. This is defined as

a management process for the systematic collection, recording, and feedback of information regarding the status of goals, objec-

Exhibit 8-5 PERT Network for Development of Open Heart Surgery Unit

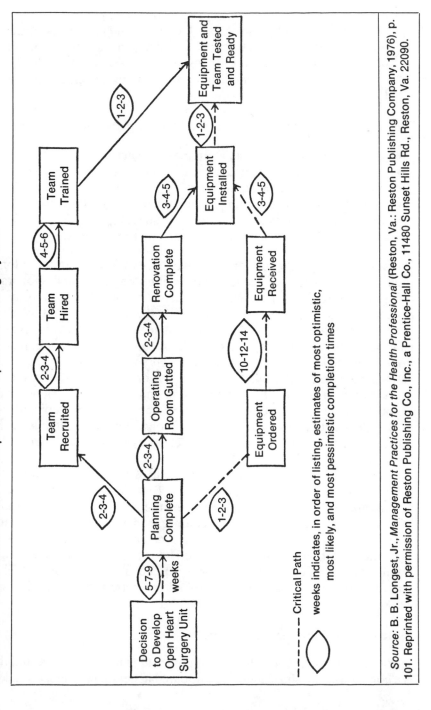

Source: B. B. Longest, Jr., *Management Practices for the Health Professional* (Reston, Va.: Reston Publishing Company, 1976), p. 101. Reprinted with permission of Reston Publishing Co., Inc., a Prentice-Hall Co., 11480 Sunset Hills Rd., Reston, Va. 22090.

tives, and actions in the . . . Plan and projects, plans and activities which relate to those goals, objectives, and actions. A tracking system provides a structure to record and document on an ongoing basis, the progress being made in moving towards the objectives and in accomplishing the actions specified in the Plan."[23]

The tracking or monitoring system enables the planning agency to

- identify successful actions, strategies, and actors
- note the progress being made in the achievement of objectives
- signal problems in the action plan
- measure how well it is doing in its implementation tasks
- provide a recorded document to use in developing reports to federal officials, to its own volunteer boards, and to the general public

Basically, the reporting system tells who does what, when, how long it took, its costs, progress made in completion of action and short-range objective(s), and any problems that arise. Generally, two forms are needed. One form presents an overview of the actions needed to accomplish the objectives (Exhibit 8-6). The first section lists the objectives and major actions to be accomplished. In the second section are recorded the priority of the objective, who is responsible for performing the requisite actions, the personnel needed in person days or months, and the estimated dates on which the actions will begin and end. The actual dates are also recorded on this form so that they can be compared to the predicted dates. In the last section, the status of the actions, e.g., on schedule, behind schedule, or terminated, is listed, as well as evaluative comments about the process.

Exhibit 8-7 is a more specific statement of all the tasks required to achieve milestones and the final action. Tasks and their recommended actions are described and aggregated to ensure that there is no overlapping. Where one task may be used to effect more than one action, code numbers might be assigned to indicate which tasks can be combined.

A tracking or monitoring system feeds directly into plan development. It indicates which objectives of the plan are being achieved and which are not. It also permits an evaluation of all the actions to determine what worked and why.

Evaluating the Implementation Plan

With a major shift from plan development to plan implementation, there is a commensurate shift in what is evaluated in health planning agencies.[24]

Exhibit 8-6 Agency Work Program—Status Report

Agency:
Original ☐, Revision ☐ No.
Date:

FUNCTIONAL AREA:
TOTAL PROFESSIONAL STAFF DAYS:
TOTAL PROFESSIONAL STAFF COST:

PERCENT OF TOTAL:
PERCENT OF TOTAL:

OBJECTIVE/MILESTONE*	Priority	Responsibility	Person Days	ORIGINAL Dates Start	Stop	ACTUAL Dates Start	Stop	** Status	STATUS REPORT COMMENTS

* Milestones are tasks noted with an asterisk.

**On Schedule = OS; Behind Schedule = BS; Terminated = T

Source: Health Resources Administration, *A Course on Resource Development and Implementation* (Hyattsville, Md.: U.S. DHHS, undated), p. D-13.

Exhibit 8-7 Short-Range HSA Implementation Tasks

AIP Actions	AIP Page Ref.	Implementation Tasks			
		First Implementation Task Associated With the Action	Second Task Associated With Action	Third Task	Etc.
Title or Brief Description of Action					

Source: Alpha Center for Health Planning, "Guide to Resource Estimation," mimeographed (Bethesda, Md.: May, 1979), p. 67.

During the plan development stage, evaluation focused on the process of plan development and other major agency functions, such as data management, regulatory activities, public involvement, and coordination. In contrast, evaluation during implementation focuses on outcome. Planning agencies are now being evaluated according to their capacity to improve the population's health status and the health systems services in their areas, the impact their activities have had on the community, and their success in containing the costs of medical care. Examples of indicators suggested by the Bureau of Health Planning for measuring impact are[25]

- health status
  —infant mortality rates
  —death rates
  —cause-specific death rates for ten leading causes of death
  —preventable communicable disease rates
- health systems
  —hospital beds/1,000 population
  —percentage of hospitals with occupancy rate over 80 percent
  —percentage of pediatric units with at least 20 beds
  —percentage open heart surgery units with 200 + procedures per year
- community impacts
  —percentage population in medically underserved areas
  —percentage population enrolled in HMOs
  —number of primary care physicians/1,000 population
  —percentage population served by community mental health centers
- cost
  —community hospital expenses per capita
  —community hospital expenses per admission
  —increase in total hospital expenses per admission from year to year
  —average hospital charge per aged discharge
  —percentage approved certificate-of-need expenditures for projects specified in health plans
  —amount of capital not expended due to agency certificate-of-need decisions or actions

Evaluations must now focus on the impact the actions have on such health indicators as those noted.[26]

Evaluation is undertaken to determine if the plan is on the right track and to justify past and future expenditures. On the other hand, evaluations are also used for negative purposes; e.g., to cover up a planning agency's weaknesses, to eliminate unpopular programs, or to delay vital decisions. Whether their purposes are positive or negative, they tend to be feared and seen more as a threat to the agency or certain professionals within it than as a means to improve a program or an agency's performance.

ISSUES AND OPPORTUNITIES IN HEALTH IMPLEMENTATION

Antitrust Legislation and Implementation

In response to a request from the Central Virginia Health Planning Agency for a ruling, the Department of Justice's Antitrust Division (a) concluded that a planning agency's review functions (reactive implementation strategy) were exempt from antitrust liability, but (b) questioned whether proactive implementation strategies that involved coordination of health providers and consumers in pursuing a common action and objective were also immune.[27] As Curran has noted, "the Federal Government has for many generations since 1890 been dedicated under the Anti-Trust Laws to competition among enterprises and to the prevention of business monopoly and monopolistic practices."[28] He goes on to note that PL 93-641 has moved in the opposite direction by determining the rates, availability, and quality of services to be offered to consumers. The efforts of health planning agencies to involve health care providers in voluntary cooperative actions to implement health planning goals and objectives are being questioned as collusive and contrary to antitrust laws. The Department of Justice claims that, while PL 93-641 explicitly authorizes health planning agencies to carry out certificate-of-need and Proposed Uses of Federal Funds (PUFF) review activities, it does not authorize proactive, collusive actions that would have the effect of reducing competition and fostering monopoly among health institutions.

In its response to the Department of Justice's opinion, the Department of Health and Human Services (HHS) cites evidence in both the law and congressional debate that clearly establishes Congress' intent that health planning agencies be exempt from antitrust laws in carrying out their proactive implementation strategies. HHS' letter to the Department of Justice points out the following evidence:

- Section 1513(c)(1) "*requires* that each . . . agency shall seek, to the extent practicable, to implement its . . . [plans] with the assistance of individuals and public and private entities in its health service area."[29]

- Section 1502 of the 1979 amendments to PL 93-641 stated: "For health services, such as inpatient . . . and other institutional health services, for which competition does not or will not appropriately allocate supply consistent with health . . . plans, . . . health planning and development agencies should in the exercise of their functions under this title take actions . . . to allocate the supply of such services."[30]
- Finally, in the debate on the 1979 amendments to PL 93-641, the House Committee on Interstate and Foreign Commerce set forth its understanding of the relationship between health planning and antitrust laws:

> The committee believes that the antitrust laws should be aggressively enforced to ensure a vigorous and competitive economy where there is reason to believe that business will in fact compete on the basis of price, quality, and service. However, . . . the committee believes there is currently little, if any, competition based on price among institutional health services. For those services unfettered competition could further aggravate existing health system problems—duplicative and unnecessary services and facilities and rapidly rising costs.
>
> While the application of the antitrust laws to promote competition is and should be the general rule, the committee believes that a practical and realistic analysis of the health care industry argues for exceptions to the rule.
>
> . . . Congress required health planning agencies to carry out specific functions and established a financial penalty for States which failed to comply with the requirements. Those statutory requirements and penalty indicate that *Congress did not expect the antitrust laws to be applied to agency actions which might otherwise be in violation of the antitrust laws, if those agency actions were necessary to carry out the prescribed functions.* (H.R. Rep. No. 96-190, 96th Cong. 1st Sess. 54-55 (1979). (Emphasis added.)[31]

While the Department of Justice has not come to a final opinion about the legality of planning agencies using proactive implementation strategies to achieve their objectives, the prevailing opinion appears to be that the Department of Justice failed to make "a careful and accurate analysis of its mandate" before making its decision.[32] Health planning leaders see the Department of Justice's position as a major hindrance to health planning if the opinion is allowed to stand.

Confrontation between Health Planning Agency and Health Provider

What follows is an illustration of how a coalescing of forces, some planned and some unplanned, resulted in a hospital's reluctant agreement to change its mission in the community from providing acute care inpatient services to 24-hour ambulatory services. It particularly illustrates the positive impact of combining reactive and proactive implementation strategies to obtain a desired outcome.[33]

> The agreement in September 1978 to close the 100-year-old Winchendon Hospital capped nearly five years of discussion and negotiation by the hospitals in the Winchendon area of Massachusetts, Blue Cross, and the Central Massachusetts Health Systems Agency (CMHSA).
>
> This case describes how CMHSA, by developing an institution-specific Health Systems Plan, served as a catalyst for the closure of Winchendon Hospital and its conversion to more appropriate ambulatory and long-term care services. It also notes how the local Blue Cross plan used its reimbursement power to create pressure to implement CMHSA's recommendations.
>
> In 1973, Winchendon Hospital, a 40-bed acute care facility located in the old mill town of Winchendon about 35 miles north of Worcester near the New Hampshire border, came before CMHSA's predecessor CHP agency with a proposal to build a $9.2 million, 26-bed replacement facility and long-term and ambulatory care centers. Based on its analysis of the Winchendon situation, the planning agency not only recommended that the application be denied but also noted that there was no adequate justification for the continuation of the existing acute care facility in light of the declining population, the historical difficulty in retaining physicians, and the availability of two other acute care facilities 11 and 17 miles from Winchendon.
>
> Shortly thereafter, the Public Health Council of the Massachusetts Health Department took a similar position and denied Winchendon Hospital its certificate of need. As a result, the citizens of Winchendon succeeded in having a bill introduced before the State Legislature, granting the Hospital a certificate of need and a license. The bill was passed and vetoed by the Governor. The veto was overridden.
>
> The State Health Department still refused to grant a certificate of need, however, arguing that the Legislature had transcended the bounds of its authority. The State Supreme Court, in the land-

mark Besse Burke decision to which Winchendon Hospital was a party, found in favor of the plaintiff, thus clarifying the Legislature's authority to override regulatory agencies and to grant determinations of need under the State's CON [certificate-of-need] statute.

As a result, in January 1976, Winchendon Hospital finally received a certificate of need. It contained a three-year deadline for beginning construction. During the next two years, however, the Hospital was unable to secure financing.

In late 1977, CMHSA released a draft acute care plan for proposed inclusion in its Health Systems Plan. The draft plan stated specifically that, in accordance with State planning standards, rebuilding Winchendon Hospital would waste scarce resources and proposed that two neighboring acute care facilities had more than adequate capacity to meet the area's need.

The specific recommendation was that Winchendon Hospital close its acute care component, affiliate for acute care services with the 153-bed Henry Heywood Memorial Hospital in Gardner, 11 miles away, and replace its facility with an ambulatory care center. It also recommended that a nursing home be developed to serve the large number of elderly citizens in the Winchendon area.

Again, the Hospital rejected this proposal. The community also reacted heatedly. Petitions opposing the closure of the hospital drew some 5,000 signatures. More than 600 people attended the public hearings on the issue, and several hundred sent letters to various senators, congressmen and HEW officials, protesting CMHSA's recommendations and claiming that CMHSA was denying them their right to adequate health care. There was a barrage of newspaper editorials calling for the closing of the HSA. Even the A-95 Agency voted for two years in a row not to fund CMHSA because of the Winchendon Hospital issue.

Simultaneously, however, Blue Cross of Massachusetts announced that it would endorse CMHSA's draft acute care plan and would support it through its selective contract mechanism. More specifically, it would not reimburse for health care services that were in violation of the Health Systems Plan.

CMHSA utilized the Blue Cross commitment to bring the situation to a head. It secured a firm commitment from the plan that services at Winchendon would no longer be reimbursed for.

In May 1978, the Joint Commission on Accreditation of Hospitals (JCAH) visited Winchendon. At the time of the site visit, the Hospital had lost both its Administrator and its Director of Nursing and was being run by lay citizens in the community. Within a month after the Joint Commission visit, the State Department of Public Health also conducted a validation survey.

Winchendon Hospital was now faced with a multitude of pressures: the imminent Blue Cross termination of reimbursement; the prospect of suspension of State approval for surgical services resulting from the validation survey, and the possibility of problems from JCAH. In addition, its certificate of need was due to expire at the end of the year, and it had been unable to obtain federally guaranteed construction loans to finance its construction because of CMHSA's opposition.

Winchendon Hospital was forced to take action. In July 1978, it signed a 90-day management services contract with Burbank Hospital, a 222-bed acute care facility in neighboring Fitchburg. Burbank immediately took over the administrative operations at Winchendon. It quickly secured a 90-day delay of Blue Cross's reimbursement termination order and began to work out a new master plan. A joint committee of the HSA, the Hospital and its directors and several Winchendon residents was established to examine solutions to the Hospital's problems.

Finally, in late September 1978, after a series of meetings, which included State representatives whom Winchendon had now asked for an extension of its certificate of need, verbal agreement was reached by CMHSA, the State Health Department and Winchendon, represented by Burbank. The agreement, which was contingent on Winchendon's phasing out major surgery immediately and minor inpatient surgery over a one-year period, was that Winchendon would be permitted to amend its CON application to remove the acute care component; an ambulatory care facility, including physicians' offices, a 24-hour-a-day primary care center and limited ambulatory surgical services would be developed in its place. The CON would also provide for construction of a nursing home. The acute care facility would be closed within 30 days of the nursing home's opening.

Because the HSP had identified the need for ambulatory and long-term care services in the Winchendon area, approval of the agreement was considered likely by the full HSA and by the State Public Health Council.

In October the Assistant State Commissioner for Health confirmed that he would recommend approval of the amended CON to the State Public Health Council if the Hospital agreed to the prompt and orderly phase-out of its existing acute care services.

On November 1, the Winchendon Board voted to delete the acute care bed portion of its CON application and to apply for approval to build a new facility that will serve both as a 24-hour-a-day primary care center and a skilled nursing unit with 40 beds. It also voted to extend the shared management contract with Burbank to three years, with the Winchendon Board remaining autonomous.

CMHSA, acting in support of the agreement, wrote on November 8 to HEW to request that the Winchendon area be designated as a Health Manpower Shortage Area to assist in the establishment of the primary care facility. And on November 28, it approved the request for a one-year extension of the certificate of need.

The Winchendon community, influenced by CMHSA's argument that health care is not necessarily hospital care, has now accepted the decision to close its Hospital. So instead of an inappropriate new hospital the town of Winchendon will have a new long-term and comprehensive ambulatory care center as a result of the combined efforts of CMHSA, the State, and Blue Cross.

Closing Hospitals

One of the main targets of health plans is the planned elimination of thousands of unused acute care beds. Developing action plans to achieve this objective calls for a combination of reactive and proactive strategies. As McClure has stated,

> The chief barrier to reduction is the absence of any climate of public support. . . . How far and how fast excess hospital use and capacity can be reduced may largely depend on whether the public and providers can be educated to accept some trade-off between the more lavish level of hospital care to which they have become accustomed, and their desires to free resources for other purposes more productive of health and well-being."[34]

In other words, eliminating or reducing beds in a hospital is a sociopolitical issue.

When hospitals are forced by circumstances to make changes in their complement of beds, the outcome cannot always be predicted. In a study of a number of hospital closings in Philadelphia, Texas, Maine, California, and New Mexico, Friedman found a number of factors had made it necessary for institutions to act. In Philadelphia, the main forces were an aging municipal hospital, loss of patients to voluntary nonprofit hospitals after the passage of Medicaid and Medicare, and the heavy expense of maintaining a teaching program.[35] Elsewhere, inability to secure a physician to operate a small rural hospital, competition from a new hospital, a refusal of a federal agency to grant a safety code waiver, and financial inability to construct an overly ambitious health center were all factors that led to the closing or merging of institutions. It appears that the demise of each institution was caused by its own set of circumstances. Of interest is the fact that, except for the failure to obtain a safety code waiver, none of the closings was a planned action of a health planning agency, partly because most of the closings antedated the development of health plans. These were independent actions taken by hospital officials acting out of necessity. Friedman draws "hard lessons" she learned from her study.

- Communication among all parties affected by the closing/merger must be started early and maintained. This includes hospital officials, employees, patients, and the general public. Failure to do this, for example, created bitter feelings in the Philadelphia closing.
- Agreements must be specific so that hospitals left to care for patients of the closing hospital know what is expected of them. In one instance, the remaining hospital was responsible for the care of an undue number of indigent patients for whom the reimbursement rate was much lower than the hospital could tolerate, yet the county claimed that no special subsidy for the indigent patients was called for in the agreement to close the county hospital.
- Employees of closing hospitals in most instances find other positions because of the expansion of services in the remaining hospital and/or the conversion of the closing hospital to other medical functions.
- When a hospital is closed, it is often put to other medical use, e.g., an ambulatory surgicenter, a nursing home, or an ambulatory care center. This, in fact, was the chief issue in the Winchendon case.
- When a hospital closes, "what is also left behind is a community of patients, trustees, physicians, and local residents, and their actions, if not conducted in good faith and with the utmost care, can turn the best-planned and smoothest hospital closing into a tragedy."[36]

In all these situations, the hospitals were forced to close, reduce, or merge. What happens when a hospital plans its own salvation?

In 1975, the chairperson of the Hospital Association of New York State stated in a letter to constituent members that "a shrinkage of our hospital system is necessary."[37] There simply was not enough money to pay for the continued expansion of the system. Therefore, quality of care was to be emphasized. This theme was echoed in many other parts of the United States in the mid-1970s. Hospital officials concluded that it is better for them to take the initiative in reducing the system than to leave the decisions to chance or federal mandate via goals in health plans. Friedman discussed four ways hospitals have successfully decreased utilization.[38]

One solution to low occupancy was the use of "swing beds" to meet changing needs. These are beds that can be used to meet alternate needs as they arise, rather than being assigned to only one hospital unit and its needs. A Utah experiment with this technique resulted in an increase in occupancy rates of more than 40 percent, accompanied by a 30 percent reduction in the average length of stay in 25 rural hospitals. In Ohio, rural hospitals reduced their length of stay from 8 to 5.3 days and increased their occupancy rates by using swing beds. Such beds not only stabilize the daily census and staffing patterns, but also improve hospital finances.

In Baltimore, the conversion of one hospital's acute care unit into a psychiatric inpatient unit of 30 beds led to an increase of 3,500 patient days per month and converted a deficit into a profit. In this instance, conversion was supported by the health planning agency and rate review commission.

Hospitals have also been forming consortia for a variety of purposes; for example, they have been sharing laboratory services, trading off under-used services to increase capacity for both, or developing emergency psychiatric networks. Two of the most far-reaching consortia are in Rochester, New York, and in the state of Michigan. Rochester's hospitals have formed an integrated plan that, to the surprise of most, required only four of its six hospitals. As one administrator stated, "Hospital administrators must take the leadership and rise above their own institutions."[39] Rather than each institution planning for its own needs, all are planning for the needs of the community by means of a systems approach. Emphasis is on meeting the needs of the community and identifying those institutions that can best meet those needs. In the past, the needs of the hospitals came first.

In Michigan, a broad-based coalition that included hospitals developed a plan to reduce the number of hospital beds. After a 14 months' moratorium, during which the regional planning agencies developed their institution-specific plans for elimination of unneeded beds, the certificate-of-need process is being used to ensure compliance with the plans. Reductions are planned by closure or consolidation of hospitals, mergers of major clinical services, or closure of such services within individual hospitals.

In a more recent study of hospital closures, McClure found evidence to support two major conclusions:

> The principal cause that forced retirement of hospital capacity was financial pressure, not planning pressure. However, in the absence of financial pressure, planning decisions to close hospitals provoked intense opposition and were difficult to sustain.[40]

Tight rate controls, combined with a population decrease in an overcrowded market, were responsible for a number of hospital closings.

> Planners and regulators were most effective in reducing excess hospital capacity when they created and coordinated financial pressure and adverse publicity on hospitals they identified as unnecessary.[41]

McClure showed how a climate was created in which the hospital itself took the final action to close. State rate review bodies refused to give relief to the "unnecessary" hospital; inspections of the hospital's plant for violations were increased; and the problems of the hospital were leaked to the press so that physicians referred patients elsewhere and creditors demanded payment of outstanding debts. In the end, the hospital trustees closed the institution. McClure further notes that the hospitals closed tended to be small and to have a decreasing occupancy rate, a deteriorating plant, failing leadership, and a weak constituency.

A major implication of McClure's study is that a full range of reactive and proactive actions is required to implement an objective. A second implication is that a planning agency should be prepared to use conflict strategies, because every institution will struggle to survive.

Finally, regardless of the implementation process used, planning agencies must learn to be creative and flexible in the use of tactics, resources, and legal means available if they are to achieve their objectives. There is no one way or best way, only a general guide that permits a myriad of alternative, imaginative routes agencies can take to reach their goals.

NOTES

1. Murray C. Ross, *Community Organization Theory and Principles* (New York, N.Y.: Harper & Row, 1955).

2. Kurt Lewin, *Field Theory in Social Science,* ed. Dorwin Cartwright (New York, N.Y.: Harper & Brothers, 1951).

3. Robert Morris and Robert H. Binstock, *Feasible Planning for Social Change* (New York, N.Y.: Columbia University Press, 1966).

4. For further information on this model, see parts of the following works: Warren G. Bennis, Kenneth D. Benne, and Robert Chin, eds., *The Planning of Change* (New York, N.Y.: Holt, Rinehart and Winston, 1964), pp. 201–234; Fred M. Cox et al., eds. *Strategies of Community Organization* (Itasca, Ill.: F. E. Peacock Publishers, Inc., 1970), Chapters 4, 6, and 8; Robert R. Mayer, *Social Planning and Social Change* (Englewood Cliffs, N.J.: Prentice-Hall, Inc., 1972), Chapter 1.

5. Bennis, Benne, and Chin, *Planning of Change*, pp. 235–249.

6. Lyle S. Schaller, "Conflict over Conflict," in Cox et al., *Strategies of Organization*, pp. 171–177.

7. *Ibid.*, p. 174.

8. See Robert Chin, "The Utility of System Models and Developmental Models for Practitioners," in Bennis, Benne, and Chin, *Planning of Change*, pp. 201–214; Robert Morris and Martin Rein, "Emerging Patterns in Community Planning," in *Urban Planning and Social Policy*, eds. Bernard Frieden and Robert Morris (New York: Basic Books, 1968), Chapter 2; Robert R. Mayer, "Planning and Change," Chapter 1.

9. Health Resources Administration, *A Course of Resource Development and Implementation* (Hyattsville, Md.: U.S. DHHS, undated).

10. *Ibid.*, p. C-17.

11. *Ibid.*

12. See Herbert H. Hyman, *Organizational Response to Urban Renewal* (Ann Arbor, Mich.: University Microfilms, 1967), Chapter 7; Robert Morris and Robert H. Binstock, *Social Planning: A Feasible Approach* (New York, N.Y.: Columbia University Press, 1966).

13. Edward C. Banfield, *Political Influence*, 2nd ed. (New York, N.Y.: Free Press, 1961) p. 3.

14. *Ibid.*, p. 312.

15. Jacob Getson, "Implementing the State Health Plan: Some Views from Massachusetts," in Alpha Technical Assistance Memorandum #22 (Bethesda, Md.: Alpha Center for Health Planning, March 11, 1980).

16. Alpha Center for Health Planning, "Guide to Resource Estimation," mimeographed (Bethesda, Md.: May 1979), p. 49.

17. Health Resources Administration, *Resource Development*, pp. C41-54.

18. Alpha, Workshop: Tools and Tactics of Implementation (Newark, N.J.: April 17–18, 1980).

19. *Ibid.*, p. 7.

20. Health Resources Administration, *Resource Development*, p. C-47.

21. Health Resources Administration, *Program Policy Notice: Guidelines for the Development of Health Systems Plans and Annual Implementation Plans*, No. 79-05 (Hyattsville, Md.: Bureau of Health Planning, February 23, 1979), p. 28.

22. Alpha, *Resource Estimation*, p. 84.

23. Alpha, *Workshop: State Plan Implementation* (Newark, N.J.: October 10–11, 1979), pp. 3, 4.

24. Health Resources Administration, *Program Information Letter: Draft Impact Performance, Standards and Health Planning Program Measures* No. 80-16 (Hyattsville, Md.: Bureau of Health Planning, August 8, 1980), pp. 8/9.

25. *Ibid.*, pp. 54–63.

26. For a discussion of the evaluation process, see Allen D. Spiegel and Herbert Harvey Hyman, *Basic Health Planning Methods* (Rockville, Md.: Aspen Systems Corporation, 1978); Health Resources Administration, *Resource Development*.

27. Harry P. Cain, Letter to Sanford M. Litvack of the Department of Justice (Washington, D.C.: American Health Planning Association, May 23, 1980).

28. William J. Curran, "The Confrontation between National Health Planning and the Federal Anti-Trust Laws," *American Journal of Public Health* 70, no. 4 (April 1980): 425.

29. Joel M. Mangel, Letter to John Poole of Department of Justice (Washington, D.C.: Office of the General Counsel, DHHS, June 2, 1980), p. 1.

30. *Ibid.*, p. 4.

31. *Ibid.*, pp. 4/5.

32. Cain, Letter to Litvack, p. 7.

33. Health Resources Administration, *Health Planning in Action*, HRP-0150101 (Hyattsville, Md.: Bureau of Health Planning, October, 1979), pp. 15–17.

34. Walter McClure, *Conversion and Other Policy Options to Reduce Excess Hospital Capacity* (Hyattsville, Md.: Bureau of Health Planning, Excelsior, Minn.: InterStudy, September 1979).

35. Emily Friedman, "The End of the Line: When a Hospital Closes," *Hospitals* 52 (1978): 68–75.

36. *Ibid.*, p. 75.

37. Emily Friedman, "The Hospital System Takes a Look at Shrinking Itself," *Hospitals* 52 (1978): 90.

38. *Ibid.*

39. *Ibid.*, p. 95.

40. McClure, *Conversion and Policy Options*, p. 48.

41. *Ibid.*, p. 49.

Chapter 9

Issues in Comprehensive Health Planning and Implementation

Many basic issues affect the capacity of health planning agencies to plan. Although several of these issues have been identified in earlier chapters, the following also have important implications for health planning in the United States:

1. Who has jurisdiction for health planning?
2. Can autonomy, coordination, and innovation exist at the same time in a planning agency?
3. Will private or public needs be met?
4. Will planning be pragmatic (opportunistic) or comprehensive?
5. When regulation and planning are both functions of the same health planning agency, which predominates?
6. Which health planning agency takes the lead: regional or state?
7. What should be emphasized in health plans: prevention or treatment?

Who controls the planning process is a powerful factor in determining whose health needs will be met. On the other hand, how much autonomy the various health actors have in how planning takes place influences whether the planning emphasis is on pragmatic or comprehensive planning.

RESPONSIBILITY FOR PLANNING

In political science, the concepts of power, authority, and influence are the key factors that determine who has power to make decisions. The actor or actors who make the decisions in the final analysis influence the outcome of any matter that comes before them. Power is generally defined as the capacity of one actor to influence another actor to do as he or she desires. Thus, the executive director of a health planning agency can compel a staff member to carry out certain functions for which that person was hired under penalty of being fired, demoted, or discredited.

345

Where this power is lodged in a legal or contractual relationship, the actor has power that stems from authority to act in certain ways. PL 93-641 mandates or authorizes health planning agencies to have at least 51 percent of their board members composed of consumers. However, if the legislation had not specified what percentage of the board should be consumers, then it would have been left to the discretion of each agency to decide what percentage of consumers should be on the agency's board. Those who make such decisions, not embedded in law, are considered to have power distinct from authority.

Yet, it is well understood that the power of informal decision making operates when actors have at their disposal certain resources with which they can compel and influence others. These sources of influences are usually money, friendship, knowledge, votes, status, and access to mass media. These resources become effective with varying circumstances. Thus, in many congressional elections, candidates, wishing to avoid the taint of being "bought," refuse contributions of more than $100 from any donor. A wealthy donor able to give large campaign contributions would have found this source of influence upon the candidate diminished compared to his power in previous campaigns. However, if the donor and candidate shared similar viewpoints on many issues, it might be possible for the donor to influence the candidate on issues where the donor had superior knowledge. Therefore, resources as sources of influence are highly flexible factors for which there are no rigid formulas in their application. Each situation involves different strategies and combinations of influence sources.[1] With the three concepts of power, authority, and resources of influence, it should be possible to analyze the question of who has jurisdiction in the health planning field.

A review of PL 93-641 and its amendments and an analysis of the manner in which it has been implemented by health experts reveals the following:

1. The influence of values affects the involvement of the private sector in policy making, planning, and implementation of activities that occur in the health care field.[2]

2. There is no community or areawide dominant central decision-making body in the health field.[3]

3. PL 93-641 gives no powers or authority to health planning agencies to operate programs.[4]

Taken collectively, these statements offer a short diagnosis of how the power relationships are arranged in the health field.

Influence of Values on Private Sector

The first factor to consider is the influence on the health field of the private sector. The friendliest critics of the private or voluntary health sector, particularly its hospital and medical school core, Brown and Somers, point out how this sector has failed to provide the leadership needed to create a necessary integrated and coordinated health system.[5] Glasser goes further, noting that the private sector has worked to prevent any real efforts at coordinating or implementing plans that involve its functions.[6] The one experiment in which the private sector itself has been the controlling actor in an effort to achieve coordinated planning has proved to be a failure. Somers pointed out that in the areawide health facilities planning councils (the predecessor to PLs 89-749 and 93-641) "one of the striking facts about the voluntary bodies is that many of them do not want responsibility for real decision making."[7] They feared being criticized for imposing a master plan on a community.

One of the significant reasons for this is the value system that pervades American society and is reflected in the health care field. Competition, self-reliance, and individualism are strongly held values that are not conducive to the collectivism and cooperation required by health planning. It is these values of collectivism, voluntarism, and cooperation that have been fostered by PL 93-641 and have come in conflict with the dominant values of self-reliance and individualism reflected in the private physicians' concern with "solo" practice of medicine and their highly valued regard for the confidentiality of the physician-patient relationship. Consequently, there has been resistance by the private health sector to voluntary, collective, or government-sponsored health planning endeavors.

It is, therefore, not surprising that Somers finds critics who accuse those largely voluntary planning bodies of placing too much emphasis on the beds and not enough on ambulatory services, of favoring the status quo and discouraging innovation, and of relying on federal funds to support them rather than using their own funds.[8] Thus, owing to these highly cherished values of self-reliance and individualism, the resistance by the private health sector to changes in health care has prevented the adoption of many significant institutional or integrated changes. Their major concern has been on quality of care and the rapid assimilation of new medical technologies, whether or not the efficacy of these technologies has been demonstrated.

Fragmented Decision Making in Health Planning

The second factor that has to be taken into account is that the health field is so highly fragmented that no one health institution dominates the actions of others. Several of the health experts noted have reported how the proliferation of health facilities and services has increased the fragmentation of the field.[9] It is characterized by a pluralistic power structure in which many small spheres of influence are exercised by hospitals, clinics, neighborhood planning bodies, etc., but none of these is strong enough to compel or persuade others to carry out its decisions. A number of reasons have been offered for the fact that these diverse pluralistic power bases are unable to act together. First, Hilleboe and Schaefer have noted how representatives from various health agencies basically mistrust each other. They attended meetings to protect their "sacred jurisdictions of nontrespassable territories."[10]

Second, several health analysts have concluded that a significant government objective is "the promotion of private interests."[11] An acceptance of this objective by those in the private health sector has led them to focus their energies on tapping the huge resources of the federal, state, and local governments in their behalf. With billions of dollars flowing into the various institutions and little accountability of their activities, there is minimal incentive to cooperate to improve the network of services. Only when faced with a crisis that finds the health institutions impotent have they reluctantly consented to work together. When such a crisis occurred in the late 1950s, at the time when many hospitals were running into high deficits, they agreed to form the many areawide health facilities planning councils. This cooperation lasted as long as the financial crisis persisted, but when monies began to flow into the hospitals through Title XVIII and XIX funds, the coordination attempt again fragmented, with each going its separate way.[12]

A third factor that limits cooperation, and therefore planning, is the rapid change that takes place in the organizations themselves. Because of changes in size, ownership, managerial stewardship, and functions, agreements reached at one time are less valid at another time. Promises of cooperation become meaningless as new leaders reject recommendations made by their predecessors. Under conditions such as these, it is difficult to bring together the diverse clusters of health institutions to plan future changes over which they will have little control.

No Operational Authority

PL 93-641 provides no "seed" money as an incentive to encourage the autonomous health actors to cooperate. The resources of influence in the form of positive inducements and persuasion are too slim to make a difference. The federal government had already learned that the substantially larger carrots they were offering through Medicaid, Model Cities, and the antipoverty programs were too insignificant to influence the health, welfare, and education institutions to make fundamental changes and better serve the residents of low-income urban communities. In time, the federal government provided a negative sanction in the form of legislation to induce compliance with respect to the construction of health facilities. However, the private sector's many years of experience in dealing with state Hill-Burton agencies to obtain approval for new or expanded health facilities served them well in transferring their influence and sometimes control to the certificate-of-need/1122 regulatory bodies; in effect, they continued to regulate themselves. Brown stated it clearly when he said,

> One thing we have learned in this country is that voluntary planning has not worked and will not work. If health care planning is left to the individual institution or voluntary planning agency, then the system grows to meet the desires of the most aggressive and sometimes least altruistic institutions.[13]

What this all means is that no one really has jurisdiction for planning in the private or public sector. The authority given to the health planning agencies has been too limited and has depended too much on good will, voluntary action, and cooperation for carrying out their functions. The agencies' resources of influence required to persuade others to comply have also been too limited to have an impact on the individual institutions.

COORDINATION

The Need

In addition to the usual demands for planning on a comprehensive and integrated basis, the effort to avoid duplication, and the need to serve the whole person, there are other equally important reasons for coordination.[14] Coordination is needed to overcome the mistrust that frequently develops in the absence of contact, as well as the misunderstanding of motives arising from a lack of dialogue.[15] The concept of "creative federalism" has as one of its basic values the promotion of leadership to meet the responsibilities with which health care institutions have been entrusted by the general public. By this process, these institutions should be able to strengthen their ability to meet their problems in a collective way not possible when they act alone. Section 1502 of PL 93-641 calls for coordinated actions in the development of "multi-institutional systems" of health services, development of group practices coordinated with institutional health services, and arrangements for the "sharing of support services." Coordination and cooperation are also needed to provide a higher quality of service by reducing excessive health services. For example, it was said that New York City had 5,000 excess acute care beds in the 1970s. Through a series of certificate-of-need and rate review actions, most of these beds have now been phased out of service. Friedman notes both the difficulty of cooperation and coordinated effort and the surprise benefits that can be gained by it.[16] Thus, coordination is needed to plan rationally, to overcome a communication gap, and to reduce mistrust among health care providers and planners.

Coordination Defined

In an in-depth study on model cities, Warren, Rose and Bergunder attempted to analyze how coordination came about.[17] In their review of the literature, they were surprised to note that the term was always assumed to be understood and defined. It is important to recognize the difference between interorganizational and intraorganizational coordination. The first assumes that coordination takes place among the independent and autonomous actors without the presence of any centralized decision maker. The second assumes the presence of a central decision maker, a board, or a chief executive who can mandate coordination within the organization. PL 93-641 is primarily concerned with interorganizational coordination. Warren et al. define this type of coordination as "a structure or process of concerted decision making or action wherein the decisions or actions of two or more organizations are made simultaneously in part or in whole in some deliberate degree of adjustment to each other."[18] In brief, two autonomous organizations agree to adjust to each other in order to achieve some goal. They may both gain the same thing from the goal, such as more patients, or different goals from the same action, such as one hospital gaining the patients of the other hospital, which in turn can maintain its solvency by giving up an expensive and poorly utilized service. One of the primary tasks of the health planning agency is to help negotiate such outcomes to the benefit of the actors involved and the public interest.

It was further concluded that there are two basic types of coordination: structured and ad hoc goal-oriented. In the structured type of coordination, the health actors agree to meet together on a regular and routine basis for the purpose of coordinating activities "without reference to any specific objective other than coordination."[19] In other words, coordination provides a communication medium whereby any problem, issue, goal, or activity can be discussed with the purpose of doing something about it. Among the four types of planning models, this definition would most accurately describe the partnership type. Through regular meetings of the whole and in committees, an entire range of matters is discussed and improvements are made.

In ad hoc goal-oriented coordination, the health groups come together to solve a specific problem or to achieve a specific goal. Once that is accomplished, the group breaks up and another group with a different configuration of actors comes together to work on another issue. They might meet on such issues as deciding what type of national health insurance bill to support, or how to improve the ambulatory referral system between public and voluntary hospitals. In this type of coordination, if a core group of actors remains together and includes other health institutions on relevant issues, the alliance model is the likely planning model for this type of coordination. The core group, such as an ambulatory care committee, invites different health institutions to participate in health matters relevant to them. While the core group remains the same, the pattern of the committee changes as new actors enter and leave the group when the issues of interest to them are discussed, solved, or tabled.

In a second type of ad hoc coordination, one actor brings together others in order to solve a problem in which he or she requires assistance and continues to coordinate the activity of the other actors until the problem is solved. This model of planning conforms most closely to the individual action type. Thus, if a committee of the health planning agency perceived a need to seek support for the passage of an environmental bill, it would take the initiative in obtaining the assistance of the agency's public relations committee to prepare press releases, the executive committee to ask prestigious persons to testify in behalf of the bill, and the executive director to bring together other institutions concerned with the bill to plan strategy for its passage. As can be seen, coordination is a complex concept, the nature of which cannot be taken for granted.

Constraints

If coordination has all these powerful benefits (trust, open communication, integrated services, more efficient use of scarce resources, and higher quality of services), what are some of the obstacles encountered when efforts are made to achieve these worthy goals? The most important constraint to the effective promotion of coordination is the very autonomy of the numerous health actors who are concerned with producing and distributing health services. This autonomy produces the fragmented services, the discontinuity among the services, and the variety of eligibility standards that permit some persons to be served while others have been rejected. Underlying this drive for autonomy and independence of action is the basic American stress on the values of individualism and self-reliance. Willard has pointed out that those widely accepted values, as practiced by individuals and institutions in every walk of life, represent the strongest barrier to the values of cooperation and altruism that foster coordination of services to help people.[20] The competitive motivation to go it alone collides with the cooperative imperative underlying PL 93-641. Under these circumstances, the health planning agency becomes a meeting hall where attempts are made to find compromises between the individual needs and interests of the autonomous providers, consumers, and government officials on the board and the public interests of the community.

A number of researchers have identified the difficulties in finding these compromises. Hilleboe and Schaefer noted that among equals none will submit to the coordination leadership of the other.[21] They seriously question whether any feasible coordination mechanism exists. In many communities, serious competition took place among health and welfare councils, hospital facilities councils, health planning councils, government, and consumer groups for control of the health planning agencies. One of the major issues in the organizational process was determining the representation on the board.

Hink and Arnold have noted that the excessive amount of energy needed just to be involved in the activity of coordination dissipates the energy needed to take actions on those aspects in which there is agreement. Furthermore, there is difficulty defining the nature of issues to be solved, identifying health needs that require attention, and solving the problems defined.[22] When staff time is limited and everyday crises intervene, it becomes difficult to put too much emphasis on coordination unless a health institution desires some goal and takes the initiative in ad hoc goal-oriented coordination.

But, probably the greatest difficulty in the coordinating process is the lack of authority and power within the regional health planning agencies. Not until PL 93-641 gave them certificate-of-need and Proposed Use of Federal Funds (PUFF) review activities did they gain some power to influence health providers. Yet, even this authority was diluted because most of the regional health planning agencies had only the power to review and recommend on proposals rather than review and approve authority; the authority to approve (or disapprove) has traditionally been vested in the state health planning agency. Thus, there was initially little reason to take the actions of the regional agencies seriously. Even a negative review could be and has been overturned at the state level. With the development of regional and state health plans, however, there has been a very high degree of consensus between regional and state health planning agencies on review decisions. Therefore, the health providers can no longer lightly dismiss the decisions of the regional health planning agencies even if they carry only advisory power.

Strategies

Coordination is most likely to take place on those specific issues in which all parties to the action stand to gain by mutual adjustment. The example cited of one institution gaining patients while another reduces its financial burden is an illustration of this strategy. Second, coordination is also possible when all parties stand to gain from their contributions. This is especially true when agencies need data that are located in a number of different agencies and can benefit by a single agency's collecting and disseminating it. This data bank becomes a much more powerful tool than it would if the data remained fragmented and each agency duplicated another's efforts. Third, coordination can reduce the communication gap among health actors by informing them of policy, staff, and service changes. It gives the health institutions an opportunity to improve their referral system, or to learn of policy changes that may be beneficial to their clientele or the public at large. Fourth, coordination is highly successful in quid pro quo, or log-rolling, situations. In any type of representative body, trade-offs have to be made. Through coordination, the nature of the trade-offs can be identified so that different actors involved can benefit. Thus, an actor interested in developing an ambulatory health center votes for another who desires to have a surgical suite expanded. While this coordinating strategy may not lead to the development of a better allocation of the most needed services, it does increase services for certain segments of the community. As more certificate-of-need decisions are based on goals of health plans, the status quo desired by health providers is maintained so that no one appears to be worse off than the others, even though the unique needs of each are being met. This process also decreases the uncertainty that usually frustrates health administrators if they are not aware of the actions being taken by their colleagues and potential competitors.

Finally, there is the competitive or contest strategy involved in coordination. Warren et al. explode the myth that coordination always involves cooperation and/or collaboration among health actors. They noted that competition by different actors striving to achieve a goal, such as winning a large federal contract, often leads to a best choice for the benefit of the public good because the public is in a position to influence the outcome by favoring one proposal over another. While one actor may benefit at the expense of other actors, it is the public that benefits most of all. Yet, in other matters, the competitors can still find ways of working together or even supporting each other.[23]

Effect on Innovation

Coordination is essentially a system-maintaining function. The sensitive balance among health actors in terms of their domain and resources is usually maintained through coordination. Legislators, who pass new laws and allocate funds for new and/or expanded services and facilities, are very conscious of this delicate balance. As Hink and Arnold noted, "Innovative program changes that require reallocation of resources within an agency are more likely to be questioned by legislative bodies than is repetition of previously accepted sets of activities."[24] Yet, even if legislators did not maintain this status quo orientation toward allocation of resources, can one assume that innovation ipso facto is a public good and to be automatically encouraged? Warren et al. challenge this assumption by noting that innovations are of benefit to some at the expense of others. For example, government sponsorship of health maintenance organizations (HMOs) initially benefited the middle and working classes at the expense of the poor, who were forced to use low-quality and often unacceptable outpatient clinics.

On the basis of their study of innovations in the model cities program, Warren et al. discovered that there were, in fact, three types of innovation. What they called "primary innovation" emphasized changing the system rather than the individual. It posed the greatest threat to the legitimacy of established organizations and the maintenance of their status quo. The other two types, "secondary innovation" and "gross innovation," are more concerned with adaptations in the existing behavior of the individuals using health services or minor changes in the way those services are rendered; the basic institutions and their orientations remain essentially unchanged. The latter two types of innovation were merely differences in degree rather than distinct from each other. The implication of these findings is that secondary or gross innovations were highly compatible with coordination that maintained the balance of the status quo. In this study, the overwhelming number of innovative activities were found to be of the secondary or gross type.[25] The real threat to the status quo thus resides in primary innovation. This coincides with the remarks attributed to Hink and Arnold earlier in this discussion. Warren et al. pointed out that, by preventing issues from arising, innovations are maintained within the acceptable framework of the health institution's basic orientation and established way of operating.

Outcome of Coordinating Efforts

In the final analysis, whether one analyzes studies on decentralized neighborhood government in New York City, health and welfare councils, health facilities planning councils, or even the first years of the health planning agencies, the effort required to achieve benefits through coordination has not been commensurate with the costs. For every critic who maintains the need for coordination, other critics

> claim that the voluntary planning movement has been too negative, with too much emphasis on saying "no" to unneeded facilities rather than on helping the hospitals to develop needed facilities and services; that it tends to favor minor needs . . . rather than major needs . . .; that it has tended to favor the status quo and to discourage innovation . . .; that the councils are too heavily representative of the providers and not enough of consumers. . . .[26]
>
> Studies of community action indicate that community-wide planning for the coordination of services, particularly in the larger urban areas, has only been sporadically successful.[27]

If the results are as meager as these quotes indicate, then why is so much effort devoted to coordination?

Why Coordinate in the Face of Limited Results?

It has already been made clear that coordination is one of those functions that presents health institutions with a basic dilemma. When it does not take place, then the outcry is for coordination. When it occurs, as in comprehensive health planning, the efforts of those involved in the process are criticized for producing too few results for the time expended. Yet, Warren, Arnold, Krause, and others point to the strongest motivation for the continuation of this process. Warren et al. stated it most strongly:

> A realistic and inclusive consideration . . . might indicate that the advantages to the coordinating organizations which accrue through the side effect of effectively disbarring new, competing, alternative organizations with different strategies for combating the city's social problems may far outweigh the purported advantage of effecting economies or improving service delivery.[28]

In summary, the major thrust of coordination is the maintenance of the status quo, and this is accomplished mainly by keeping competitors outside the system. All other benefits are secondary, whether they be exchanging information, trading favors, or keeping costs down. Under these circumstances, the systems model of planning poses the greatest threat because it is geared to goal-oriented coordination, primary innovation, and changes in the health system and in its pattern of delivery. The partnership planning model, on the other hand, is most conducive to structured coordination and secondary/gross innovation in which the emphasis is on maintenance of the status quo.

THE PUBLIC AND PRIVATE INTERESTS IN HEALTH PLANNING

One of the major recurring issues the health planning agency board and staff face is the determination of whose interests are served. This is a frequent subject of debate in political circles in terms of the majority versus the minority voice. In recent years, the court has been the most vocal supporter and corrective force on behalf of minority rights when these have been unfairly affected by the rights of others. A major thrust of health planning agencies' efforts is in discovering the balance between the public and private interests as represented in majority and minority positions on different issues.

In this section, Banfield and Meyerson's definition of public and private interests will be used. "A decision is said to serve special interests if it furthers the ends of some part of the public at the expense of the ends of the larger public."[29] Thus, in the recent use of funds to build HMOs, was the public interest served by allocating most of these funds to hospitals and other medical bodies that served a primarily middle-class constituency rather than the much needier minorities of the inner cities? Has the passage of PL 93-641 with its emphasis on private, nonprofit health systems agencies been in the public interest if it effectively reduces accountability to the general public and particularly representation of the grass roots minority citizens on their potentially self-perpetuating board structure? Neither of these are simple questions because they imply that, by meeting the needs and interests of the middle class, the largest constituency in the planning regions, the greater needs of the poor for both service and representation are being sacrificed. Would the meeting of these minority needs represent a private or public interest in view of the fact that they are numerically a minority constituency? On the other hand, these authors state that a decision "is said to be in the public interest if it serves the ends of the whole public rather than those of some sector of the public."[30]

To help answer such questions, Banfield and Meyerson identify two major ways of viewing the public interest. The first, the unitary conception, conceives of the public interest in which "the whole may be conceived as a single set of ends which pertain equally to all members of the public."[31] According to this conception, both questions posed previously would be answered affirmatively as being in the public interest because the end of both the middle- and low-income classes would be synonymous. However, in the implementation of the HMO concept and the health system's agency's board structure and representation, the ends would be nullified if all parties were not treated equally in terms of who received HMO services and who was represented on the health agency's board, because this would distort the systems conception of the public interest. Unfortunately, idealistic principles are seldom transplanted into reality to benefit all persons and groups in society equally. Even among "equals," some are more equal by virtue of their added status and resources of influence than others. A physician is more equal than a Puerto Rican shopkeeper, even though both may have the same voting strength on a board. Thus, the systems conception refers both to the identification and to the actual carrying out of an idealistic intent in which all groups share equally.

The second conception of the public interest is individualistic whereby "the ends of the plurality do not comprise a single system" and the "ends of the plurality 'as a whole' are simply the aggregate of ends entertained by individuals, and that decision is in the public interest which is consistent with as large a part of the 'whole' as possible."[32] This means that numerous groups in society have different agendas, ideas, and strategies on how they plan to achieve the items on their agendas. However, if several of these self-interest groups were able to agree on an objective, even if for different reasons, then this combined power represents a plurality of intent that is then held to be in the public interest. For example, there is at this time no plurality so strong that it can be said to represent the public interest in terms of the kind of national health insurance package that would be most beneficial to the American people.

In essence, the basic question underlying the public-private interest issue is who benefits by actions taken in health planning. Unlike PL 89-749, which stated that all the people should benefit equally and thus assumed a systems conception of the public interest, PL 93-641 takes an individualistic approach because it identifies groups of people, such as the urban and rural poor, who should benefit most from plans. But, the real question is whether the beneficiaries of health planning are those identified in PL 89-749 or in PL 93-641.

PL 93-641 identified three major constituencies that had to be included on the boards of the health planning agencies. These are the providers of health service, consumers, and government officials. Providers are typically physicians, hospital administrators, presidents of medical societies, or other professional medical associations, and the chief officials or their representatives of prestigious health institutions of various types. Consumers are representatives of two types—the consumer elite who represent the middle- and upper-class points of view and the consumers who represent the working class and the low-income users of tax-supported medical services. Government officials are executives or their surrogates from both health- and nonhealth-related agencies. The question is which of these groups benefits most from its involvement in health planning?

Prior to the era of consumer involvement in publicly sponsored programs, most of the consumers on boards were members of the consumer elite. Occasionally, a union official would represent the working man, but almost never was a low-income minority consumer found on any board. For the most part, health providers controlled health planning and programs; thus, the Hill-Burton legislation was dominated by state hospital officials. Yet, because every federal dollar was matched by two local private dollars, the government officials, according to Somers, were unable to control either what happened to non-Hill-Burton construction funds or to Hill-Burton funded projects.[33] This permitted the individual hospitals practically to control the type of new and expanded facilities built. In addition to lack of control by the Hill-Burton state agencies over private facilities' expenditures, the private health institutions by their membership on the voluntary health facilities planning councils also controlled the decisions made in these bodies. Seldom were their applications for facility expansion denied. The councils and the Hill-Burton bodies were created to represent the public interest, yet their boards were largely composed of members from the individual institutions who were mainly concerned with their private interests. It takes no imagination to conclude that the private interests would benefit by manipulating and controlling the public interest orientation of the boards. The result of such control is that there is no real distinction between the public and private interests because the private interests define their interests as the public interest. Morris stated this very well: "Every voluntary social agency is likely to express the predominant interest of one major group in a community, even though other groups are represented on the governing board of trustees."[34]

Haldeman, president of the now defunct Health and Hospital Planning Council of Southern New York, provided further evidence of the individual hospitals' dominance when he stated:

> The fact that there have been remarkably few recommendations for disapproval during the years the legislation has been in

effect is . . . tangible evidence that we have been able to bridge
the gap between areawide planning and individual hospital planning without trespassing on the rights and responsibilities of
individual hospitals to plan their future destinies.[35]

Yet Somers reacted to this by questioning how effective this emphasis on
the private interests of the individual institutions is in meeting the needs
of the total population.[36]

In this competition between the public and private interests, some
observers have seen a potential counterforce represented by the power of
the federal government. One critic views the federal government as dominant because it sets the rules and has the resources and staff to have
"developed a dominance in health affairs it will not relinquish."[37] According to this view, the health planning agencies are deliberately kept weak
so that, in any conflict situation, they are guaranteed to come out second
best. Another writer, while calling for a true partnership between the
government and the private sector, expressed fears that the public sector
would overwhelm the private sector as it funded ever greater portions of
the health bill and expanded its planning and regulatory controls over the
private sector.[38]

Yet, other voices have noted with equal eloquence the lack of power of
health planning agencies and the relatively minor role played by the consumers, particularly the grass roots consumers, on the agency boards. One
writer calls consumer representation a "political gimmick" because consumers represent, not the public interest, but special interests. As for the
representatives of the poor, they seldom attended meetings and did not
understand the issues being discussed.[39] Another writer identified a conflict between the health planning agency's mandate to improve the organization of health services and the physician's control of those services. He
pointed out, for example, how a typical surgeon in 1964 controlled ten
hospital beds, each of which was worth $4,500 annually to that surgeon.
In return, he or she provided some "free" medical service. With the
inception of Medicare and Medicaid, the surgeon no longer provided any
charitable services, in spite of the fact that the community was providing
very expensive equipment and hospital facilities.[40] In this conflict, the
private interests of physicians and hospital institutions have received the
greatest benefits because of the lack of power of the consumer representatives.

Although federal officials have attempted to influence and control health
planning agencies through guidelines and evaluations, this influence has
not only failed to strengthen their public interest role, but also has undermined their capacity to cope with the private, self-interests of the health

establishment. This has occurred because the law failed to give agencies the authority and power required to compel local health institutions to implement their policies and goals. One critic summed up this situation quite strongly:

> Basically, both hospital and health and welfare planning coun-
> cils are restricted purpose agencies without public mandate. Both
> are somewhat elitist in structure, lack procedures for due process
> and effective implementation of proposals, suffer from insecure
> funding bases, are dominated by special interests, and offer unex-
> ceptional track records of achievement.[41]

This writer concluded that there were no real differences between the government officials and the special interest groups in the communities, particularly identifying the academic medical elite and the practitioner-community hospital elite. He found that they had the same goal, which had been the "perpetuation of profits and the maintenance of their existing power and control over the system."[42] Smith found the same relationship between the National Institutes of Health's funding patterns and the universities and professional associations that formed "an enormously powerful and politically legitimate constituency of able, energetic people in frequent communication, sharing a common goal and interests. . . ."[43] He characterized these funding patterns as subsidies with few strings attached.

Who Benefits?

The consumers, as board members on health planning agencies, have had little voice in determining the public interest. They have either been ineffective, or they have largely found themselves in agreement with the health providers. Although they are the most logical representatives of the public interest, they have generally acted as junior partners.

The government sector, which one would expect to be either the mediator between the consumers and providers, or the voice of the public interest, has served two functions. At the areawide level, the legislation has given the health planning agency itself limited staff and authority but weighty responsibilities and heavy functions. Thus, they have not been able to achieve what the legislation promised. The government representatives have not played an overly aggressive or significant role in the agency's activities.

It is the government role at the federal level that is decisive. On the one hand, its regulations have overburdened the agencies with responsibilities they could not adequately perform. In this regard, it has undermined their capacity to perform while maintaining for itself the dominant role among the three levels of government. Whether by design or unwittingly, the federal level has so effectively minimized the capacity of the health planning agencies to perform that they, in effect, guaranteed the maintenance of the status quo. Yet, it was the status quo that comprehensive health planning was supposed to alter.

The representatives of health providers, whether acting as board members of health planning agencies or as officials of the independent health institutions, have maintained their self-interested position with respect to health planning. This has been done by their directly controlling the decision-making boards that pass on programs and projects of interest to them. Even disagreements among various factions of the health providers as between the American Medical Association (AMA) and the American Hospital Association (AHA) have not prevented the individual institutions from achieving what they have set out to do. This is not to assert that the health providers have acted against the public interest or their achievements have not produced necessary and vital health services. Rather, it is to suggest that, according to the individualistic conception of the public interest, each of the institutions acted to benefit its own interests regardless of the impact of its actions on the overall needs of the public. In these actions, the most powerless groups of people, such as the elderly, the minority groups, and the rural and urban poor, have generally failed to benefit.

Collaborative efforts of two or more health institutions that could have produced better services, even for the populations they were serving, have usually been rejected. This, of course, is in keeping with the dominant American values of individualism and self-reliance, as opposed to the public interest values of humanism and cooperativeness.

Finally, the health institutions have always done what has been in their own best interests, regardless of the mechanism developed to stimulate a coordinative, integrated, and comprehensive approach to the use of scarce health resources. Whether it was the Hill-Burton, the Health Facility and Planning Council (HFPC), the Regional Medical Program (RMP) or the Partnership for Health Act, the outcome has been the same. Neither voluntarism nor the use of financial incentives has made a difference with respect to the individualistic actions of the health institutions. They have acted alone and in their own self-interest. However, with the passage of PL 93-641, stronger regulatory functions have been built into the law, which, if carried out as designed, may reduce somewhat this overly strong influence of health providers.

What Strategies Are Available?

There continue to be exhortations for improving health services and delivery through cooperation, coordination, or partnership. Even the health providers and their representatives echo these values. In response to these challenges, some health analysts have proposed solutions they believe would realistically improve the voice of the public interest.

Hink and Arnold have advocated the development of competition among health providers in line with the way the private sector of the market operates. This would be done by offering the consumers an adequate range of choices so that the producers of services have to improve their health products in order to capture their share of the consumer market, stagnate, or go out of business. With regard to planning, Arnold particularly advocates competitive health planning committees, each working on the same type of problem or issue, one with a consumer or public interest orientation, the other with a provider or private interest orientation. In the competition, the public would have a greater voice in determining what and how health services would be provided to the people.[44] Since this was proposed, amendments to PL 93-641 have given much greater emphasis to developing competition among health providers, especially by means of HMOs.

Based on an economic model, Bailey recommends that the federal government itself become the "collective consumer," or "monopsonist," and serve as a countervailing force to the health providers to ensure quality care at reasonable cost. As the federal share of the health dollar grows larger, the self-interest of the government becomes more important because it is put under pressure by the tax-paying consumer to get the most for its dollars. With the impending passage of a national health insurance bill, this responsibility becomes even more important and makes its role as a viable partner in the public-private relationship more significant.[45] Under pressure to promote cost containment, the Health Care Financing Administration has taken a much greater initiative in setting rates for Medicaid and Medicare benefits consistent with the services provided. Further, the Professional Standards Review Organizations (PSROs) have placed greater emphasis on efficiency in the use of health services by their efforts to reduce inappropriate services and unneeded care. Both are examples of the federal government's attempts to carry out its role as a "monopsonist."

Krause recommends the creation of a Federal Health Commission outside existing agencies to undertake research to expose the too familiar relationship between federal officials and private health producers. By focusing on these activities, which are not in the interests of the public, he believes the needs of the public would have a better opportunity of being identified and implemented.[46]

Somers recommends strong federal controls with incentives to the health producers to guarantee the most enlightened regulatory mechanism for ensuring the public interest. She rejects both the public utility and the "for profit" model of self-regulation as not likely to work in the public's interest.[47]

The final recommendation came from Congress itself. PL 93-641 provides much stronger authority, as well as more powerful sanctions and incentives to stimulate health planning. While the role of the consumer is reduced in this bill, the centralization of the fragmented, federally sponsored health programs provides the power needed at the local level, which has been absent in all preceding efforts. Through this centralization of power, congressional legislators hope the public interest will have a greater chance of being realized under PL 93-641.

PRAGMATIC VERSUS COMPREHENSIVE PLANNING

In an important article on rational planning in 1959, Lindblom made a distinction between comprehensive planning and what he later called disjointed incrementalism.[48] The distinctions he drew are summed up in Table 9-1.

Lindblom basically argued that neither man's intellect nor the use of computers had developed sufficiently to comprehend all the available theories and their values, means, and outcomes to derive a best plan. Consequently, a comprehensive plan, based on rational thought, could not be developed. He then examined how decisions were made in real situations by administrative officials. He discovered the process that is outlined in the pragmatic, or disjointed incrementalist column; namely, only those incremental changes were considered that would resolve the immediate problem. There was a simultaneous emphasis on the ends to be achieved and on the means to achieve them, and if other policy analysts agreed, then it would be considered for adoption. No attempt was made to seek all the possible alternatives that could or should be considered. If they came to mind they would be given attention. Nor was any thought given to theory. If the proposed change seemed to have some chance for success, its application in actual practice would determine its suitability. If the change worked, it would replace the previous activity. In turn, it was expected that this new program would also be replaced in time by another.

So strong and closely reasoned was Lindblom's argument, that many planning theorists, while accepting its validity, felt uncomfortable with its implications, namely, the acceptance of the status quo. Lindblom's eval-

Table 9-1 Planning Types

Comprehensive	Disjointed Incrementalism (Pragmatic)
1. Clarification of values or objectives is distinct from empirical analysis of alternative policies.	1. Selection of value goals and empirical analysis of the needed action are intertwined.
2. Policy formulation is approached through means-end analysis. First ends are isolated, then means to achieve them are sought.	2. Since means and ends are not distinct, means-end analysis is often inappropriate.
3. The test of a good policy is that it can be shown to be the most appropriate means to desired ends.	3. Test of a good policy is that different analysts find themselves directly agreeing on a policy.
4. Analysis is comprehensive; every relevant factor is taken into account.	4. Analysis is very limited: a. Important alternative outcomes are neglected. b. Alternative policies are neglected. c. Affected values are neglected.
5. Theory is often heavily relied upon.	5. Succession of comparisons greatly reduces or eliminates reliance on theory.

uation was primarily reactive rather than forward-looking in nature. Consequently, planning theorists have sought a middle ground, somewhere between incrementalism and comprehensive planning. This school of thought came to be represented by such planners as Meyerson, Davidoff, and Bolan. Unlike Lindblom, these planners felt that a planning process could be developed that would take into account future time dimensions as well as means and ends.[49] The significance of this discussion for comprehensive health planning is obvious. A perception based on Lindblom's thinking would have raised serious doubts as to the validity of the comprehensive health planning concept, whereas others have recognized that even partially future-oriented planning could have some positive impact on a fragmented health system suffering a variety of afflictions. Arnold summed it up in these words:

> To develop a planning society, one of the most difficult bonds we will have to shed is that of our orientation to the present in our problem-solving. We must begin to think of an evolving, conditional future.[50]

Yet, there were others who raised questions about the rationality or feasibility of such future-oriented planning. They maintained that there are so many points of view and value conflicts in planning goals and objectives, that in the end decisions are made based on political feasibility.[51] While no one denies the political aspects of decision making in health planning and the ultimate plans, it is thought that improved data and identification of a wider range of alternatives, under the scrutiny of cost-benefit analysis, produces better decisions than would occur in the absence of such knowledge. It is for this reason that many have come to understand and to stress the interrelationship among the technical, theoretical, and political aspects of planning. How a plan is implemented and which goals and objectives are given highest priorities are as important to a health planning agency board and its staff as the development of the goals' statement and the cost-benefit analyses that went into them.

Under the Partnership for Health Act, health planning agencies practiced the Lindblom model of pragmatic or disjointed incrementalism. At that time, funding applications were replete with descriptions of meetings held, coordination efforts made, projects reviewed, crises responded to, and occasional policy statements written on some narrow aspects of health services or the delivery system. Under PL 93-641, however, a major shift has taken place. Comprehensive five-year plans, similar to the middle-range plans advocated by Davidoff and Meyerson, have been completed for both the regions and the state, in addition to all the other activities. Nevertheless, until these plans have been implemented over several years and their effect has been evaluated, it is too early to determine whether they are fully developed, action-oriented plans or only public relations documents. The next five years will tell the story.

REGULATION OR PLANNING?

In recent years, regulation of health facilities has been receiving much attention. The most pervasive reason given for this is the rising cost of health care. Of all the sectors of health care, the expenditures for hospitalization take the largest piece of the health dollar. It is not surprising therefore that cost conscious health officials and congressional leaders are paying the closest attention to the rising costs of hospitalization. The idea is that, if new health facilities or the expansion of existing facilities can be curbed, the cost of hospitalization might be eased. Underlying this effort at cost containment of unneeded hospital services is the push being exerted by many forces, including consumers, medical societies, congressional leaders, and federal officials, for the passage of some form of national health insurance. Legislators are very mindful of the inflationary impact the passage of Medicaid and Medicare had on the cost of medical services, especially physician fees and hospital rates, in the 1960s. If nothing more is done than was done in the 1960s, then the inflationary push of national health insurance will be three to four times greater. While there has been much thought given to the necessity for restructuring the health system,[52] the major mechanism used so far to achieve cost control has been regulation.

Certificate of Need

In Chapter 7, there was a discussion on the nature of certificate-of-need legislation and the passage of Section 1122 of the Social Security Act, which gave the states that had not already passed certificate-of-need laws authorization to review and approve requests for health facilities and programs that involved federal funds. Certificate-of-need legislation requires a health institution to obtain a certificate from the state to show its need before it can build a new facility or expand its institution. Because less than half the states had passed such legislation and a number of others had rejected such legislation, Congress passed PL 92-603 in 1972 to ensure the efficient use of its scarce health funds. It also hoped by this move to spur the remaining states to pass legislation that would also require similar review for nonfederally funded projects.

Some critics at that time felt that certificate-of-need legislation was really too limited in scope to have much impact in containing costs. They strongly believed that, in addition, there ought to be regulation of personnel needs, of special types of services (e.g., renal dialysis and open heart surgery), and of existing services and facilities. PL 93-641 has taken into account some of these past shortcomings by mandating that all states must enact certificate-of-need laws by 1981 and must include review and recommendations pertaining to existing health services and specialized services. Personnel needs are being regulated under another law that sets fiscal constraints on federal funding of personnel training and education. Yet, Somers has pointed out that regulation of hospitals is in fact widespread. The problem, she felt, was that it was too fragmented and uncoordinated to have a positive effect on the operations of the hospital.[53] She identified 68 different hospital programs or facilities affected by direct government controls. These involve regulation of personnel, reporting systems, working conditions, and the physical plant, among others. Thus, there is a plethora of regulatory controls over existing health services personnel and facilities as well as for new services, personnel, and facilities under certificate-of-need and Section 1122 legislation.

Benefits of Regulation

One would expect that so much regulation and control of health services would be a liability for the health institutions. This has not been the case at all. Hospitals have grown and prospered, even as regulation of its functions has proliferated. A partial reason for this is the fact that, because such legislation is on the books, the public believes that the public interest is being protected. The assumption is usually made that only those requests for new or modernized health facilities will be approved in order to maintain state standards. While the public expects that its paid hospital monitors and regulators are doing their jobs, it more usually is the case that the largest and strongest of the health institutions are generally shown great deference by health planning agencies and health councils in consideration of their past achievements, status, and power. This same deference is shown by courts to physicians and health officials on various legal issues that come before them. Somers has noted that these health institutions "have usually received the benefit of every legal doubt."[54] This makes the health planning agencies, health councils, and state health departments very wary before they reject an application from most of the large health institutions because of potential challenges to procedures in court.

But, not only have the institutions themselves benefited by regulation. The health planning agencies and the public have also benefited. The passage of certificate-of-need and Section 1122 legislation has in many instances merely formalized what they had been doing informally. One of their major functions had been to review requests for federal funds. Legalizing the process made it more open to the public. Instead of only friendly health providers reviewing proposals as in the health planning councils, the health planning agencies and their consumer representatives also have had an opportunity to participate. This benefits the institutions because they can uncover consumer resistance before large expenditures of time and money are made on a project. This also gives the staffs and boards of health planning agencies a feeling of making important decisions on the future well-being of health care in their communities. Finally, certificate-of-need and Section 1122 legislation have given the agencies the feeling that they have gained a handle on the activities occurring in their areas with the aim of bringing about some rational use of facilities and services in place of the fragmented and uncoordinated "system" that has existed. In order to deal with the numerous requests for reviews, the staff and boards of health planning agencies have had to develop logical procedures, time tables, and criteria for reviewing the proposals. It has forced a tightening up of administrative procedures to ensure that reviews were completed within the specified time limits. In such ways, health institutions, health planning agencies, and the public have benefited from the regulatory function.

Limitations and Deficiencies of Regulation

As a tool to contain the inflationary impact of costs on health care, regulation has not succeeded very well (see Chapter 7). Regulatory procedures such as certificate-of-need review lack control over other factors, such as overspecialization and its attendant high fees, incentives to hospitalize rather than to treat in less costly outpatient facilities, and the institutions that determine what services are offered and to whom.[55]

This ambiguity of what regulation is supposed to do produces some unfortunate results. It can easily lead to approving the construction of hospitals in high-cost urban centers where the concentration of poor are located, thereby raising the cost of construction and the resultant rates for service. It can lead to rejecting proposals for more efficient and effective health care services on the grounds that services already exist for a target population even though they are more inefficient and costly. It does not take into account the high cost of maintaining the facility, which is estimated to be the equivalent of the facility's construction cost for each 18 months of operation.[56] The long-term operating costs of the facility are a much more significant factor in containing inflationary costs of medical care than the capital costs of the facility itself.

Finally, certificate-of-need legislation has a built-in cost mechanism that guarantees the high cost of medical care. Once constructed, health facilities tend to be used. This is evidenced by two communities in Canada with widely different numbers of "acute beds" per 1,000 population. The community with 7.5 beds/1,000 claims that it needs more beds just as much as does the community with 4 beds/1,000.[57] When there are empty hospital beds, there is an incentive to use them because of the emphasis on hospital treatment in third party insurance contracts. This incentive produces a high bed occupancy rate. However, because of the overproduction of beds in the 1960s and 1970s, a number of older hospitals, particularly small institutions located in poor communities that are no longer able to attract patients, are slowly being eliminated.

Furthermore, as the occupancy rate decreases, two significant side-effects occur. First, the number of patients using different specialty services is reduced. This in turn reduces the quality of care. As Cherkasky attested with respect to cardiac surgery centers, infrequent use of specialized skills dulls their effectiveness.[58] Second, the lowering of an occupancy rate tends to increase the per diem cost of the facility because rates are determined by the average number of patients in the hospital census, which is in turn related to gross costs of operating that facility. Thus, the paradox of the goal sought by regulation is often the payment of higher costs for less effective services. On the other hand, if the beds do become used to capacity, this produces its own self-fulfilling prophecy and continuation of the cycle. A dilemma is thus created for which the regulatory function has no solution. If occupancy rates are high, the result is a clamor for more facilities and continued high-quality services. If the occupancy rate is low, the quality of care goes down while the hospital rates go up. In either case, the cost of health care increases, nullifying the objective of the regulatory function.

The regulatory function, whether embodied in state certificate-of-need legislation or Section 1122, has severe limitations in its capacity to achieve even its own limited goal of cost containment. In fact, it tends over time to produce the opposite effect. While there is a necessary place for regulation, its function is definitely more limited than the emphasis and attention it has been given by health economists, public administrators, and legislators.

Relationship of Planning to Regulation

In a major study of certificate-of-need legislation and its relationship to health planning, the Macro Systems consultants came to the conclusion that planning is "indispensable not only to certificate of need but to all programs regulating resource allocation."[59] It is required to determine what facilities are needed, where they should be located, and whom they should be serving. It is needed to identify the gaps in services and the redirection of resources to fill those gaps. It is needed to advocate for the public interest as opposed to reacting to the proposals of the private health interests. It is needed as a mechanism that is sensitive to the changing needs, usages, and priorities of health services in a community, a sensitivity that is lacking in the regulatory function with its emphasis on efficiency and costs and the use of narrow criteria that determine the approval or rejection of proposals.[60]

These factors point out the major distinction between comprehensive health planning and regulation. Planning is long-range and forward-looking, and it uses a systematic process for developing what is needed to improve the health care system of a community. On the other hand, regulation is a means-oriented function, used to implement the goals of an areawide health plan. As such, it is reactive, efficiency-oriented, conservative, and bound by rules and regulations that prescribe what should be approved or rejected. In this respect, planning should normally precede regulation. Once plans have been implemented, however, the regulatory function provides a feedback mechanism for evaluating the impact of the plan's goals and objectives on the costs of health care and on the health status of its target population. It is this evaluation that provides a new assessment of the health climate in a health service area. This is used in an analysis for deciding what new steps are required to improve the health care system in the next cycle of planning. Thus, both planning and regulation are necessary to produce a positive health system that serves people. But, what happens when regulation is given the more prominent role in a planning agency?

Impact and Dangers of Regulation on Planning

Although health planning is beginning to carry out the function expected of it, a number of voices in Congress and the executive branch are being raised to question the significance of planning as a cost containment tool. In order to understand what happens when regulation is given more emphasis than planning, it is important to examine what occurred under the Partnership for Health Act, when regulation was the primary agency function.

Then as now, health planning agencies were severely understaffed. Under the Partnership for Health Act, most functions such as developing health plans, motivating citizen involvement in planning, collecting, and disseminating health data, and setting broad policies all appeared to have no specific time by which they must be accomplished. In short, they were not time-bound. On the other hand, the "review and comment" process had determinate time periods, usually 60 days, within which the review must be completed. Given the facts of meeting ongoing "review" deadlines with limited staff, one of the negative consequences of the "review" process was to give precedence to the regulatory function over the planning function.

A second negative consequence that follows from this was that the orientation of the staff and board of the agencies changed from a positive, forward-looking, long-range planning stance to a short-range, reactive, often negative planning orientation. Regulation was often viewed as the major component of the planning process and became a substitute for planning. The agencies began to plan by being "against" or "for" a proposal or project they were asked to review. They became less aggressive in taking the initiative in identifying what was in the best interests of the community. They gave up their catalytic role of helping other components of the health system to improve their services, especially those services that were identified during the planning as being especially crucial to achieving the goals and priorities of the community.

By defining their priority function as regulation, the health planning agencies changed their primary constituency from the interests of the broad community to the special interests of health providers who serve only a narrow segment of the community. Without a plan and its goals and priorities to set guidelines of how it should react to the multiple proposals being submitted to it, the agency staff and board judged each proposal on a set of arbitrary subjective judgments that were open to challenge in courts of law. Desiring the good will of health providers, the staff and board, many of whose members were also representatives of the health providers submitting proposals for their approval, generally looked favorably on the great majority of proposals. In the process, the agencies were "captured" or coopted by the health providers. This is a common way for federal regulatory agencies to work out their relationships with the firms they are supposed to regulate. One of the reasons for this outcome was that the agencies were required to match up to 50 percent of their federal funds for agency operation with local contributions. Since most of the agencies were incorporated as nonprofit, private bodies, they looked to the corporate and private sector for a significant portion of the matching funds. It was usually the same financially strong health providers who sat on the boards, contributed the matching funds, and submitted proposals for review. Referring to the impact of the "review and comment" function on health planning agencies, the OSTI report concluded "we think that even formal provisions for the submission of advice to the state agency might jeopardize agencies' independent existence as long as they depend on matching funds."[61] Under PL 93-641, both to avoid a conflict of interest and to make it possible to render certificate-of-need decisions on an objective basis, health planning agencies are not permitted to accept funds from health providers.

These negative consequences of the regulatory functions on health planning agencies resulted in some unfortunate outcomes. They rendered the agencies ineffective in their efforts to plan because of their insufficient staff. They put the agencies in the position of defending themselves in courts of law over challenges by the health providers whose proposals had been rejected. Because of the inability of the agencies to forecast the outcome of these judicial challenges, rather than jeopardize their jurisdiction over the "review" process, they often made private settlements under the threat of a court challenge, usually in favor of the health provider. Finally, all of these factors undermined the most precious value the agencies worked to achieve and maintain—their credibility in the eyes of the public and the legislative decision makers. If a large segment of the public viewed the agencies as the captives of the health providers, their goals and priorities were perceived as prejudiced in favor of the health providers.

On the other hand, if the agencies antagonized the health providers by their "review" decisions, then their plans were unlikely to be implemented by the very health providers who viewed the agencies as their adversaries. Thus, as Gottlieb pointed out, while it is possible for planning and regulation to coexist in the same agency, ". . . it is difficult to predict that they will coexist."[62]

Table 9-2 Selected Functions of Organizational Units Created under PL 93-641: Nature of Relationships among Units[1]

Functions	HSA	SHCC	SHPDA
Planning			
Data activities	C	—	C
HSP/SHP development	C	C	C
Annual implementation plan development	U	—	—
Facilities plan development (Title XVI)	C	C	C
Resource allocation			
Development fund grants and contracts	U	—	—
Approval of uses of federal funds in an area	U[2]	—	—
Approval of state categorical plans	—	U[2]	—
Approval of facilities projects (Title XVI)	C	—	C
Regulatory			
New institutional services review and recommendation[3]	C	—	C
Approvals of C/N applications	—	—	U
Findings on continued appropriateness	C	—	C

[1]As established by provisions of the law only.
[2]Varies in single HSA states.
[3]This is viewed as a planning function in congressional intent. It is included here because of its close relationship with C/N review.

Source: National Governor's Conference, *Making the National Health Planning Law Work: The State Perspective* (Washington, D.C.: February, 1977), p. 33.

STATE OR REGIONAL HEALTH PLANNING

At this time, nearly all the regional and the majority of the state health planning agencies have developed their health plans. A review of many of these plans reveals that there is little similarity between them, although state health plans are supposed to be the result of an integration and coordination of the regional health plans. This requires a common format. Certificate-of-need decisions must be based on comparable criteria and procedures to ensure uniformity between the decisions of state and regional planning agencies, and spheres of authority should be clearly delineated so that coordination and decision making flow smoothly among autonomous planning units. Table 9-2 describes the functions and organizational units involved. Complementary functions (C) are those involving two or more of the planning units, and unique functions are those performed by one planning unit. An examination of three areas (planning, regulation, and coordination) reveals some of the problems that have surfaced over who has control of what in planning and implementation.

Planning

There are two main problems in planning: the development of a common planning format and the sharing of data. Development of this format is a major responsibility of the Statewide Health Coordinating Council (SHCC), but it also involves state and regional planning agencies in the process (Sec. 1524(c) of PL 93-641). However, while the mandate is clear, its implementation has been confusing. Regional planning agencies were officially appointed and had begun to carry out their planning functions well before most of the state health planning agencies were operating. Consequently, the regional agencies were forced to develop their own formats of how a plan should be structured. In one eastern state, where regional planning agencies met on a regular monthly basis, no two agencies developed similar planning formats. Probably because of their drive to maintain their own independence, regional health planning agencies are reluctant to give up this power to the state or to each other. Yet, because there is no common format, certain problems arise:

1. It is difficult to integrate regional plans into a state plan.
2. It is difficult to compare the plans for content, progress in goal accomplishment and consistency with national or state priorities.
3. It is difficult to develop a state data bank that can be used by all regional agencies not only because their data needs vary, but also because they need data aggregated in different ways.

An example of the outcome of each agency maintaining its independence is seen by the order of priorities established by the Central New Jersey and State of New Jersey's health plans:[63]

Central New Jersey	State of New Jersey
1. Develop long-term care services and facilities.	1. Improve the services of local health departments through regionalization and copurchase of services.
2. Develop mental health, drug and alcoholism treatment services with emphasis on prevention.	2. Emphasize preventive/early detection services re mothers, infants, and life styles.
3. Promote multiinstitutional health services.	3. Work with regional health planning agencies to regionalize services of local health departments.
4. Provide physicians in medically underserved communities.	4. Require family planning, family living, and sex education in public schools.
5. Improve emergency medical services.	5. Fluoridate public water supply.

Not one of the five highest priorities of the regional agency corresponds to a high-priority goal of the state agency. A report by the National Governor's Conference in 1977 predicted this sort of conflict when it stated, "Major points of potential conflict in health plan development include HSA [health systems agency] nonacceptance of statewide needs and priorities as identified by the state agency."[64] Likewise, this same report advocated that the states collect all data and make them available as needed by the regional planning agencies. Because of the numerous differences in format, priorities, and content of regional plans, it is unlikely that state agencies have the capacity or funds to serve as central depositories of all data. Nor would the regional agencies want to depend on state agencies for information when they may need it in special formats and in a timely manner.

Regulation

To carry out certificate-of-need reviews, comparable criteria and procedures are required. PL 93-641 and its amendments specify in Section 1532 the minimum requirements, but states and regions may be more stringent in developing their criteria and procedures. After the publication of national guidelines and standards related to acute care hospitals and high-cost medical technologies, state and regional planning agencies were required to take these into account in developing their criteria for specialized medical services. A study of the acceptance and use of these national standards stated,

> Approximately 50% of all field site HSAs and SHPDAs did not have review criteria consistent with resource standards regarding: (1) obstetrical services; (2) neonatal special care units; and (3) pediatric inpatient occupancy rate.[65]

Planning agencies showed greater consistency in setting their standards with federal hospital occupancy rates and computerized axial tomography (CAT) scanners, but less acceptance of national standards with respect to cardiac catheterization, radiation therapy, and open heart surgery. There is thus some reluctance on the part of state and regional health planning agencies to accept federal guidance in setting standards for acute care and specialized hospital services. It should be noted that, despite the great potential for differences between state and regional agencies over setting of criteria and procedures, regional agencies still tend to let the state take the lead in this matter. This is shown by the fact that 95 percent of all certificate-of-need reviews are approved by both state and regional agencies, implying a use of common criteria and procedures. Where they differ, the state's decision almost always stands.

Thus, though the regulatory function could have been a source of conflict between state and regional agencies, the regional agencies' acknowledgment of the preeminence of the state's role in setting regulatory standards has to a large extent avoided such problems. Even with respect to federal standards, differences may result from the difficulty of state and regional agencies in securing the data on which to set standards consistent with federal recommendations, rather than from disagreement with those standards.

Authority

Table 9-2 shows that six functions require coordination between the regional and state agencies. The Governor's Conference report clearly expressed a concern with the potential loss of authority to the regions in carrying out these six functions. Because regional agencies had a substantial head start in their development, the state agencies feared that they would be forced to accept regionally developed guidelines, plan formats, and even health plans before they had an opportunity to organize themselves. While PL 93-641 mandates this coordination, it provides "relatively little concrete direction on the specifics of the relationship to be developed."[66]

An illustration of this concern is noted in the Southern Regional Council's comment on the development of the Central Texas Health Planning Agency. Even though most regional planning agencies were making satisfactory arrangements with the states in the South, this was not the case with Central Texas. The report states:

> The Central Texas and the other Texas HSAs are forced to operate under state restrictions and controls that preclude effective health planning. . . . The role of the Governor is extremely important . . . because the major decision-making powers reside with the state agencies and the governor's office. This has proved to be one of the most serious constraints on the HSAs, for it means that the HSAs must please those state agencies which are controlled by and accountable to the governor.[67]

The governor was so unsympathetic to the development of regional agencies that he placed road blocks in the way of developing the SHCC. His efforts aimed at controlling the regional health planning agencies: "state agencies feel that the HSAs must be controlled so that they do not overstep their boundaries."[68] Owing to the concerns such as those raised by the Governor's Conference and noted by the Southern Regional Council, Congress sought to resolve some of these potential ambiguities regarding power and authority in the amendments to PL 93-641. Those amendments substantially boosted the authority of the governor's office in making decisions and overturning regional health planning agency decisions that may conflict with state policy or plans. For example, the governor may now overturn a regional health planning agency's PUFF decision made under formula grants; the state agency has clearly been given the lead in appropriateness reviews; and the governor has the option of selecting the chairperson of the SHCC. While substantial consultation and coordination with regional agencies are expected, it is clearly the state and the governor's office that have been given the greatest authority.

PREVENTION OR TREATMENT

Health prevention and health promotion have received increased attention in the past 15 years. Much of this was initially in response to the sense of alienation felt by certain groups about the manner of treatment offered by the medical profession. Others have seen it as the desire of individuals to wrest control of what happens to their body from the professionals.

This movement was given strong congressional sanction in the citizen participation movement in the 1960s. More recently, the federal government has become aware that greater emphasis on prevention and promotion may be a cost containment strategy that will pay large dividends. This is seen by the prominence given to prevention in the Public Health Service's *Health: United States* annual reference documents and its "Forward Plan for Health." Its most important publication is the Surgeon General's report, *Healthy People,* a report on health promotion and disease prevention.[69] These social, psychological, and economic factors have coalesced to make certain strata of the American people more conscious of their own responsibility for their health. Consequently, a focus on health promotion and disease prevention has found its way into health planning, particularly after Lalonde demonstrated that three other factors were more important to improving health status than medical intervention: environmental, biological, and behavioral.[70] Finally, the experiment in California showed that, as a person observes more of the seven simple rules to improve living habits, his or her longevity was commensurately increased.[71]

Promoting, controlling, or expanding a movement that is underway is not easy. A 1977 conference on consumer self-care in health identified a number of issues requiring research.[72] These include questions about the efficacy of the various health promotion or disease prevention activities; who in the population practices self-care; what their relationship, if any, is to traditional medical practice; what types of medical personnel might be replaced by these various activities; and whether a favorable cost-benefit relationship exists to contain costs of medical care. It appears that, as of the late 1970s, these various alternative health promotion/self-care methods were being practiced mainly by the upper middle class, precisely because they could afford the services and also because they could fall back on traditional medical practice if the methods failed to produce the desired results. However, whether these activities can be packaged to appeal to the working and middle-income classes remains a question.

Furthermore, there is a lack of conceptual clarity in the definition of the movement. Terms such as *disease prevention, holistic medicine, alternative medicine,* and *self-care* are used almost interchangeably. Proponents of different factions within the movement tend to define themselves with special terminology in order to establish their distinctiveness. Without a precise definition of the movement and an exact description of its activities or methods, it is difficult to know whether it represents a real change, a supplementary method of traditional medical pratice, or an alternative to it.

The very first edition of the *American Journal of Health Planning* was devoted to "wellness" or positive health.[73] While all the articles carried important messages with respect to "wellness," Carlson's article in particular identified a number of obstacles health planners would have to face if they were to support this movement.[74] Among those cited are:

- The economic incentives in favor of traditional medical care may simply be too great for adherents of holistic medicine to overcome.
- The medical care system, because it is a major employer, will find many allies if sustained attacks are made on it.
- The movement might be coopted by those more concerned with cost containment than with improvements in the health of the population.
- The "danger that many of the promising approaches and techniques might be 'oversold' as so much 'snake oil,' and the concept of holism tarnished as a result."
- Medical practitioners and researchers must be educated in the concepts of holism to abort medical schools' efforts to produce medical practitioners in a traditional way and thus to impose their concepts on this new movement.

In addition to traditional medical practitioners, there are others who find serious fault with the whole movement.[75] Health promotion/disease prevention/holistic medicine is perceived as a form of victim-blaming, i.e., the individual who fails to achieve the improved health status is blamed for not trying hard enough or accused of giving up too soon. Members of this school of thought believe there are factors in the environment over which they have no control that, in spite of their individual efforts, produce disease. Dangerous highway construction, high noise levels in the workplace, dangerous chemical pollutants in the air and water, and high levels of work- or poverty-induced stress are factors that may have more to do with disease and poor health than the actions taken by individuals to change their life style. The Surgeon General's report, *Healthy People,* recognizes this need to take collective action to reduce such dangers in the environment; it recommends both levels of activity, since one does not preclude the need for the other. Even if the environment were improved, people would still drink to excess, overeat, take dangerous drugs, and drive recklessly.

All of the factors cited can confuse health planners and their community decision-making boards. With uncertainty about the efficacy of the holistic movement and the real rewards of health promotion and disease prevention, it is not surprising that health plans often indicate an ambivalent attitude. The importance of these activities is usually acknowledged in the introduction to the health plan. In some instances, they are used as the basic philosophy behind the high-priority goals in the body of the plan. The plans may even have a section devoted to health status in which improvements in death rates for specific conditions, such as heart disease or cancer, are given heavy emphasis. In some cases, chapters on disease prevention in which emphasis is on preventing venereal disease, reducing cigarette smoking, and ensuring high levels of child immunization rates are included. However, the ambivalence of the health plans manifests itself in the body of the plan. There, after the articulation of disease prevention, health promotion, and the importance of improving health status, the greatest emphasis is given to cost containment efforts through reduction of unnecessary capital expenditures and use of lower cost medical procedures. Prominence is given therefore to acute care, long-term care, and specialized medical technology. A second emphasis is on the improvement of the quality of care through increasing the number of primary care physicians and their assistants, adding community mental health services, and improving the uneven distribution of home health services. Both of these strategies are based on the assumption that the current medical care system works well and needs only to be made more efficient by raising its quality and making it more accessible to underserved populations.

On the other hand, the plans contain very few recommendations on ways to attack the causes of diseases, and they seldom specify which populations will benefit from the improved medical services. In short, while the health planning agencies recognize the need for prevention and promotion strategies, either the treatment/disease orientation of traditional medicine overwhelms them or the adherents of holistic medicine are not specific, articulate, or numerous enough to promote their own case; in the final analysis, treatment services are given greater attention in almost all health plans than is prevention.

This emphasis on treatment has been reenforced by the Public Health Service. Even while it has produced the Surgeon General's report, *Healthy People,* it has published national health standards that deal exclusively with acute care and specialized medical technology. Further, federal health planning guidelines also promote these standards by urging planning agencies to consider them in their health plans. In the event that the agencies either do not agree with the standards or fail to address one or more in their plans, the agencies are required to provide a rationale for these differences. The health planning guidelines state that each regional and state health plan after a stated date "must be consistent with the resource standards."[76] In a previous section of these same guidelines, the four "essential core elements" that must be part of all health plans are identified: acute care, emergency medical services, long-term care, and mental health services. All of these are treatment-related and have little or no relationship to disease prevention or health promotion. Thus, while one arm of the Public Health Service is discussing healthy people, other arms are planning to improve services for sick people.

The health plans contain the officially sanctioned goals and priorities for the future of the states and communities that produced them. If the treatment orientation is highly emphasized, as it is, and promotion and prevention are given only passing mention, as they are, it can be anticipated that treatment will be promoted over prevention services for many years to come.

NOTES

1. For discussion of these concepts, see Robert Morris and Robert Binstock, *Feasible Planning for Social Change* (New York: Columbia University Press, 1966); Edward C. Banfield, *Political Influence* (New York: Free Press of Glencoe, 1961); Robert Dahl, *Who Governs?* (New Haven, Conn.: Yale University Press, 1961); and Nelson W. Polsby, *Community Power and Political Theory* (New Haven, Conn.: Yale University Press, 1963).

2. See Elliott A. Krause, "Health Planning as a Managerial Ideology," *International Journal of Health Services* 3 (1973): 445–463; and Roger M. Battistella, "Rationalization of Health Services: Political and Social Assumptions," *International Journal of Health Services* 2 (August 1972): 331–348.

3. Douglas L. Hink and Mary Arnold, "Agency Problems with Community Health Planning," in *Administering Health Systems*, ed. Mary Arnold et al., (New York: Aldine-Atherton Press, 1971).

4. William R. Willard, "CHP: Diverse Factors in RMP," *American Journal of Public Health* 58 (June 1968): 1026–1030; and Albert Metts, *Relationship between Comprehensive and Environmental Health Planning*, Public Health Reports 84 (1969): 647–654.

5. Anne R. Somers, "An American City and Its Health Problems: A Case Study in CHP" *Medical Care* 5 (1967): 129–141; and Ray E. Brown, "Health Facilities and Health Services," *Inquiry* 10 (March 1973): Supplement, pp. 17–22.

6. William A. Glasser, "Experiences in Health Planning in the U.S.," mimeographed (New York: Bureau of Applied Social Research, Columbia University, June 1973).

7. Anne R. Somers, *Hospital Regulation: The Dilemma of Public Policy* (Princeton, N.J.: Princeton University Press, 1969), p. 141.

8. *Ibid.*, p. 140.

9. See notes 6 and 7 on this point.

10. Herman Hilleboe and Morris Schaefer, "Administrative Requirements for CHP at the State Level," *American Journal of Public Health* 58 (1968): 1043.

11. Glasser, "Experiences in Planning," p. 42; and Krause, "Managerial Ideology."

12. Somers, *Hospital Regulation*, Chapter 1.

13. Brown, "Health Facilities," p. 19.

14. See C. Rufus Rorem, "Objectives and Criteria for Area-wide Planning," *Hospitals* 38 (June 16, 1964): 66–67; Albert E. Heustis, "The Role of the Community Health Planning Agency," *Bulletin of N.Y. Academy of Medicine* 42 (December 1966): 1185–1192; Avery M. Colt, "Public Policy and Planning Criteria in Public Health," *American Journal of Public Health* 59 (September 1969): 1678–1685.

15. Hilleboe and Schaefer, "Administrative Requirements"; and Robert M. Symond, "Health Planning," *Medical Care* 5 (May/June 1967).

16. Emily Friedman, "The Hospital System Takes a Look at 'Shrinking' Itself," *Hospitals* 52 (November 1978): 90–92; and Emily Friedman, "The End of the Line: When a Hospital Closes," *Hospitals* 52 (December 1978): 69–75.

17. Roland L. Warren, Stephen M. Rose, and Ann F. Bergunder, *The Structure of Urban Reform* (Lexington, Mass.: Lexington Books, D.C. Heath, 1974).

18. *Ibid.*, p. 68.

19. *Ibid.*, p. 67.

20. William R. Willard, "Report of the National Commission on Community Health Services—Next Steps," *American Journal of Public Health* 56 (November 1966): 1828–1836.

21. Hilleboe and Schaefer, "Administrative Requirements," p. 1043.

22. Hink and Arnold, "Agency Problems."

23. Warren et al., *Urban Reform*, p. 74.

24. Hink and Arnold, "Agency Problems," p. 297.

25. Warren et al., *Urban Reform*, Chapter 5.

26. Somers, *Hospital Regulation*, p. 140.

27. Hink and Arnold, "Agency Problems," p. 283.

28. Warren et al., *Urban Reform*, p. 79.

29. Edward C. Banfield and Martin Meyerson, *Politics, Planning and the Public Interest* (Glencoe, Ill.: The Free Press, 1955), p. 322.

30. *Ibid.*

31. *Ibid.*, p. 323.

32. *Ibid.*, p. 324.

33. Somers, *Hospital Regulation*, p. 136 and rest of section for discussion of weakness of councils in curbing activities of its members.

34. Robert Morris, "Basic Factors in Planning for the Coordination of Health Services," *American Journal of Public Health* (Parts I and II, February 1963, and March 1963, p. 471).

35. Haldeman, quoted in Somers, *Hospital Regulation*, p. 148.

36. *Ibid.*, p. 141.

37. Ellen Z. Fifer, "Hang-ups in Health Planning," *American Journal of Public Health*, May 1969, p. 768.

38. Lester Brewlow, "Political Jurisdictions, Voluntarism, and Health Planning," *American Journal of Public Health*, July 1968, pp. 1147–1153.

39. Fifer, "Hang-ups."

40. Pierre de Vise, "Planning Emphasis Shifts to Consumers," *Modern Hospital* (September 1969) pp. 133–136.

41. Krause, "Managerial Ideology," p. 458.

42. *Ibid.*

43. David G. Smith in Arnold et al., "Emerging Patterns of Federalism: The Case of Public Health," *Administering Health Systems*, Chapter 8, p. 138.

44. Mary Arnold, "Philosophical Dilemmas in Health Planning," *Administering Health Systems*, eds. Mary Arnold, Vaughn Blankenship, and John Hess (New York: Aldine-Atherton Press, 1971), Chapter 9; and Hink and Arnold, "Agency Problems," Chapter 17.

45. *Ibid.*, Chapter 14.

46. Krause, "Managerial Ideology," pp. 461–463.

47. Somers, *Hospital Regulation*, Chapter 9.

48. Charles E. Lindblom, "The Science of Muddling Through," *Public Administration Review* 19 (Spring 1959): 79–88.

49. See Edward Banfield, "Ends and Means in Planning," *International Social Science Journal* 11 (1959): 361–368; Paul Davidoff and Thomas A. Reiner, "A Choice Theory of Planning," *Journal of American Institute of Planners*, May 1962, pp. 103–115; and Richard Bolan, "Emerging Views on Planning," *Journal of American Institute of Planners*, July 1967, pp. 233–245.

50. Arnold et al., *Administering Health Systems*, p. 222.

51. Richard Sasuly and Paul Ward, "Two Approaches to Health Planning: The Ideal vs. the Pragmatic," *Medical Care*, May/June 1969, pp. 235–241. Also, Arnold, et al., *Administering Health Systems*, Chapter 10.

52. Paul D. Ward, "Health Care Regulation," *Hospitals* 46 (April 1, 1972): 101–105.

53. Somers, *Hospital Regulation*, Chapter 2.

54. *Ibid.*, p. 193.

55. Irving Leveson, *Financing and Regulation of Health Services*, Office of Program Analysis, Planning and Budgeting, mimeographed (New York City: Health Services Administration, November 1973).

56. Joseph L. Dorsey, "Certificate of Need Laws," *Architectural Surgery* 1 (June, 1973): 765–769.

57. *Ibid.*

58. Martin Cherkasky, "Resources Needed to Meet Effectively Expected Demands for Services," *Bulletin of New York Academy of Medicine*, December 1966, pp. 1089–1098.

59. Marco Systems, Inc., *The Certificate of Need Experience: An Early Assessment* 1, summary report (April 1974).

60. See Symond R. Gottlieb, "Certificate of Need: Potential Threat to Planning," *Hospitals* 45 (December 16, 1971): 51–53.

61. OSTI, *Surveys of Selected 314 (a) and 314(b) CHP Agencies* (Newton, Mass.: April, 1972), p. 75.

62. Gottlieb, "Certificate of Need," p. 53.

63. Central Jersey Health Planning Council, *1980–1984 Health Systems Plan* (Hightstown, N.J.: undated), pp. 8–16.

64. National Governors' Conference, *Making the National Health Planning Law Work: The State Perspective* (Washington, D.C.: February 1977), p. 37.

65. Analysis, Management & Planning, Inc., *Executive Summary: Evaluation of Criteria Being Used in Conducting Project Reviews by HSAs and SHPDAs* (Cambridge, Mass.: November 30, 1979), p. 15.

66. National Governors' Conference, *State Perspective*, pp. 31–32.

67. Southern Regional Council, *Placebo or Cure? State and Local Health Planning Agencies in the South* (Atlanta, Ga.: 1977), p. 60.

68. *Ibid.,* p. 61.

69. U.S. DHHS, *Healthy People: The Surgeon General's Report on Health Promotion and Disease Prevention* (Washington, D.C.: U.S. Government Printing Office, 1979).

70. Marc Lalonde, *A New Perspective on the Health of Canadians* (Ottawa: Government of Canada, April 1974).

71. Lester Breslow, "Risk Factor Intervention for Health Maintenance," *Science* 200 (4344) (May 1978): 908–912.

72. Health Resources Administration, *Consumer Self-Care in Health* (Washington, D.C.: National Center for Health Services Research, August 1977).

73. American Association for Comprehensive Health Planning, *American Journal of Health Planning,* July 1976.

74. Rick J. Carlson, "Planners and the End of Medicine," *American Journal of Health Planning,* July 1976, pp. 32–37.

75. Howard S. Berliner and J. Warren Salmon, *The New Realities of Health Policy and Influences of Holistic Medicine* (Amherst, Mass.: University of Massachusetts, Health Administration Program, undated). Working Paper #79-1.

76. Health Resources Administration, *Program Policy Notice 79-05: Guidelines for the Development of Health Systems Plans and Annual Implementation Plans* (Hyattsville, Md.: Bureau of Health Planning, February 23, 1979), p. 16.

Chapter 10

The Citizen Actors in the Planning Process

Citizen participation is not a new concept. Traditionally, it has been limited to the political arena, primarily through the tools of letter writing, voting, and campaign activities. This traditional form of participation is defined by Verba as "acts by those not formally empowered to make decisions—the acts being intended to influence the behavior of those who have such decisional power."[1] The emphasis was on the ability to influence rather than the actual involvement of citizens in the decision-making process.

The 1960s witnessed a demand for a new form of citizen participation that saw citizens not only influencing decision makers, but directly included in the planning, administration, and implementation of policy. The demand was raised by numerous political and social organizations from civil rights activists to consumer-oriented Nader's Raiders.[2] Frequent demonstrations and "sit-ins" by "out" groups were typical activities illustrating the demand for inclusion in the decisional processes.

The "Great Society" legislation was a response to these new pressures and such programs as the Office of Economic Opportunity (OEO), the Regional Medical Program (RMP) and Model Cities were the result. It would appear that the purpose of such legislation was to offer something to everyone and to introduce the concept of "maximum feasible participation."[3]

This new participation has been studied, analyzed, and primarily discredited. There has been criticism of professional cooptation of the uneducated and inexperienced as well as complaints that social issues have become so technical that direct citizen participation is no longer possible. Further criticisms have been directed at the inability of most citizens to persevere and remain motivated in the pursuit of goals. Experience has shown that, too frequently, citizens may be stimulated to action during a perceived crisis, but tend to diminish their level of interest over time, leaving the participatory process in the hands of an interested hard core few.

Verba summarizes the fundamental obstacle to implementing participation in the following statement: ". . . all societies are characterized by inequalities in intellectual material and social resources, in motivation, and in the availability of social structures through which one can participate."[4] Given the existing inequalities, the achievement of true citizen participation without the cooptation of one group by another remains a challenge. The special significance of the recent movement has been its focus on urban areas, the poor, the ethnic minorities, the politically disenfranchised, and on the incorporation of participation as a legislative or administrative mandate.[5]

Consumer participation in the planning of health facilities and programs had been initially provided for by the Comprehensive Health Planning Act of 1966, which specifically called for each state and territory to designate an agency to do comprehensive health planning and to select a council comprised of providers and consumers of health services. With the passage of PL 93-641 in 1974, the general requirements of the 1966 act were replaced by the more specific requirements regarding consumer and provider members, their representation on the governing body, and their functions and responsibilities. Experience of the governing bodies in the ensuing five years led to further clarification of the citizen role in the 1979 amendments.

CITIZEN REPRESENTATION IN HEALTH PLANNING

Burke notes that there are four types of decision-making structures: mass participation, monolithic, polylithic, and pluralistic models.[6] Mass participation refers to the town meetings in which all citizens participate and therefore represent themselves. In the monolithic structure, a small elite group of influential citizens agree among themselves and make decisions in their own interest. However, within the monolithic structure, there are different individuals with particular interests to whom the rest defer when issues relating to those interests arise. The polylithic model differs from the monolithic in that, on each major issue, there are separate groups of influential citizens who control the decisions within these areas, such as health, education, or automobile production. Within each issue area, citizens with specialized interests have differentiated levels of influence. Within the health area, some citizens would be influential because of their special concerns for hospitals, others for home health care, and still others for environmental or mental health. Thus, there are both general and specialized areas of interest, each with its group of influential citizens. Finally, the pluralistic model is based on the fact that within a community there are a number of influential citizens with relatively equal status and power. As different issues arise, varying combinations of these influentials coalesce around each issue, whether it is building a hospital or closing an unneeded elementary school. These influential citizens are generalists rather than specialists; they slide from one issue area to another, depending on their interests and the time they have available when an issue arises. Such pluralistic models are typically found in homogeneous communities, such as suburbs, agricultural communities, or university towns.

Thus, it can be seen that there is no one community decision-making model that holds true for all communities or health planning service areas. Because most health service areas have a minimum of 300,000 persons with a range of socioeconomic population classes, it can be expected that they will engage in decision making consistent with the polylithic model, in which the health services community represents only one of the many series of interest sectors within it. Further, within the health service sector, a number of actors are ready to champion separate health issues, such as mental health, primary care, and nursing homes.

Given the mandate of health planning agencies to plan so that most of the major health areas are taken into account, it becomes essential that their governing bodies be broadly representative. Providers, consumers, and government officials should logically be included on such a governing body. Marmor and Morone point out, however, that PL 93-641 failed to make a major distinction between what they call accountability and participation on the one hand and representation on the other.[7]

Accountability means "answering to" or "having to answer to" some other group. Elected officials are answerable to the voters just as health planners are answerable to their executive director and/or governing body. "The crucial element in each case is that accountability stems from some scarce resource desired by the accountable actor."[8] Elected officials want their constituents' votes, and the health planners need continued support and supervision to do their work. In contrast, participation refers to the direct involvement of the citizen in public decisions and is exemplified by the mass participation model. In a complex democracy, it is not possible for 300,000 persons to congregate to discuss health issues. Others must represent them. The main direct participation of the people is then reduced to choosing representatives to serve on the health planning agency's governing body. It is their representatives who directly participate in planning. Thus, who these representatives are and what their accountability is to the general public and the constituencies who elect them become key issues.

The form of representation of the governing body members thus becomes important. Marmor and Morone, as well as Peterson and Greenstone, distinguish among three forms of representation: formal, descriptive, and substantive.[9] Formal refers to the method by which the representatives are chosen and controlled, i.e., election or selection. Thus, the American Hospital Association (AHA) might select from its membership one or more persons to represent the association on the health planning agency, or it might have its nominees compete with other health provider groups or individuals through a general election for membership to the governing body. Similarly, consumers could be elected or selected.

Descriptive representation is based on the characteristics or qualifications members of the governing body should have. How many are to be senior citizens? or women? How many are to be from the low-income or high-income group? How many are to reside in metropolitan or nonmetropolitan areas of the community? These are characteristics that describe who the consumers should be. Likewise, providers are described as to whether they are to be physicians, hospital administrators, health insurors, health researchers and teachers, or spouses of health care providers. In essence, the objective of selecting or electing people based on their characteristics is an attempt to mirror the composition of the general public. "The assumption is that if a representative resembles his constituency, he will act as they would, were they to make decisions."[10] If governing body members are chosen only on the basis of their descriptive characteristics, they are not necessarily accountable to any specific constituency or organization in the community. Members of governing bodies are sometimes directly accountable to organizations that chose them, but as often they are not accountable to any specific group. Their accountability, if any, is to the governing body itself.

Substantive representation goes one step further than descriptive representation. It requires members to represent and be accountable to the group that chose them. A representative should think and feel the way his or her constituency does, report back to it, and obtain guidance on the issues coming before the governing body. This guidance need not be in the form of specific voting instructions, but rather should define broad parameters within which the representative can vote for or against an issue and be consistent with the constituency's general orientation. Thus, a representative of the Consumer Health Coalition knows the organization favors some form of national health service. A health planning body considering this issue may not be able to propose a goal fully consistent with that policy because of the strong opposition of providers. Instead, it proposes a more general goal that supports the right of all people to quality health care without stating the form it should take. The coalition's representative should have enough freedom to support this concept without reporting to the group. In addition to accountability, the representative should have some influence on the outcome of issues that affect the group's special concerns. Substantive representation requires efficacy and effectiveness from the representative. It is not merely whether the representative voted, but whether the representative was able to influence the way others voted.

Because the general public is interested in health care as only one of numerous other concerns, health is not always the most important issue on the public's agenda. A person selected from the general public as an at-large representative may find it difficult to know just what the general public thinks about a particular health planning issue. Indeed, the public may be deeply divided or totally indifferent. There may well be no public body that the representative can consult on how to vote. Consequently, members chosen through descriptive representation do not always know what the public wants or thinks important about all the issues. This places the representative in the position of speaking as an individual and that voice may or may not reflect public opinion. When the members are formally selected by the governing body itself, they are under heavy pressure to vote as the leadership desires or lose their chance to be reappointed when their terms expire. This self-appointive mechanism can even undo substantive representation when such representation is not mandated by the agency's bylaws. For example, the representative of a respected consumer organization was not reappointed because "the HSA [health systems agency] board and staff were displeased with the way our representatives voted."[11]

To ensure that democracy can function in a situation where representatives are often in conflict on various issues, substantive representation may well be the fairest way of selecting consumer and provider members of the governing body. It may also be the best way to ensure that all issues concerned with health matters in the community will be aired and to guarantee accountability of representatives to their various health constituencies. Furthermore, failure to vote in a certain way will not result in a loss of future representation. Thus, a democratically developed governing body includes representation from all the major and many of the minor consumer and provider health interests in the community. This guarantees accountability (representatives would have to vote in a manner consistent with their group's orientation), a democratic interaction among the representatives (bargaining and negotiation would be required to secure enough votes to decide an issue), and efficacy (those championing a certain position would give up something in return for future considerations). It would enable both rational/technical and political/value factors to come into play. As Mott asserts,

> The rational decision model is politically naive, because it presents planning as essentially a technical process in which the experts choose or provide others with an objective basis for selecting means, if not end. It fails to recognize that in the real world the determination of objectives as well as the causes of action, is a highly subjective process, especially the selection of objectives.[12]

THE LAW AND CITIZEN PARTICIPATION

In the 1960s, three major health planning acts were passed. Initially, none of them called for a consumer majority for regional health planning agencies. Both the RMP and the Hill-Burton Program were largely dominated by health providers. While the Comprehensive Health Planning Act called for a consumer majority at the state level, it was not until the act was amended two years later that such a majority was mandated for the regional agencies. In his testimony supporting such a consumer majority, James Brindle, then president of the Health Insurance Plan of Greater New York, stated in his testimony:

> The principal decision-making role should be reserved to people who truly represent the general public as consumers of health services, rather than people who might be expected to have more parochial views of planning. Ultimate responsibility for resolution of broad questions of social policy should remain free from identification with the limited and sometimes specialized interest of any particular health profession or the prevailing philosophy in the hospital industry.[13]

With the passage of PL 93-641 and its subsequent amendments, the language describing the citizen role was made more specific. At least a majority, but not more than 60 percent, of the governing body is required to be composed of consumers. These consumers must represent the social, economic, linguistic, racial, and handicapped elements of the population. Consumers with knowledge of mental health issues and major purchasers of health care must also be included as members. Further, consumer majorities are required for the agency's executive committee, its subcommittees, and its advisory bodies. All board members are to receive in advance expenses (taxis, baby-sitting, meals) as needed to enable them to attend. This is particularly aimed at alleviating the hardships that attendance may place on the poor, the handicapped, the elderly, and mothers of young children.

At least 50 percent of provider members must provide direct health care service to patients, such as physicians, nurses, dentists, podiatrists, physician's assistants, and optometrists. In addition, administrators of health care institutions, health care insurors, health care educators, and those connected to the allied health professions must be included among providers, with a special emphasis on the inclusion of those knowledgeable about mental health services. The governing body must also include elected officials and other representatives of local government units. Finally, it must have a percentage of nonmetropolitan members at least equal to the percentage of nonmetropolitan residents in its health service area.

This specification of the composition of the governing body is limited, however, to socially descriptive representation. It tells who shall sit on the governing body, but not their accountability or degree of influence. As noted earlier, substantive representation refers to the selection of representatives to ensure that they truly speak for a constituency. As Marmor and Morone state, "Acting in the public interest is not—in itself— enough. . . . Constituents must have the 'final say' if government action is to be attributable (and *accountable*) to them."[14]

Initially, the health planning agencies were given complete freedom in choosing the members of their governing body. However, the Senate Committee deliberating on amendments to PL 93-641 was "concerned that as a result of the current law, these agencies, which are supposed to be open and accessible, can become closed with a handpicked board providing policy direction, unsupported by the general public."[15] To prevent the governing body from becoming self-perpetuating, the amendments require that one-half the body be selected by a mechanism other than appointment by the existing members. No specific means are suggested, but the mechanism must be documented and approved by federal officials. The agency should further show how it will reach out to previously unrepresented consumer and provider groups and involve them in the selection process. Depending on the formal mechanism chosen, the selection process can result either in a descriptive representative board that is not accountable to a specific constituency or in an accountable, substantive representative board. For example, if all persons from different consumer and provider groups congregate at a specified time and place to elect half the governing body, the members so chosen may not be accountable to anyone, even though the descriptive requirements of the act are met. On the other hand, if identified consumer and provider groups are permitted to select their own representatives and are guaranteed future representation, this would be substantive representation with accountability to a constituency. Thus, while the amendments inhibit a self-perpetuating governing body, Congress has not yet taken the next step to ensure true accountability and substantive representation.

Currently, about 50,000 consumers and providers volunteer their time to the activities of health planning agencies. Around 9,000 persons are members of regional agencies, 53 percent of whom are consumers. Another 2,000 serve on the Statewide Health Coordinating Councils (SHCCs). In addition, 16,000 members volunteer their time on subarea councils, and another 25,000 serve as members of committees and task forces of regional planning agencies.[16] This is a substantial involvement of volunteer time and energy.

Table 10-1 offers a partial description of the composition of 135 health planning agency boards as of 1976. The following are important highlights of this table:

- Direct providers comprise 76 percent of all providers. PL 83-641 called for a minimum of one-third direct providers. Although this was raised to 50 percent by the 1979 amendments, it appears direct providers were already well represented, a major intention of Congress.
- Females represent 26 percent of the membership. This is well below their 50 percent ratio in the general population.
- Twenty-five percent of consumer members of regional planning boards are minorities, 75 percent of whom are blacks. This indicates they are well represented on agency boards.
- The average governing body size is 44 members, slightly smaller than their predecessor boards of 51 members. This is a reflection of the law's mandate to keep the size of the board manageable.

With each new legislative act and amendments, Congress has set more precise requirements for health planning agencies to ensure that they function in an open process and maintain democratic representation. In support of this congressional intent, Presidential Executive Order 12160 (Exhibit 10-1) requires all federal agencies to take steps to ensure positive and active consumer involvement in federal program activities. A Consumer Affairs Council, composed of members of 12 major departments of the executive branch, was created to coordinate and monitor implementation of this executive order. Basically, the order sets forth five basic functions required of all federal departments. Together, the legislative and executive branches of government are working to increase the public's involvement in federal activities.

Table 10-1 Selected Characteristics of HSA Governing Boards and Executive Committees

	Governing Boards		Executive Committees	
	No.	Percent	No.	Percent
A. *Consumer-Provider*				
Consumer members	3,072	52	690	53
Provider members	2,808	48	617	47
TOTAL	5,880	100	1,307	100
B. *Providers*				
Direct	1,786	64 76	459	76
Indirect	573	20 24	158	24
Not classifiable	449	16 —	—	—
TOTAL	2,808	100 100	617	100
C. *Consumer Minority Members*				
Blacks	598	76	157	82
Hispanic	128	16	19	10
Native Americans	45	6	14	7.5
Asians & Pacific Islanders	13	2	1	0.5
TOTAL	784	100	191	100
D. *Sex (All Members)*				
Male	4,343	74	991	76
Female	1,537	26	316	24
TOTAL	5,880	100	1,307	100
E. *Providers by Category*				
Physicians (Incl. DOs)	637	23 27	137	22
Dentists	135	5 6	24	4
Nurses	164	6 7	37	6
Subtotal (Category I)	(936)	(34) (40)	(198)	(32)
Health care institutions (II)	862	31 37	155	25
Health care insurors (III)	142	5 6	37	6
Health professional schools (IV)	157	7 7	37	6
Allied health professionals (V)	233	8 10	190	31
Not classifiable	448	16 —	—	—
TOTAL	2,808	100 100	617	100
F. *Public Officials*				
Consumer members	594	68	155	72
Provider members	277	32	60	28
Elected officials	472	54 62	107	50 60
Appointed officials	294	34 38	70	32 40
Not classifiable	105	12 —	38	18 —

Table 10-1   Continued

	Governing Boards		Executive Committees	
	No.	Percent	No.	Percent
State officials	72	8 9	15	7 8
Local officials	669	77 87	162	76 82
Other officials (e.g., COG)	25	3 3	20	9 10
Not classifiable	105	12 —	18	8 —
TOTAL	871	100	215	100

NOTE: The above information and breakdown reflect the governing board and executive committee membership of those 135 HSAs that were designated and funded by July 1, 1976, *and* for which such data were made available shortly thereafter.

As will be noted, several of the breakdowns include significant "not classifiable" categories. In those instances, two different percentages are shown. One includes the "not classifiable" category, and the other excludes it. In item B, for example, 449 (or 16 percent) of the total 2,835 provider members were "not classifiable" as either direct or indirect providers. As a result only 64 percent of that overall total are direct providers and 20 percent are indirect providers. Since those percentages could be misleading another set of percentages is shown to the right restricted to those 2,359 provider members who could be definitely identified as either direct or indirect providers.

Source: Bureau of Health Planning/Office of Evaluation and Legislation, Health Resources Administration, February 2, 1977.

Exhibit 10-1   President's Executive Order on Consumer Affairs (No: 12160)

Extract from Guidelines published in the Federal Register, February 4, 1980

1–4. Consumer Program Reforms.

1–401. The Chairperson, assisted by the Council, shall ensure that agencies review and revise their operating procedures so that consumer needs and interests are adequately considered and addressed. Agency consumer programs should be tailored to fit particular agency characteristics, but those programs shall include, at a minimum, the following five elements:

(a) *Consumer Affairs Perspective.* Agencies shall have identifiable, accessible professional staffs of consumer affairs personnel authorized to participate, in a manner not inconsistent with applicable statutes, in the development and review of all agency rules, policies, programs, and legislation.

(b) *Consumer Participation.* Agencies shall establish procedures for the early and meaningful participation by consumers in the development and review of all agency rules, policies, and programs. Such procedures shall include provisions to assure that consumer concerns are adequately analyzed and considered in decisionmaking. To facilitate the expression of those concerns, agencies shall provide for forums at which consumers can meet with agency decisionmakers. In addition, agencies shall make affirmative efforts to inform consumers of pending proceedings and of the opportunities available for participation therein.

(c) *Informational Materials.* Agencies shall produce and distribute materials to inform consumers about the agencies' responsibilities and services, about their procedures for consumer participation, and about aspects of the marketplace for which they have responsibility. In addition, each agency shall make available to consumers who attend agency meetings open to the public materials designed to make those meetings comprehensible to them.

(d) *Education and Training.* Agencies shall educate their staff members about the Federal consumer policy embodied in this Order and about the agencies' programs for carrying out that policy. Specialized training shall be provided to agency consumer affairs personnel and, to the extent considered appropriate by each agency and in a manner not inconsistent with applicable statutes, technical assistance shall be made available to consumers and their organizations.

(e) *Complaint Handling.* Agencies shall establish procedures for systematically logging in, investigating, and responding to consumer complaints, and for integrating analyses of complaints into the development of policy.

1–402. The head of each agency shall designate a senior-level official within that agency to exercise, as the official's sole responsibility, policy direction for, and coordination and oversight of, the agency's consumer activities. The designated official shall report directly to the head of the agency and shall apprise the agency head of the potential impact on consumers of particular policy initiatives under development or review within the agency.

CITIZENS' ROLES AND RESPONSIBILITIES

Burke views the term *role* as a behavioral concept that "signifies what a person occupying a specific position actually does. The position, in other words, is a definer of the role."[17] He further notes that the person occupying the position may define the role in personal ways. For example, one chairperson of a health planning agency may take very aggressive actions to inform the public of the agency's positions, while another may prefer to emphasize the regulatory function of the agency. While the position itself is passive, the actions of the person filling the position make the role a passive or active one.

Responsibility connotes a board member's sense of accountability to the mission of the health planning agency on one hand and to the organization he or she represents on the other. Such dual allegiance can create conflicts for the board member when the policy advocated by the planning agency is at variance with the position of the organization. When the agency's policy is consistent with the organization's position, it can reenforce the member's commitment to the agency goal or policy. Further, if the members have guaranteed seats on the board by virtue of the bylaws, then the way they carry out their assigned roles will be as much determined by how they view their position as by the degree of congruence between the agency's and the organization's positions on policy issues.

Roles played by board members of the health planning agencies are defined by the functions they are required to perform:

- plan development
- review of proposals for certificates of need
- review of existing institutions for appropriateness of their services
- implementation of plan goals and objectives
- advocacy of a plan's goals and objectives
- education of the community about its health services
- adoption of positions on public health issues

In carrying out these roles, board members share their political and social status with the agency, provide expert information on a variety of technical subjects, and give advice on alternative strategies for achieving the agency's goals. To be effective, board members must educate themselves about health matters, such as costs, utilization of services, quality, access, and availability of services, and their own organization's point of view on health issues.

Stating what the roles and responsibilities of board members are and carrying them out may lead to role confusion. Lack of clear federal or state guidance, differences of opinion on which roles and responsibilities should be emphasized, and dilemmas caused by their dual accountability all contribute to the confusion board members often feel about their roles and responsibilities. A few examples can illuminate the problems.

In a study of 15 subarea health planning councils, Arthur D. Little Consultants found substantial variance in the degree of involvement board members played in carrying out their roles respecting plan development, review, implementation, community education, and public issue involvement. Of these five roles, the councils placed their greatest emphasis on implementation and their least on plan development.[18] Part of the reason for this stems from the fact that the health planning agencies did not want the subarea councils to be involved in plan development, but only to support their efforts in implementation, even though some of those actions were not related to priority goals of the agencies' long-range plans. Clearly, the area councils have only advisory responsibilities compared to the decision-making roles and responsibility of the planning agencies. Often, the planning agencies have little interest in what their councils do as long as they are not in conflict with major agency policy goals. Implementation was a particularly attractive role for the councils. They carried out this role by:

- maintaining their close contacts with local government
- building support for programs by using their extensive local contacts
- negotiating and facilitating activities with providers, especially hospitals
- assisting in developing grant proposals that brought funds and new programs into their council area
- lobbying with local and state government for special programs or changes in existing policies or programs[19]

The report concludes:

> much of the implementation activity does not grow specifically out of the annual implementation plan but is either a continuation of pre-existing activities in the subarea or a response to locally generated issues. . . . Health planning agency policy seems usually to be one of allowing the subarea to choose those objectives that its volunteers are most interested in pursuing.[20]

A number of reasons were offered by Little Consultants for the active involvement of subarea councils:[21]

- provider self-interest. Health providers are particularly concerned with protecting their positions and the quality of their work.
- local pride. There was a strong desire to provide the best health services possible, and health planning and implementation activities were viewed as two major roles that could help bring about this goal.
- defense against outside control. Consumers and providers are concerned that the federal government and even their own health planning agency may make decisions that will be detrimental to the provision of health services in their communities. By serving on subarea councils, consumers and providers feel they can protect themselves from any adverse effects of projected policies.
- consumer self-interest. Consumers are particularly concerned about losing good services and are eager to extend the scope of services in their communities. They consequently take active, advocate roles in behalf of special constituencies in their community, such as the poor and elderly, and their health services.
- capacity to bring about change. Volunteers see councils as vehicles to bring about changes they perceive are needed in their own communities. Through both reactive and proactive strategies, volunteers feel they can influence health services in their community. Unlike planning, which is conceived as general, abstract, and future-oriented, implementation, review activities, and public issue involvement are all concrete activities that can produce quick outcomes.

An analysis of the Little study indicates that citizens favor active roles that produce results. Although their legal function is only an advisory one, subarea councils, often with the blessing of the central planning agency, play an authoritative, decision-making role and act as though they were autonomous bodies. This reduces the board members' dilemma of dual accountability and permits the activism associated with the activities found by Little in these subarea councils. In those councils in which such freedom was not extended by the central agency, role conflicts often took place. This, however, occurred in the minority of cases.

The following shows what happens when consumers, not accountable to any specific constituency, decide on whether to raise the fee schedule of a New York City hospital.[22] One consumer, JF, is a 30-year-old white woman who is single with no children, earns $4000 per year working part-time, and is very active on consumer health boards. A second consumer, ML, is a 35-year-old black man, who is married with two children, owns his business, and has an income of $30,000 per year. They are two of the members appointed by the hospital to represent the consumer point of view in the operation of the hospital's ambulatory clinic. They have advisory power only, but their decisions are generally accepted by the hospital trustees and administration. The following dialogue is mainly between these two participants, although many more actually participated. JF is asking the hospital to produce a financial statement to show why an increase in the fee schedule is necessary.

ML: So what would the revenue statement prove?

JF: I believe that it would prove that hospitals pay very little for direct costs and a great deal for costs allocated from administration. The costs allocated for supervision of interns and residents are unbelievably high. The fact that the hospital refuses to provide us with this public information in a form which would be useful to us leads me to be suspicious and take this stand even more forcefully. They should not raise the rates of the fee schedules!

ML: Look here, Jackie. No matter where the costs come from there's a deficit. The hospital can't be lying about that and they really need the increased income to cover the deficit.

JF: The statement will certainly show that the revenue from self-pay patients is not significant and that the proposed fee increase for these patients will be ineffective in reducing the deficit. We are not talking about enough money to do the hospital any good, but it is enough money required from patients to do harm to them. The primary impact of the increase will be to reduce access to care and decrease the number of patient visits, further decreasing even that small income.

ML: But since the fee is what a person can afford to pay, as stipulated in the contract, why are you beefing?

JF: The fee is NOT affordable! I thought I made that quite clear!

ML: But if the patients are asked to pay what they can afford—

JF: Excuse me for interrupting, but the patient is asked to pay the fee, NOT what they can afford. The fee is set by the contract and is *supposed* to reflect what the patient can afford.

ML: You can't tell me no one can afford to pay $10.00 to see a doctor!

JF: The income for category A is $2,901 to $3,999 for a family of one. Can that person who makes $55 to $75 a week before deducting social security and taxes, afford $10 for a clinic visit when that's 10 to 20 percent of his salary?

ML: No one makes only $55 to $75 a week. They can get on Medicaid if they do.

JF: I make that much, and I can *not* get on Medicaid.

ML: I think you have to try and look at it from the hospital's point of view, so that you can be fair. The hospital's costs have gone up, so they have to charge more. Everyone else does. Besides, you're a board member. Don't they do favors for you? My hospital lets me and my wife in free because I'm on the board.

JF: That sounds like a pay-off to me.

ML: Certainly not. I do for them on the board, and they do for me and my wife in the clinic.

JF: I'm angry. You don't know how your own program works. You don't understand the way the fee schedule works. Yet, you're willing to create hardships for people that you're supposed to represent on this board and in this meeting!

ML: I *do* represent my board, and my board represents the hospital. After all, there are hospital people on the board.

JF: But consumers are supposed to be the majority on the board. And if your board doesn't represent the consumers, who does? Your hospital already has its representatives. It seems your personal interest and that of the patients could not possibly coincide. That's one reason why we're not progressing at all. Neither reason nor facts have made any impression. I guess it's time to stop this agony and take a vote.

The vote of the majority was in favor of raising the fee schedule and not to request any financial or other information from the hospital.

This scenario clearly illustrates the effort of JF, chairwoman of the committee, both to educate and advocate in behalf of the poor constituency. Although none of the members had been selected by specific organizations to serve on the board, they tended to support and represent those generic constituencies with whom they identified. There was no substantive representation with accountability, but the businessman, ML, could sympathize with the hospital's deficit; as a businessman, he would seek income from any source, however small, to close the deficit. The fact that special favors are accorded to him and his wife only add to his own strongly felt views. Implied in his own beliefs is that the poor could earn more income than they do. By charging patients according to what they could afford, he felt he was being fair to those who had little income while holding to his belief that a person should be as self-reliant as possible.

JF, who works only part-time in order to continue her activities to improve health services for the poor, strongly identifies with her constituency because she lives at the same economic level. She has felt the hospital overcharges in the ambulatory care unit by adding overhead costs that, in her opinion, properly belong to other cost centers of the hospital.

Since the outpatient service represents the community physician for most of the poor, any charges beyond their ability to pay cause them to postpone care until a crisis occurs. Although she does not represent a specific organization to whom she is accountable, JF has a generic constituency who expect her to protect and promote their rights and views. As chairwoman, she has the responsibility of leading the discussion. However, she played the role of educator (showing how the poor would be affected by the rate increase) and advocate (promoting the status quo while revealing the limited knowledge base on which the hospital supporters were making their case). The committee as a whole was acting as a review body in advising the hospital board of trustees on its proposed increase in the fee schedule. The committee gave a consumer legitimacy to the hospital's proposal by voting in favor of the rate increase. Thus, the committee members played several roles in rendering a decision on this issue.

In this case, it appears that JF failed to heed a basic community organization principle: "education precedes action." She failed to educate ML before the meeting, out of the glare of the public spotlight. As Roche states—talking about health planning agencies—

> staff and volunteers must be oriented and prepared to intervene prior to the actual need for intervention. If a solid intellectual and emotional foundation for intervention does not exist . . . prior to the need for action, the likely result will be confusion, intense . . . squabbling about the "appropriateness" of acting, or a tendency to "pass the buck" for action to some other entity.[23]

Because she had not obtained the budgetary information in advance and analyzed it in a businesslike manner, JF could not intellectually convince ML to support her case. Her appeal to emotions fell on deaf ears because ML strongly believed in the value of people making it by their own labor just as he did. Only if JF could show that the ambulatory services overcharged to pay for deficits in cost centers in other parts of the hospital might she have made her case with ML and those who supported his point of view. Since they did not have this information, both relied upon their own basic values and the policy orientation of those constituencies they felt they were representing and voted accordingly.

In order for citizen volunteers to understand their roles and responsibilities, it is necessary for them to understand the distinction between public and private interests. Public interests are typically represented by government bodies that carry out programs enacted by legislatures. As such, any program that is implemented is said to be in the public interest. On the other hand, Burke notes that private interests are quite different:

> A group of citizens come together around a common cause. They recruit others and persuade them to identify with their interest. They may even try to make their group "representative" of the total population . . . to provide sanction and legitimacy. The group, however, is still an interest group organized to achieve a cause that it alone feels is desirable.[24]

The private group needs consensus in any actions it intends to take because it alone carries out the actions it desires. A legislative body requires merely a majority vote because it expects others, either in the executive branch of government or in the private sector, to carry out its will. Private interest groups are dependent on good will to implement their goals. Finally, a private interest group has no authority to compel others to do its bidding. For this reason, they are termed "powerless" by Burke. "The power of an interest group is the conviction of its case and the influence of its members."[25]

Health planning agencies are an anomaly. They are neither purely public nor purely private interest bodies. They represent what has recently been termed "the third sector," since they take on the characteristics of both the private and public sectors. Like the public sector, health planning agencies have been delegated some authority by legislative bodies to plan and make review decisions; but, like the private sector, they cannot compel health care institutions to carry out their goals. Like those in the public sector, their boards are intended to be representative of all sectors of the public and health provider communities; they resemble legislative bodies in that a majority vote is sufficient to determine a goal. Yet, like a private sector body, they need a consensus vote from their members in order to obtain the good will and community support to implement their goals.

In essence, this means that a third sector agency is effective only if it acts like a private interest body. However, the representativeness required of the health planning agency is such that only in special circumstances are the board members likely to have common values and thus to succeed. Medeiros notes that planning is a rational, systematic process that assumes like-minded decision makers.[26] Yet, a health planning agency requires a constant information exchange and, therefore, an open-ended capacity to change goals as new information emerges. To carry out these goals, planning agencies must intervene in the health system to change them consistent with the goals. "To the extent that planning agencies intervene, the schizoid tendency of rational/institutional integrity versus working in an open-ended health system will be apparent and will require careful monitoring."[27] Thus, third sector agencies are in a dilemma.

An example of what happens when a health planning agency tries to act like a private sector agency and ignores the delegation of authority is seen in the demise of the Los Angeles health planning agency. A General Accounting Office (GAO) report found irregularities in the election procedures, in payments made for legal counsel, and in the hiring of staff and top agency officials.[28] Subsequently, the staff and certain segments of the governing body formed a coalition against the providers so that, for all practical purposes, the providers were unable to represent their constituents.[29] This conflict came to a head in a chaotic meeting of the governing body in which the chairman refused to allow certain members to speak. A member who managed to seize the microphone asked for the dismissal of the chairperson. This member was ruled out of order, as the item was not on the agenda (it had been deliberately omitted by the staff). When a vote was taken to have another member run this particular meeting, chaos broke out and the meeting was declared adjourned. The effectiveness of the chairman to lead was severely impaired, however, as a majority of the governing members refused to attend future meetings called by him. Further, without membership involvement, the board was unable to discuss how to meet the stringent conditions laid down by the regional office of the Department of Health, Education, and Welfare (HEW). Consequently, because of the paralysis of the board, among other reasons, the agency was phased out by HEW. A new governing body is in the process of development to reestablish the agency.

It is clear that an agency must maintain its legitimacy by the representativeness of its governing body. The capture and operation of the agency by the staff and a minority of the governing body converted the agency from a third sector into a private interest agency and cost the agency its legitimacy. The roles of providing education and advocacy were assumed by a minority of the leadership group, while the majority were relegated to a dissident role. Yet, needing a consensus to plan and review proposals, the governing body was paralyzed when the majority refused to follow the chairman's lead. Thus, an agency's legitimacy is based on its capacity to maintain its broad, public sanction so that it can assume its roles of planning, review, implementation, and public issue advocacy.

In another study, it was found that role ambiguity is a danger that third sector bodies such as health planning agencies must guard against. A study of two mental health planning boards was made in a state where the law was not specific with respect to the role of the area boards.[30] It was discovered that, although one board had a broad base of citizen members, most lacked any knowledge of mental health; there was consequently a tendency toward inaction while they educated themselves. On the second board, all members were experts in mental health, and the board took an activist role in planning and promoting the interests of the mental health agencies within their planning area. In short, the board members seized the ambiguity of the law to interpret their role as they saw fit. One took a passive, inactive role; the other took an active, advocate, leadership role. The active area board, in effect, had converted itself into a private interest group, since most of its members and committee chairpersons were professionals from the mental health field. Their legitimacy came from the mental health agencies that the members represented rather than from the broad base of public interests. To the extent that community interest groups were indifferent to the board's activity, the board would be able to act as a private interest group with no role conflicts. If it were challenged, as in the Los Angeles example, its legitimacy would eventually be nullified if it failed to take these other interests into account. In that event, it would probably behave more like the passive board, which had a broader, more representative body.

It can be seen from these illustrations that determination of roles and responsibilities is a complex process that involves a number of factors: the mandate of the agency, the type of board (public, private, or third sector), the type of representation (socially descriptive, formal, or substantive), and the emphasis placed on certain roles over others (planning and review over implementation or public issue, or vice versa). All of these factors determine how responsible and accountable the board becomes in playing its roles. Because there is no best model of what roles and responsibilities a health planning agency board should play, the board would do well to reflect on this matter before it plunges into its activities.

OBSTACLES TO CITIZEN PARTICIPATION

Two types of obstacles prevent full and effective citizen participation: administrative and structural. Studies reveal that these obstacles affect mainly consumer activity.

Administrative Obstacles

Administrators of health planning agencies either inadvertently or consciously place obstacles in the way of consumers. They may fail to provide access to information, consumer health education relating to health planning, staff expertise to advocate a consumer point of view, and assistance with the costs of participation.

Access to Information

Health planning is becoming increasingly technical in nature. Vast quantities of information are required if the planning models and formulas are to be used. Agencies often lack much of the information required for making decisions. As a result, both the planning agencies and the consumers often must make decisions based on an inadequate base of information. Consumers may have an additional problem of not understanding the implications of the information they do have. In the heat of plan development and certificate-of-need review meetings, there is limited, if any, time to explain to consumers the meaning of the information presented to them. Even more important, unless told what data are missing, consumers may not even know that there are deficits in their information base. In a report to the National Council on Health Planning and Development, Shannon states the problem very explicitly:

> The overriding general problem facing consumers on HSA governing bodies and SHCCs is a relative lack of knowledge concerning the functioning of the health care system, the wide array of health care programs, statutes, and regulations, and permeating both of these areas, an accompanying jargon that is difficult for a lay person to understand. The nature of HSA activities and functions and the substance of a health care systems plan are geared to a sophisticated knowledge and background that are more likely to be found among the ranks of the providers and planners.[31]

After an extensive review of consumer participation literature, Checkoway concludes that consumers' lack of knowledge and expertise makes it difficult for them to relate their ideas and concerns to providers and planners.[32] In their survey of HSA consumer members in four large urban areas, the Consumer Commission on the Accreditation of Health Services found that 86 percent of the respondents felt the need for more information.[33] Lack of complete information and inability to interpret the information available in regard to the issues under discussion are the most pressing problems of consumer participants.

In contrast, provider members have no such problem. They have their professional associations, their institutional experts, and the health planners to provide and interpret data for them. Because of their medical and scientific backgrounds, they are usually comfortable handling raw data and statistical analyses. One writer found that an excellent strategy for dealing with the consumers' demand for data is not to withhold it, but to drown them in it so that they cannot tell the "forest from the trees." As this writer states, "The more information provided, the more difficult it will be for consumers to learn anything important and the more the executive can point with pride to his/her attempts to inform the board."[34] Thus, not only does the provider have a greater abundance of data, but also has the greater capacity to understand its meaning.

Lack of Consumer Health Education

The problem consumers have in understanding the data given them can only be overcome by educational training from sympathetic health planners, but it has been pointed out by the experts noted that planners find it easier to communicate with health care providers than with consumers. Consumers therefore require their own technical experts who respond to their needs and partially counterbalance the experts who are readily available to providers. It is difficult to find such experts for consumers, however, because most health planners have been trained and educated by health care providers and often have had internships in health provider institutions before they became health planners. Further, it is thought that, if consumers have access to such expertise, "their participation is expected to cause delays in action, to expand the number of conflicts, and to increase the cost of operations."[35] While it is acknowledged that providing such expertise to consumers may allow them to make more enlightened decisions, it may indeed take more time to reach decisions, since decisions cannot be made as quickly when all parties with their varying points of view have a comparable knowledge base. Consumers, in particular, require continuing education to achieve this parity with providers and planners.

In response to Executive Order 12160 and the 1979 planning amendments, the Bureau of Health Planning and health planning agencies are now required to assign high-level planners who devote their time to providing technical assistance to consumers. These planners are expected to provide health education seminars, information requested by consumer members of the board, and to advocate the consumer position in agency and board affairs.

Costs of Participation

Participation takes time and energy on the part of volunteers. The argument has been made that providers engage in board work as part of their professional assignment; they are paid for attending meetings, allowed travel expenses, and given time off. They participate to protect or promote the interests of their institutions; they receive backup support, such as secretarial services, development of policy positions, and data analysis.[36] On the other hand, consumers do not gain such benefits from their participation. More often, their costs far outweigh any tangible benefits. In analyzing the costs of consumer participation in the Los Angeles health planning agency, Cooper identifies these costs:

> In actual fact, participation requires an expenditure of time, effort, and money in order to attend hearings, become involved in planning workshops, respond to questionnaires, be interviewed, write letters to officials, secure information about the issues, and take part in advisory committees.[37]

Consumers consciously take such costs into account when they make decisions about attending a specific agency event. What are the benefits in exchange for the time, baby-sitting, parking and automobile expenses involved, for the tensions generated at the meeting, and for the follow-up activities? Health planning agencies can make the costs high or low, depending on their interest in consumer involvement. They can schedule meetings at times and places that make it easy or difficult for consumers to attend. They can pay expenses in advance or reimburse out-of-pocket costs only long after the event has passed. They can raise unrealistic expectations about the importance of consumer participation or put it in proper perspective, e.g., they are advising the governing body or serving as a feedback mechanism in an open public hearing. Unlike providers, whose certificate-of-need proposals are to be reviewed or whose goals represent important future opportunities for their institutions, consumers seldom have such direct benefits for their involvement. They must be satisfied with better services for their community and the psychological rewards that come from having served their community's health needs. Newcomers to the health participation field are not as apt to perceive or accept these intangible rewards as sufficient inducement to continue. Those who have long been involved know of the rewards that come from winning small victories (prevented a hospital from expanding its obstetric service or secured a primary care physician for their neighborhood), and have learned the value of patience, persistence, and perseverance. Typically, this hard core group of consumer experts are generally overcommitted and pay a high cost in psychic energy. Thus, consumers often find the costs of involvement to be a real obstacle to their continued participation, and many begin to reduce their efforts.

Structural Obstacles

While administrative obstacles are generally under the control of the agency's administration, structural obstacles are not. Among such obstacles are the lack of a consumer constituency, the nonexistence of a consumer network of health organizations, poor communication among consumers, and lack of access to the community's health decision makers. The common theme behind all these obstacles to effective consumer participation is the domination of health planning and service institutions by provider members of the agency's governing body. Unless a countervailing force of active consumers and their organizations can be developed, the structural barriers will remain too difficult for consumers to overcome.

Consumer Constituency

Marmor and Morone have previously pointed to the fact that consumers are generally selected to meet the socially descriptive requirements of the law. This means a consumer can be chosen because she is a black female who lives in a nonmetropolitan section of the health service area. She may have no constituency who actually named her and to whom she is accountable. She is, in effect, a consumer at-large with the whole nonmetropolitan community as her constituency. Lacking a specific institutional base, she has no one to support her decisions, to provide her with information, or to tell her the parameters within which she must vote; she is her own autonomous decision maker. As such, she has no power or influence; she brings only the political/social status she has in her own right to the position, but these latter characteristics are incidental. Shannon would say that she lacks an organizational base, that she lacks accountability to an organized consumer body. In contrasting this type of consumer representative to the provider, he would say that "providers usually have a particular interest to represent, whereas consumers' interests are as fragmented as the portion of the population they represent."[38]

Such consumers can be readily captured by the more vocal and sophisticated provider members of the board. For example, in one Illinois health planning agency, a consumer member who was a business executive voted consistently to create additional, unneeded services even though "most business groups have taken public stands supporting the official cost containment efforts."[39] A low-income representative, a minister, voted with the hospitals who wanted minimal or no monitoring and little publicizing of the Hill-Burton regulations that required hospitals to provide free care to indigents, in spite of the fact that his constituents would be most affected.[40] Both of these consumers could vote against their generalized consumer interests because they were not accountable to a specific organization.

Lack of a Consumer Network

Providers are said to have powerful associations and professional groups who meet regularly and provide guidance on how they should vote. Such organizations may support each other's proposals and goals. In contrast, consumer groups are highly fragmented. They are small, underfunded, work hard just to survive, and generally do not know or get together with their counterparts on issues in which they have a common concern unless a major crisis occurs, such as the elimination of a substantial number of hospital beds that have been serving the poor. Health planning agencies have been particularly lax in recruiting strong representatives among the poor for the governing bodies, according to Shannon. In urban areas where the poor's health services have been jeopardized by fiscal crises, it is generally non-health planning agencies that have taken the lead in opposing cuts in service. Consumers have been passive supporters at most.

While one way to overcome this lack of community support is to develop a network of consumer health bodies, this requires staff support and at the same time must counteract the general public's belief that providers are the only ones who know what is best in health care. Furthermore, compared to crime and inflation, health care is a less immediate concern for most members of the general public. Forester believes that only as consumer health groups widen their constituency to include citizen organizations such as labor unions, women's groups, or community citizen bodies will they be able to ensure that the items on the health planning agency's agenda include issues other than the ones providers consider important.[41]

A recent study of committee selection in a large urban health planning agency showed that a handful of members sat on six or more committees and served as chairpersons of these committees, while 19 members (14 consumers and only 5 providers) were assigned to no committees. Most of those who had not been assigned to committees were newer members. Except for the governing board and executive committee, consumers were often in the minority, in spite of the mandate calling for consumer majority on all legally constituted meetings of the agency.[42] The implication was that consumers had been shunted aside while providers and their consumer allies ran the agency as their own. Thus, a network of consumer constituencies and their friends is essential if the consumer members are to have a somewhat equal influence and reflect their majority representation in developing agency agenda and determining planning policy.

Poor Communication among Consumers

While a consumer network is almost a precondition for improved communication among consumers, the fact is that consumers champion a wide variety of values. This makes it difficult for consumers to speak with one voice. The Consumer Commission survey found that 80 percent of those interviewed ranked the establishment of good communication among consumers as a very important issue.[43] However, there are a number of problems in developing this communication. First, consumer groups must accept their differences and the fact that no one group can speak for all of their diverse interests. Even among provider groups there is no one voice that speaks for all the professional groups. Second, independent consumer groups are fearful of being swallowed by any superbody that purports to represent their interests. Consumer groups may support each other's point of view, but they do not want others speaking for them through a larger body. Finally, consumers on health planning agencies may well resent any external health body that attempts to determine what their major goals should be. After all, that is the role and mission of the agency. These consumers may find it difficult to accept leadership from an outside group. Thus, while the Consumer Commission and other leading health consumer bodies champion some form of national consumer network, the obstacles are quite formidable.

A study by Grossman of the voting preferences of consumers and providers on a large midwestern health planning agency regarding certificate-of-need proposals produced an unexpected finding. It was anticipated that voting would be divided along consumer and provider lines. However, analysis found that consumers and providers tended to vote for the same type of projects. In this case, they supported mainly public health service projects, such as community mental health centers, health maintenance organizations (HMOs), and health promotion projects, and disapproved hospital and nursing home projects. The truly surprising finding, according to Grossman, was that consumers displayed greater solidarity in their voting patterns than did providers: ". . . there is evidence that consumers and providers are different with respect to voting solidarity, and consumers appear to exhibit greater solidarity in their voting behavior than do providers."[44] For example, in disapproving hospital proposals, an average of 94 percent of the consumers tended to vote the same way on these projects, while only 46 percent of the providers did so. Respecting public health projects, 88 percent of the consumers and 70 percent of the providers voted the same way. They were about equal with respect to nursing home projects, 69 percent voting in the same direction.

These findings challenge the long-held beliefs of provider solidarity and influence on how consumers vote on health projects. The author suggests that, as consumers become more sophisticated in the rationally oriented methods of health systems planning, they rely less on political conviction and more on facts to determine their decisions. While this is only one study, it does indicate another dimension to provider-consumer relationships. It also raises some doubt whether consumers really have such poor communication that they cannot come to a common understanding of what projects and goals are in the best interests of their community.

Access to Community Decision Makers

The typical health consumer lacks the capacity to deal with community health decision makers regarding a wide number of issues that may affect them. Consumer board members may have contact with those health care providers who sit on health planning agencies and, to the extent that these providers are the true decision makers, can establish a superficial relationship with them. Whether they can carry on a dialogue relating to the poor's accessibility to prestige hospitals, expansion of ambulatory services to serve ethnic and minority groups, or more referrals to home health agencies is open to question, however. Issues of this type are conflict-laden, because of differing conceptions of how health issues should be dealt with, and involve the status and prestige of health institutions affected by a health planning agency's decisions. Only if a consumer group has shown an inclination in the past to support a health provider's position on an issue are its decision makers likely to engage in a dialogue with the group.

Providers deal actively and routinely with each other as well as with political, government, and financial decision makers. This gives them an enormous head start and insight into the feasibility of various health planning goals and certificate-of-need projects that come before the agency. They can determine whom the projects will serve, the capacity of the particular institutions to finance new health services related to the plan's goals, and the feasibility of expanding existing services. These are important factors about which providers may have advance information. Consumer members are generally barred from such inside data and often are forced to make decisions based on the bits of information that health providers provide at meetings or give to the health planners for general public distribution.[45] Thus, lack of access puts consumers at a decided disadvantage in making knowledgeable decisions. It also helps to maintain the mystique of provider board members as all-knowing authorities, an image that they have fostered and that has been carried over from the physician-patient relationship.

Size of Board

Little has been said of the size of the board and its effect on the citizen's role in the participatory process. Except for the obvious fact that large boards are unwieldy, what are the consequences of board size? As Verba indicates, "if large numbers have an effect on the outcome, as in elections, the contribution of any single individual is likely to be very limited."[46] Verba goes on to say that the smaller the scale, the greater the satisfaction of input and impact. The more informal the relationships, the higher the informational content and feedback. In planning terms, the more widespread the participation, the more likelihood for compromise, less carefree planning, and the introduction of "irrationalities" in planning.[47]

If too large a board is unwieldy and fosters watered-down consensus, Blum recognizes additional effects. According to Blum, too large a board promotes the use of executive committees, forces coalitions, and results in decision making by the few, which is not the rationale behind the federal guidelines for health planning.[48] The OSTI, in fact, did find in its study of various boards that, if the boards were large and unwieldy, then the director works to ensure that members neutralize each other and that the staff assumes the responsibilities of the board.[49] On the other hand, too small a board limits the desired diversity, and if representation is too small, it affects the board's credibility.

EFFECTIVENESS OF CITIZEN PARTICIPATION

There is increasing interest in trying to determine whether citizen involvement on a health planning board has any real effect. At one extreme, there is the view expressed by Levin that citizen participation is a waste of time because the dominant orientation of health planning is based on the medical model and its emphasis on disease. However, board decisions on changing the medical delivery system will have little impact on the major chronic diseases of heart disease, cancer, and stroke.[50] He would prefer consumers to separate from health planning agency boards and develop their own broad-based consumer advocacy movement with a focus on public health solutions to health care.[51] At the other extreme, there are those who champion consumer involvement in health planning agencies, but believe that its effectiveness should be measured by process outcomes, i.e., how they involved themselves in decision making. Fearon makes a strong case for this emphasis, as she believes it unfair to hold consumers responsible for changing health indicators when many factors other than their decisions are involved in those measures.[52] Indeed, there is "little empirical evidence on the effectiveness of a governing body . . . and therefore few measures on what constitutes effectiveness."[53] Consequently, the best that can be done at this point is to identify some of the factors that might be considered in measuring effectiveness when empirical studies are done.

Outcome Measures of Effectiveness

Outcome can be conceived from two levels of accomplishment: the consumers' achievement of their objectives, such as adopting a health plan or approving a set of bylaws, or the effect of the achievement of the plan's goals on health indicators, such as mortality, disability, or morbidity. The first level indicators are generally referred to as the outputs of activity, i.e., the direct result of the consumers' involvement. They are tangible, concrete, and usually specific. These accomplishments are really a means to the second level of change, the impact the agency's activity has on the population's health status or the efficiency of the health system. However, because consumers have very little direct involvement in whether a hospital, nursing home, or mental health service changes its services to conform to the plan's goals, they cannot be held fully responsible for outcomes regarding a population's health status. Consequently, only output measures on which consumers can have an impact should be used to measure their effectiveness. In health planning, these would be the products they adopt: the long-range and annual implementation plans, bylaws, project review manuals, decisions on certificate-of-need proposals, development of an appropriateness review manual, special studies on personnel availability, or a regionalization plan, as well as the number of speeches or public appearances made by the members. These are all visible, measurable products that represent consumers' true outputs. It should be stated that, since consumers and providers are both involved in developing these products, the main problem may be to measure the consumers' share of influence on the final output. This is very difficult to measure, although Grossman's study on project review decisions, which was discussed earlier, is one way to do it.[54]

In a study of certificate-of-need decisions in New England states, the Codman Research Group came to two conclusions regarding consumer and provider involvement in those decisions:

1. Contrary to predictions at the time PL 93-641 was enacted, the new planning system has been neither captured by health providers nor an effective control on health care institutional expansion.
2. The planning system has not been captured by providers.[55]

The study based these conclusions on the fact that providers were not of a common mind with respect to individual certificate-of-need proposals. Competition among institutional providers often caused them to oppose each other on specific projects. Further, national guidelines have as strong an impact on which proposals are approved or disapproved, as do local inputs. Finally, consumers have generally been more supportive of the health planners' concern for cost containment than for cost increases stemming from providers' emphasis on quality of care improvements. These findings do not indicate that consumers are equal to providers in influence, but rather that providers do not control the process as much as had been anticipated. The output of the consumers' activity could be measured by the percentage of times they voted with the majority on decisions.

In another example, the work of Mt. Sinai Hospital with the East Harlem Tenants Council illustrates the effects of consumer involvement.[56] The council learned to distinguish between measures of efficiency and effectiveness and to apply these measures in reviewing their health center's quarterly reports and annual operational plans. They learned how to set priorities in determining center health policy. As a member of the council board stated,

> In view of our training we will now demand of the project director a systematic quarterly report in order for us to evaluate what has been done and begin to set policy based on objectives. . . . Many times we have to make decisions and/or suggestions without information.[57]

Thus, in this case, output included improved capacity to make thoughtful evaluations of the center's progress; development of policies, goals, and priorities; and the intangible output of being in control of the center's activity.

In a third example, Fearon notes the impact of consumer members of advisory committees on ambulatory care, outpatient departments of voluntary hospitals in New York City.[58] She feels that consumer demands, supported by city health planners, resulted in the hiring of full-time directors of ambulatory care, expansion of outpatient clinics into full departments of ambulatory care or community medicine, and the provision of alternative treatment to patients with nonemergency conditions who appeared at emergency medical departments. These are outcome measures of effectiveness because these consumers were directly connected to a health service rather than one step removed in a health planning agency.

These examples suggest measures that can be used to demonstrate consumer effectiveness with respect to output and outcomes. Many more empirical studies are necessary before agreement can be reached on which are the best indicators of consumer effectiveness.

Process Measures of Effectiveness

Process measures refer to the consumers' degree of involvement in agency activity. This activity may or may not be concerned with the development of agency products, such as plans or manuals. Involvement may take many forms:

- increased number of consumers participating in a planning discussion or other committee meeting
- capacity of consumers to influence providers and other consumers to accept their values, such as concern with disease prevention
- accountability, as shown by their reporting back and seeking guidance from their own organizations on a variety of issues
- greater acceptance of consumer participation by provider members of the board
- capacity to influence the agenda of a meeting
- ability to develop alliances or coalitions in support of issues that concern them

Some of these activities are easier to measure than others. For example, it would be difficult to determine the extent to which consumers influenced provider thinking, but examining the full minutes would reveal whether more consumers are making their voices heard in debates.

The combined impact of consumer involvement in process and outcome activities should give consumers greater influence in what happens to the health care system and the health status of people. Shannon sums up the real meaning of consumer effectiveness in this way.

> Effective participation has meant . . . the ability to deal on the same grounds as providers and planners . . . effective participation and its impact means *accomplishment*, the ability to achieve a desired objective. From this then flows a sense of personal power, a sense of making a real contribution to the aims of the health planning program in making the health care system responsive to the needs of people.[59]

PLANNING MODELS

Even though the four planning models applied throughout this book are hypothetical, applying them makes it possible to clarify the various roles of community boards, the primary participants and influences in decision making, the commitments that boards may have, and the effect of the size of the board on decision making.

Each model has as its premise a particular outlook or concept of consumer-provider participation in health planning. Most consumers involved in health planning boards are college-educated professionals, while most providers proved to be medical institution administrators, members of professional societies, or physicians. Similarly, government board representation deferred to the participation of the local health official. These are also the types of consumers, providers, and government representatives whose participation can be evaluated in relationship to each model. Participation of consumers, providers, and government officials can be measured on a low to high continuum. Similarly, the influence each participant has in the decision-making process as it pertains to each model can be measured from low to high.

Earlier in this chapter the myriad roles from which a board could choose were mentioned. Those roles included policy planning as it embraces the roles of planning, reactive/proactive implementation, and advocacy. In part, the role a board plays is related to the board's commitment. Is the board committed to the delivery of health care as it relates to and affects all areas and individuals? The public interest? Is the board committed to specific interests, interests that merely affect a given community or locality? A private interest?

The last board characteristic relates to the degree of board fragmentation or cohesiveness. The degree of fragmentation in turn affects the speed with which decisions are made. Table 10-2 depicts the variations in board characteristics according to the planning model used by health planning agencies.

Systems Model

Because of the technical expertise that this model calls for in planning, the most active participants on the board are those providers that deal with technical decisions in their daily occupations: the medical institutional administrators and members of professional medical societies. Consumer and government participation will tend to be low because of the technical nature of systems planning. Most consumers and government representatives are not proficient in the language or application of systems analysis.

The board functions as a policy planner because it embraces the roles of assessing health facilities and health indicators, setting priorities, and recommending policy and goals. Not only does the board initiate planning activities, but once a policy decision is reached, the board and staff become the chief advocates of that policy. It is important to note that the activities

Table 10-2 Relationship of Board Characteristics to Planning
Models

Board Characteristics	Planning Models			
	Systems	Partnership	Alliance	Individual Action
Degree of participation				
Consumer	Low	Low—moderate	Low—moderate	High
Provider	High	Moderate—high	High	Low
Government rep.	Low	Low	Low	Low—none
Roles				
Planning reactive	Policy planning	Planning	Proactive implementation	
Reactive implementation	Reactive implementation	Advocate	Advocate	
Proactive implementation Advocate				
Commitment	Public interest	Public interest	Public interest	Private interest
Decision-making influence				
Consumer	Low	Low	Low	High
Provider	Medium—high	High	High	Low—none
Government rep.	Low	Low	Low	Low—none
Staff	High	Low	Moderate	High
Degree of fragmentation	Medium—high	Medium—high	Low—medium	Low
Speed of decision making	Slow—moderate	Slow—moderate	Moderate—fast	Rapid

of the board are directed at all sectors of the health system—personal health care, environmental health, and socioeconomic health-related conditions. The commitment is broad, being based in the public interest. The board and staff are advocates of public health policy as opposed to grass roots or private health interests.

The highest degree of decision-making influence in the systems model lies with the staff because they possess the greatest degree of technical expertise. Providers' influence varies from moderate to high, depending upon their level of expertise.

Considering the number of health components that must be evaluated and planned and the comprehensive nature with which the systems board attacks the health delivery system, the board becomes highly fragmented as it deals with each component. Consequently, decision making might be very slow, since each unit must evaluate a component and come to a recommendation. The total decision-making time depends upon the quickness with which each unit reaches a decision.

Partnership Model

Unlike the systems model, the partnership model finds the consumers on the board being somewhat assertive, although the provider participation surpasses consumer participation. This is partially due to the nature of partnership planning. Planning in this model is issue-oriented, the primary focus being on the delivery of health care. When the public raises an issue such as air pollution or lead poisoning, this too becomes one of the issues on which the board will focus. As this statement implies, the roles of this type of board are reactive because policies are developed in response to health crises or community demands. The board, however, does not become involved in advocating its policies. Consequently, because the board is so removed from implementation or plans of action, this type of board's existence is the most threatened of all the models, and members become preoccupied with justifying their existence.

Because the focus of partnership planning is the delivery of health care, the providers of health care (the medical institutional administrators) are the prime decision makers. The consumer component of the board may raise an issue, but the providers decide the action to be taken. The staff may make general comments about the apparent weaknesses or strengths of the health care system, but evaluations are undertaken by the provider institutions.

The degree of fragmentation of the board varies, depending upon the number of issues with which the board is concerned—the more issues, the more committees and subcommittees to evaluate the issues. Decision-making time also varies, depending upon the number of subcommittees involved on an issue.

The most obvious example of the partnership model is the health and welfare council that has provided coordination to the human resources agencies for so many years. In these councils, seldom does a policy issue that has not already been debated and agreed upon in the committee or task forces that studied the issue come before the entire board for a decision. However, because of the many diverse points of view that must be taken into account on both the committee and the board, the policy is generally couched in broad terms so that each member of the council can give a personal interpretation of what it means. In this way, conflicts are held down while broad policy issues with high board consensus are accepted after committee deliberations. It is believed that the majority of planning agencies use this model for making decisions.

Alliance Model

The degree of participation of consumers and providers in the alliance model generally follows the same pattern as that of the partnership model. What is different are the roles played. In the alliance model, the locus of considering policy and making recommendations, like the partnership model, is lodged in the committee structure of the board. Unlike the partnership model, the committee perceives itself as an advocate for either taking initiative on issues or taking stands on public issues that affect its members and actively seeking to bring a resolution to the matter, regardless of whether it creates division within the entire board. Its sense of commitment is, therefore, greater than would exist on a policy committee in advocating for and seeking to implement its recommendations. Because of the energy involved, the alliance committee generally has time to consider only one issue at a time. When several committees act in this manner, the agency board merely serves as a "rubber stamp" of the decisions generated by the committees in order to avoid division on the board. Periodically, when committees take different positions on the same issue, the board erupts into a battleground because the commitment of the committees toward their own positions is too great for anyone to back down gracefully.

Such a model assumes that the members of the committee generally have similar values. Those who differ from the majority are either ignored or drop out of the committee. Because the main emphases of the health planning agencies have been on matters that have primarily concerned provider interests (such as project review; data collection and studies on subjects such as ambulatory care, professional personnel, or bed needs for the community; or on special studies dealing with specific medical problems) the provider has had the greatest commitment and involvement on the committees. Staff's role is mainly to provide technical and secretarial services to the committee. Because most of the decisions are made in the committees, there is both a low degree of fragmentation and a fairly rapid capacity to make decisions once the issues have been set forth and the alternatives identified.

This type of decision making is exemplified by the studies made by special task forces of the New York City agency in the 1970s on malpractice insurance and domiciliary care facilities. These task forces were composed primarily of providers who were both peers and colleagues who had known each other over the years. In a fairly short period of time, studies of the issues were made, decisions determined as to a policy and course of action to take, and the task forces mobilized both board and public bodies to support their stand in their effort to implement their recommendations. Once the issues were resolved, one way or another, the task forces disbanded.

Individual Action Model

Unlike those in the previous models, the participants in the individual action model are private issue-oriented; there is no consideration of the impact of a decision on the entire health system but rather on a segment of the system. The degree of participation of the consumer is higher than that of either the provider or the government official. Again, this is due to the nature of participative planning. This planning is concerned with project type planning that affects a small segment of the overall system. The consumers have community-based interests; they act as community educators, specific problem solvers, initiators, and advocates of a specific policy. The arrival at such a policy is usually in reaction to a health crisis or policy maker's decision. The influence of the consumer on decision making is very high, as is that of the staff who act as the technical advisors of the consumer. The provider and government representatives have little impact on decision making in this model because the consumer has made the policy decision. The board's consumer representatives are a small cohesive group, and decisions are reached rapidly.

A case in point is the consumer reaction to the New York-Pennsylvania Council's decision to close Ideal Hospital. The rallying of community members, educating the residents to the need for a hospital, brought enough pressure upon the council that the board determined not to support its task force's proposals and returned the issue for further study.

SUMMARY

What then can be expected from the actors involved in the health planning process? It would appear from current literature and recent studies that the old relationship vis à vis the "expert and the layman" persists. Can the desired outputs from consumer participation indeed be achieved? Can the relationship between board and staff foster improved program planning, better communication between consumers and providers, educate the consumer to more knowledgeable sophisticated use of services, provide for those most in need, foster professional accountability, broaden community support for programs and service, and supply the mechanism for grievance input?

According to Blum,

> Experience indicates that nearly all parties get upset, that nearly all can grow in the sense of learning what makes others tick. New ways of working together, comprehension of the basics of health care and of health promotion, ability to define what is mutually wanted and how to set about obtaining what has been defined as wanted.[60]

Concurring with Blum are the conclusions of the OSTI report which declare that, in reality, health staff and board can function together in designing policies. According to OSTI, the differences between the consumers and providers are more imagined than real, and few aspects of health care delivery are adequately understood by either group.[61] Review and comment may have been a distraction from the original intent of comprehensive planning, but it may also have served the useful function of an educating device and a catalyst around which agency consolidation could take place.

There are still the problems of board attendance, provider elitism and dominance, lack of consumer interest, lack of motivation, as well as staff attitudes that may endanger the participatory process. Yet, experience seems to be pointing toward the direction of meaningful dialogue. If not a dynamic, measurable change, the experience seems to indicate a subtle change in once rigidly held perceptions. Although it is difficult to substantiate, there is some feeling that consumers are more sophisticated and that providers are increasingly impressed with consumer knowledge, insight, and use of data.

NOTES

1. Sidney Verba, "Democratic Participation," *Annals of the American Academy of Political Science* 373 (September 1967): 55.
2. Gerald Landsberg, *Community Participation in Community Mental Health Center Policy and Decision Making,* Program Analysis and Evaluation Section, Maimonides Medical Center, January 1975, p. 2.
3. *Ibid.*
4. Verba, "Democratic Participation," p. 59.

5. William Bolman, "Community Control of the Community Mental Health Center," *American Journal of Psychiatry*, August 1972, p. 175.

6. Edmund M. Burke, *A Participatory Approach to Urban Planning* (New York: Human Sciences Press, 1979), pp. 31–32.

7. T. R. Marmor and J. Morone, "HSAs and the Representation of Consumer Interests: Conceptual Issues and Litigation Problems," mimeographed (Hyattsville, Md.: Health Resources Administration, February 10, 1978), p. 2.

8. *Ibid.*

9. *Ibid.;* see also Paul Peterson and David Greenstone, "Racial Change and Citizen Participation: The Mobilization of Low-Income Communities Through Community Action" in *A Decade of Federal Anti-Poverty Programs*, ed. Robert Haveman (New York: Academic Press, 1977). Their formulation is very similar to that of Marmor and Morone.

10. Marmor and Morone, "HSAs and Consumer Interests," p. 11.

11. Consumer Commission on the Accreditation of Health Services, "Some New Thoughts on the Issue of Consumer Representation," *Consumer Health Perspectives* VII, no. 6 (December 1980): 2.

12. Basil J. Mott, "The Myth of Planning without Politics," *American Journal of Public Health* 59, no. 5 (May 1969): 799.

13. Terry E. Shannon, *Interim Report on Consumer Participation* (Hyattsville, Md.: Health Resources Administration, April 1980), Appendix I, p. 2.

14. Marmor and Morone, "HSAs and Consumer Interests," p. 15.

15. Shannon, *Consumer Participation*, Appendix I, p. 18.

16. *Ibid.*, p. 2.

17. Burke, *A Participatory Approach*, p. 274.

18. Health Resources Administration, *An Evaluation of the Operation of Subarea Advisory Councils*, Health Planning Information Series #15 (Hyattsville, Md.: U.S. DHHS, August 1979), pp. 112–148.

19. *Ibid.*, p. 140.

20. *Ibid.*, p. 141.

21. *Ibid.*, pp. 210–212.

22. Consumer Commission, "Issue of Consumer Representation." This is a summarized, condensed version of the much longer scenario that appears in this edition of the Health Perspectives.

23. Joseph L. Roche, "Plan Implementation: A Community Organization Approach to Health Planning," mimeographed. Paper presented at annual meeting of American Health Planning Association in Boston, Mass. (W. Springfield, Mass.: Western Massachusetts Health Planning Council, Inc., June 1, 1979), p. 15.

24. Burke, *A Participatory Approach*, p. 79.

25. *Ibid.*, p. 80.

26. Clayton Medeiros, "Planning and Public Accountability," in *Health Regulation*, ed. Herbert H. Hyman (Germantown, Md.: Aspen Systems Corporation, 1977).

27. *Ibid.*, p. 143.

28. Elmer Staats, *Report of the General Accounting Office*, Report on irregularities in the operation of the Los Angeles Health Systems Agency (Washington, D.C.: Comptroller General of the United States, February 24, 1978).

29. John Carlova, "How a $7 Million HSA Flagship Sank Itself," *Medical Economics*, May 14, 1979, pp. 79–86.

30. Robert A. Dorwart, William R. Meyers, and Edward C. Norman, *Effective Citizen Participation in Mental Health: Comparative Case Studies*, Public Health Reports, 94, no. 3 (May-June, 1979): 268–274.

31. Shannon, *Consumer Participation*, p. 4.

32. Barry Checkoway, "Citizens on Local Health Planning Boards: What are the Obstacles?" *Journal of the Community Development Society* 10, no. 2 (Fall 1979): 101–116.

33. Consumer Commission on the Accreditation of Health Services, "The Development of a Consumer Health Network," *Consumer Health Perspectives* IV, nos. 4 and 5 (July-Oct. 1977): 5.

34. Allan B. Steckler and William T. Herzog, "How to Keep Your Mandated Citizen Board Out of Your Hair and Off Your Back: A Guide for Executive Directors," *American Journal of Public Health* 69, no. 8 (August 1979): 811.

35. Checkoway, "Local Health Planning Boards," p. 105.

36. Consumer Commission, "Consumer Health Network."

37. Terry L. Cooper, "The Hidden Price Tag: Participation Costs and Health Planning," *American Journal of Public Health* 69, no. 4 (April 1979): 370.

38. Shannon, *Consumer Participation*, p. 4.

39. Philip C. Chinn, "The Struggle for Consumer Control," mimeographed. Paper presented at Conference on Consumer Participation, West Springfield, Mass., Spring, 1980, p. 13.

40. *Ibid.*, pp. 12–13.

41. John Forester, "Toward Democratic Health Planning: Political Power, Agenda Setting, and Planning Practice," mimeographed (Ithaca, N.Y.: Cornell University, April 1980).

42. Gregory Muraskiewicz, "Report on the Functioning and Membership of the Committees of the Health Systems Agency of New York City," mimeographed (New York City: Community Action for Legal Services, Inc., April 23, 1980).

43. Consumer Commission, "Consumer Health Network," p. 5.

44. Randolph M. Grossman, "Voting Behavior of HSA Interest Groups: A Case Study," *American Journal of Public Health* 68, no. 12 (December 1978): 1191–1194.

45. Consumer Commission, "Consumer Health Network."

46. Verba, "Democratic Participation," p. 73.

47. *Ibid.*, p. 75.

48. Henrick Blum, *Health Planning* (New York: Human Sciences Press, 1974), p. 468.

49. OSTI, "Organization for Social and Technical Innovations," *Final Report on Contract HSM 110-71-44*, April 1972, p. 19.

50. Consumer Commission on the Accreditation of Health Services, "Health Consumers at the Crossroads: Which Way to Go?" *Consumer Health Perspectives* 6, no. 8 (February 1980): 6–8.

51. *Ibid.*

52. *Ibid.*

53. Shannon, *Consumer Participation*, p. 18.

54. Grossman, "Voting Behavior."

55. Codman Research Group, Inc., *An Integrated Approach to Evaluating the Impact of Health Planning in New England: Executive Summary*, Contract No. 291-76-003 (Hyattsville, Md.: Health Resources Administration, June 1980), p. 4.

56. Samuel J. Bosch, Rolando Merino, and Ruth Zambrana, *Training of a Community Board to Increase the Effectiveness of a Health Center,* Public Health Reports, 94, no. 3 (May-June 1979): 275–280.

57. *Ibid.,* p. 279.

58. Consumer Commission, "Consumers at the Crossroads," p. 5.

59. Shannon, *Consumer Participation,* pp. 15–16.

60. Blum, *Health Planning,* p. 455.

61. OSTI Report, "Organization for Innovations," p. 85.

Chapter 11

Training for Comprehensive Health Planning

One of the major issues that surfaced through a review of the literature with respect to citizen participation was the need for their training, especially for consumers, in the concept, functions, and planning of comprehensive health planning to ensure board effectiveness. One of the first attempts to provide such training and prepare consumers for participation on the health planning boards occurred in 1968 and 1969 when the Department of Health, Education, and Welfare (HEW) awarded some 25 grants to various institutions around the United States to perform this training. In this definitive evaluation of six of these training programs for "disadvantaged minority" residents, Cooper found that, in fact, none of the almost 300 consumers he investigated found their way onto any of the agency boards in their regions. Since this was the manifest reason for funding these training programs, he concluded that these six programs were failures.[1] The major reason he gave was that the training institutions had no coordination or relationship with the planning agencies in their regions in order to alert them to their training activities. The consumers, therefore, were being trained in a vacuum; this was the beginning effort, however, and the Bureau of Health Planning has learned something from this early experience.

PROFESSIONAL HEALTH PLANNING STAFF

Basic Requirements of the Health Planner

Under contract with the Educational Testing Service, the Bureau of Health Planning developed some fairly specific guidelines on the competencies required by executive directors, directors of planning, entry level planners, and other basic positions on the staff of a health planning

425

agency.[2] These qualities are divided into three components: (1) knowledge of a specific area, (2) skills and abilities, and (3) personal characteristics. To illustrate these characteristics, the competencies needed by an entry level health planner are cited.[3]

Under knowledge areas, the entry level planner should have at least the following:

- general knowledge of current laws and regulations related to health planning
- a broad understanding of the health care system, how the components are related to each other, and how they meet needs
- knowledge of planning theory and methods, as well as the health status of the population and its subsectors
- the capacity to describe how the public health system functions
- an understanding of the impact of economic costs and trends on the consumer and the health care system
- an ability to do research needed to carry out planning functions
- an ability to work with groups to develop plans

These competencies provide the entry planner with the basic, general knowledge needed to plan, work with community leaders, and operate within the parameters of the law and its regulations. This general knowledge provides the foundation on which the planner can build by applying this knowledge to specific problems and issues. It is a knowledge base that can be used in a variety of health planning settings, such as private industry, consulting firms, hospital planning, or government planning.

Under skills and abilities, the planner should be able to do at least the following:

- speak clearly and concisely to a variety of groups, using language in an appropriate way
- write in a logical and coherent manner with a vocabulary that is acceptable to the audience
- work well with others both in the agency and outside it
- search for, organize, and interpret a wide array of data consistent with the task at hand

These are basic skills needed for all health planning positions, whether an entry level planner or the executive director of an agency. None is unique to the health planning field. Yet, planners must develop them to a high level in order to function in a competent manner.

In addition to the general knowledge base and communication skills needed by the entry level planner, certain personal characteristics are essential:

- positive thinking and attitudes, loyalty to the agency, and a commitment and motivation to do a good job
- an ability to adapt to changing work assignments and positions in the agency
- an ability to work under pressure and take the initiative
- maturity, as shown by patience, tolerance, and tact

Because planning is a very intense profession, planners must show a coolness under pressure and must be able to work both as team members and as individuals to accomplish the many tasks of a planning agency. Through experience, planners are expected to grow—to learn more, to develop a more sophisticated capacity to use their skills, and to mature in their personality traits so that they can cope with a wider range of difficult activities while working under more trying conditions (Exhibit 11-1).

Composition of Health Planning Agency Staff

An Orkand study of 189 regional planning agencies in 1976 revealed a number of characteristics about the size, racial composition, experience, and functions of planning agency staff.[4] It indicated that the average agency comprised 7.4 professional and 3.8 support staff. They varied by region, however, with Region VIII averaging 4 and Region II, 13 professionals. Compared to the staff size of previous health planning agencies, current staffs are about 50 percent larger. Much of this is due to the funding guaranteed by HEW (now HHS) to ensure that no agency has fewer than the five basic professionals needed to carry out its planning functions.

Almost 50 percent of the staff had been employed by the predecessor planning agency. It is only logical that people with previous experience in health planning should be hired by a new health planning agency. The other staff members had come from a wide variety of previous positions, including work with the Regional Medical Program (RMP), Hill-Burton, hospitals, regional planning bodies, local governments, and universities. An examination of Table 11-1, which indicates the past experiences of professional staff in the 13 agencies in Region II (New York, New Jersey, Puerto Rico, and the Virgin Islands) as of 1980, shows that most staff have

Exhibit 11-1   Skills, Knowledge, and Personal Characteristics
Required by an Advanced Health Planner

Knowledge areas

Understanding of current legislation and government programs in the health field and relationship to agency programs and functioning; understanding of priorities of divergent interest groups within agency's constituency; in-depth understanding of the legislative process and how and when to become involved

Specific and in-depth knowledge of resources and services that impact on health, including prevention medicine, institutional planning and services, environmental services, health education, innovative delivery mechanisms, technologies, health care personnel patterns, and health care personnel training and standards

Knowledge of planning theory and alternative planning techniques and their application, including forecasting, systems analysis, simulation, information analysis; thorough understanding of the appropriate functions and skills required of staff, board, and other agencies in relation to the technical steps of health planning and implementation

Detailed knowledge of the organization and functions of the public health system, epidemiology, and vital statistics

Familiarity with health economics and finance, such as cost-effectiveness/cost-benefit analysis, projection of demand, health care costs, health care insurance, health institution financing, reimbursement

General knowledge of data collection, analysis, and management techniques as input for health plan development; familiarity with sources of data

Knowledge and understanding of theory and application of group dynamics, e.g., how to structure groups, conduct group sessions, and evaluate outcomes

Skills and Abilities

Ability to speak clearly, concisely, accurately, and persuasively in communicating orally with a wide range of audiences

Ability to write clearly and concisely, and to adapt vocabulary, style, and usage to purpose. Ability to make technical subject matter understandable to nontechnical audiences; to edit and review drafts of others

Ability to work effectively with other people to obtain cooperation and involvement, clarify issues, and influence outcomes. Tactfulness, patience, discretion

Ability to assume and maintain a leadership role in a group and to influence, convince, direct, and persuade others in order to accomplish an objective

Ability to process and organize a broad variety of information and data to extract relevant concepts and elements for the health planning process

Ability to plan and organize work, systematically schedule and allocate time and resources (both budget and personnel), set priorities, and provide for coordination of flow of work and activities

Ability to convert plans and decisions into action or implementation; e.g., activate work programs, involve and invoke support, develop strategies, and take advocacy action

Ability to be practical and objective in the analysis of problems and even-handed in dealing with situations and people

Ability to understand and work with the political process—lines of communication, control, authority, power

Ability to mobilize, organize, and involve community elements in the health planning and implementation process

Personal Characteristics

Positive attitude toward work and career, willingness to serve, dedication and interest

Mature; tolerant of imperfections in things, people, and situational annoyances; can withstand frustration

Adaptable and flexible; receptive to new ideas, different cultures, innovative approaches

Self-confident in abilities and skills; attracts and holds attention and confidence of others

Stable; can work under pressure, think on feet, respond rationally under stressful conditions

Self-starter; can identify what needs to be done and proceed on own schedule

Table 11-1   Size of Agency by Past Health Experience of
Professional Staff, Region II

| | Size of Agency by Budget- | | | | | |
| | Under $1.05 Million (7 Agencies) | | Over $1.05 Million (6 Agencies) | | Total | |
Type of Experience	No. Staff	Average/ Agency	No. Staff	Average/ Agency	No.	Average
Planning	37	5.3	68	11.3	105	8.1
Health/hospital	37	5.3	46	7.7	83	6.4
Research	17	2.4	17	2.8	34	2.6
Business/tech/fin	12	1.7	18	3.0	30	2.3
Human services	14	2.0	16	2.7	30	2.3
Data	8	1.2	14	2.3	22	1.7
Commty organization	4	.6	16	2.7	20	1.5
Education	10	1.4	10	1.3	20	1.5
Other*						

*Other includes pharmacy, law, architecture, library work, art, nutrition.

Source: Original Survey of DHHS Region II HSA Work Programs.

had previous planning and/or hospital experience. Research, business, technical, finance, and human services are also well represented. Since a health planning agency is required to carry out several different types of functions, e.g., administration of the agency, data gathering and analysis, planning, project review, and implementation, it is not surprising to find staff with expertise in a number of different disciplines.

Respecting the four basic functions required of agency staff, national statistics reveal that, in the past, 27 percent were involved in administration, 29 percent in planning, 13 percent in data gathering and analysis, and 14 percent in project review and implementation.[5] The rest were involved in other activities, such as library work, community organization, and special studies. An examination of Table 11-2 reveals a different pattern of staff distribution in Region II in 1980. It shows a lower percentage of professional staff involved in all the functions except planning, where 41 percent of the staff worked. It also shows a much larger "other" category, which is due to the greater diversity of professional functions taken on by the larger agencies. The typical agency in Region II has a higher budget than does any other region in the United States.

Minority professional staff on health planning agencies in the United States made up about 9 percent of the total staff. However, over 50 percent of the agencies had a proportion of minority staff lower than that in the population of their health service area.[6] Women made up 29 percent of the professional staff, with 77 percent of the agencies below parity with the

Table 11-2   Size of Agency by Work Assignments of Professional Staff in Region II Agencies in 1980

| Work Assignment | Size of Agency by Budget | | | | | Total | |
| | Under $1.05 Million (7 Agencies) | | Over $1.05 Million (6 Agencies) | | | | |
	No. Staff	No./ Agency	No. Staff	No./ Staff	%	No.	No./ Staff
Administration	20	2.9	23	3.8	14	43	3.3
Professional	116	16.6	146	24.3	86	262	19.3
Data	8	1.1	9	1.5	6	17	1.3
Planning	55	8.0	71	2.0	41	126	9.7
Resource develop- ment	14	2.0	17	3.0	10	31	2.4
Other*	39	5.6	49	8.1	29	88	6.8

*Other includes functions involving finances, coordination, education, library, evaluation, public relations, program specialist.

Source: Original survey of 13 HSA Work Program Applications for 1980 in Region II.

percentage of women in the general population. The median age of all agency professional staff was 30 to 34 years at the time of the survey in 1976. This indicates that many staff members were recent graduates of professional graduate schools.

The national study indicates that, as of 1976, almost 60 percent of staff had more than a baccalaureate degree, 26 percent a baccalaureate, and 2 percent less than that.[7] This would indicate that the staff is highly professionalized. In Region II, 37 people held master's degrees in hospital administration, with another 25 holding master's degrees in public health (Table 11-3). Another 24 staff had earned graduate degrees in social sciences, 23 in health planning, and 22 in urban planning. In addition, other staff members held graduate degrees in public and business administration, economics, social work, education, law, and health education. It can be seen from this diversity of professional education that a variety of specialties were represented on Region II planning agencies. This range of educational backgrounds is highly appropriate for complex series of activities required of health planning agencies. It is also an indication that many staff were involved in activities for which they had neither the education nor previous work experience. For example, the health planning agencies in Region II used 126 health planners (see Table 11-2). Yet, only 105 staff indicated they had previous planning experience and only 45 staff had any graduate education in planning. From these statistics, it would seem that

Table 11-3   Size of Agency by Professional Staff Education in
Region II Agencies, 1980

| | Size of Agency by Budget | | | | | |
| | Under $1.05 Million (7 Agencies) | | Over $1.05 Million (6 Agencies) | | Total | |
Type of Education	No. Staff	No./ Agency	No. Staff	No./ Agency	No.	No./ Agency
Health planning	5	0.7	18	3.0	23	1.7
Urban planning	9	1.3	13	2.3	22	1.7
Hospital administration	11	1.6	26	4.3	37	2.8
Public health	12	1.7	13	2.3	25	1.9
Social sciences	12	1.7	12	2.0	24	1.8
Public administration	11	1.6	9	1.5	20	1.5
Business administration	12	1.7	5	0.8	17	1.3

Others include economics (9), social work (14), education (7), nursing (1), rehabilitation (3), health education (5), law (3), community organization (3), baccalaureate (29), associate degrees (6).

Source: Original survey of 13 HSA Work Program Applications for 1980 in Region II.

81 professional staff were engaged in planning without having a previous planning degree and almost 60 of these gained their experience on the job. To the extent that staff members had graduate degrees that touched on planning in some capacity, such as those in public health, business or public administration, or architecture, the agency benefited from this diversity of skills and experiences. While no conclusion can be drawn about the competency of the staff to carry out their functions from a description of their education, questions can be raised whether a person is able to obtain even the basic professional requirements without the requisite educational degree.

Before turning to a discussion of citizen and staff training, it may be of interest to review the comments of a leading health profession educator, writing in 1972, concerning the preparation of health planners.[8] Citing the findings of the Tulsa Conference on Education Priorities in Comprehensive Health Planning, 1970, Brown notes the stress on "training generalists, not specialists or technicians, for planning," putting "process competence" above "content competence" that calls for emphasis on "interpersonal-political dimensions" in carrying out the health planning and health services administration, producing "health service generalists," and he mentions his own university's program graduate, who is "as comfortable in a planning agency as . . . in a hospital." A further benefit, Brown notes, is that planners and administrators will better understand each other if they evolved from similar roots, producing more effective planning and delivery in the future. Sketchily outlined curriculum elements place heavy emphasis on the social forces: needs, goals, change, and social planning.

Brown advocates the distinction of health planning from the "more traditional forms of planning," calling the latter "dominated by technocratic approaches and . . . more or less sterile of political and human concerns." Health planning, Brown states, "has been the product of its own experience; it has grown essentially on its own. Lacking the necessary legitimacy and power, it has depended on persuasion, planning process in individual institutions and agencies, and participation of a number of key community individuals and groups."[9] Preferring to maintain the distinctive flavor and commitment of health planning, Brown will accept "collaboration" from the functional areas, but urges the profession to retain the uniqueness of the health planning process, acquired through ten years of experience.

In summary, the staffs of the current health planning agencies have experience in a wider diversity of disciplines and a more relevant and higher level of education than did those of their predecessors. This has been made possible by federal financing of planning agencies at a level that makes it possible for even the smallest agency to carry out basic agency functions; by PL 93-641, which specifies the type of expertise required to operate the agencies; and by the increased professionalization of the health planning field.

ORIENTATION AND TRAINING OF AGENCY BOARD AND STAFF

Citizens must be provided with the skills and information needed to carry out their roles as community health decision makers. Education of health consumers, in particular, is intended to overcome the disparity in knowledge that hampers their effective participation. The 1979 amendments have given this responsibility to a senior staff member of the health planning agency. According to the amendments, the staff will provide "such information and technical assistance as they [citizens] may require to effectively perform their functions." While the amendments apply to both consumer and provider members of the governing body, they particularly single out the special needs of the consumers.

Three major methods have been used to educate and orient citizen boards and incoming staff members to their responsibilities and functions. These are education seminars offered by the technical health planning centers, by the health planning agency itself, and by outside consultants under contract with the federal government and/or the planning agency.

Education Models

Steckler, Phillips, and Burdine point to two basic models for organizing health planning boards: the conflict/negotiation and the concordance/agreement decision-making models.[10] Using different terminology, Bradley refers to these models as constructive conflict and consensus planning models.[11] The conflict model assumes

> that there are at least two competing, opposing hostile camps, each one struggling to shape the health care system into its concept of what it should be like, and both fighting the other by a variety of means, from education and persuasion to confrontation and political struggle.[12]

This model accepts that social change, in this instance change in the health care system, comes about mainly through conflict. Those in control of the system are reluctant to give up that control to those who advocate different concepts of how and what services should be rendered. Consequently, the clashing concepts and forces that are ever-present in the larger society are simply carried over into the halls of the health planning agency by members with these opposing views. The competition for power among these members is reflected in every facet of the roles and responsibilities of board members (planning, implementing, and advocating public positions on basic health issues). The board members typically reflect the concepts of the constituencies to whom they are accountable. On health planning bodies, providers generally have the power and influence and seek to maintain and reenforce it through decisions that are favorable to their concepts of medical care. The forces of change are more likely to be represented by consumer advocates who find problems with the current system and seek to rectify its deficiencies. These differences are generally observed in health planning between those who favor disease-oriented treatment facilities and those who favor preventive, education type of services. Still others find the problem in the fabric of the sociopolitico-economic structure of society, which favors a small elite over the masses of the general public.

In the concordance/agreement or consensus model, board members assume that providers and consumers all share the same goals and concept of what constitutes effective health services. Generally, differences are over means and allocation of resources among health providers, and these are generally ironed out in committees or private, informal meetings. Only consensus decisions are made public. As Bradley notes,

. . . only issues which are likely to result in widespread agreement tend to be raised. Consensus may be assured through many possible organizational strategies—coopting powerful leaders from the community, stacking committees or councils with people having known attitudes about health planning, negative selection of ideas, issues, and people, and isolation and fragmentation of representatives of groups whose interests may conflict with the status quo.[13]

An example of this was noted when the board of a large urban planning agency refused to reappoint a half dozen consumer board members who advocated views that conflicted with those held by the majority of providers and consumers.[14]

These nearly opposite models are almost never found in pure form in a health planning agency. A health planning agency is likely to be oriented toward one concept of health care over another, but there is usually a mixture of the two types of decision making. PL 93-641 is predicated on the concordance/consensus model, with its acceptance of the medical model of health services. While it gives some minor emphasis to prevention and health education, its major thrust is on preserving the status quo and improving the efficiency of the medical system. If the law produces any type of conflict, it is between the government's concern with reducing medical costs and the health providers' emphasis on improving quality of care (which generally translates into high medical costs). The law is based on the assumption that both consumers and providers would endorse the existing model of medical care.

These models of decision making have a marked effect on the type of education consumers desire. Those who favor the conflict model want to learn how to obtain power and influence, how the medical economy operates, and how to develop leadership and interactional skills. Those favoring the consensus model are more concerned with developing technical skills for setting goals and priorities, sharing information, and learning positive public relations skills. For one, the outcome is on changing the current status quo; for the other, it is improving and maintaining the current medical system.

Types of Consumer Education

Burke has identified eight basic skills that volunteer participants will find necessary in health planning. These are divided into technical or cognition skills and interactional skills.[15]

Technical Skills	Interactional Skills
General intelligence	Social-professional contacts
Factual knowledge of issue	Experience
Background knowledge	Popularity
Written communication skill	Verbal communication skill

Technical skills are needed to carry out a rational planning process that involves interpreting a great deal of data, understanding a wide variety of issues, setting priorities for a plan, and then implementing the plan's goals and objectives. These skills mainly involve the intellect and the capacity to think logically. Interactional skills involve mainly dealing with other persons and learning to influence them while appreciating and being sensitive to their points of view. Interactional techniques are also concerned with leadership skills, ability to negotiate, and use of political and social influence to advance a particular position.

Technical Model

Two models of citizen education illustrate how this technical model operates. In one example, educators helped the members of a community action group to improve their technical skills of planning and monitoring their health services program. In the other, a rational planning model was utilized to teach consumers, providers, and staff of health planning agencies to work together in resolving problems. In both cases, the consensus/ concordance model of decision making was involved.

In the first case, the Mt. Sinai (New York City) Department of Medicine was engaged to assist the East Harlem Tenants Council (a community action program financed with federal antipoverty funds) in the planning, development, and monitoring of its health center. The educators and council's governing body agreed on the following objectives over a 12-month period:

Read monthly statistical reports critically (reports containing data on the effectiveness and efficiency of the health center).

Recognize utilization and productivity trends.

Use data reports to decide among alternative technical recommendations made by the center's staff.

Critically analyze expenditures in relation to the health needs of the community and the health center's objectives and sources of income.[16]

These objectives require members of the council governing body to develop the technical skills to plan, monitor, and evaluate the operations of the health center. The board was fearful the center staff would take control because of its greater technical expertise and thereby reduce the board's role to rubber-stamping the center's recommendations. At the conclusion of the yearlong meetings, improvements in the board's capacity to understand and take initiative in setting goals, priorities, and policies for its health center were definitely noted:

1. "There was a major gain in knowledge . . . related to measures of utilization, effectiveness, and productivity."
2. "All board members definitely increased their level of participation in the group discussions." While all participated to some extent, four members of the board's executive committee were the most active participants.
3. "Substantial learning occurred in the use of appropriate terminology and in the handling of concepts related to the operation of the center."
4. "The most outstanding changes were observed in the board members' ability to extrapolate data from the management information system and request additional specific information. . . ."[17]

This is an excellent example of how the shared values of the members of the board made it possible to focus on technical skills. Through the use of an external skills-building consultant, the board was able to narrow the disparity between the knowledge of its professional health center staff and its own. This is exactly the aim of the 1979 amendments. As Shannon, in his report to the National Council on Health Planning and Development, stated,

> . . . one way to overcome the disparity in knowledge between consumers and providers and to enhance the participation of consumers . . . is to provide separate staff support to consumers.

> The focus of the staff support function should be on providing information to governing body members that they can use in decision-making.

> Training can be most effective when it concerns specific health care issues that impact on a community, as opposed to systems and process issues whose effect on the consumers' ability to obtain needed care is not always clear.[18]

If these statements are used as criteria, the Mt. Sinai educational project was quite successful. It overcame the disparity of knowledge, focused on information the board could use, and concentrated on a highly specific issue with which the board was concerned.

In the second case, Columbia University's School of Public Health Continuing Education Program was contracted by HEW to assist the newly emerging health planning agencies under PL 93-641 to develop a "system for ongoing agency education."[19] Their model for action planning has the following objectives:

1. to develop teams of staff and board members with skills in planning for change;
2. to institutionalize an agency mechanism for continuing education;
3. to build an agency system for on-going problem identification and resolution;
4. to create opportunities for broader community involvement in . . . plan development and regulation.[20]

The model is divided into orientation and action planning modules. The orientation module includes four elements:

1. assessing educational needs of the board
2. identifying trends affecting the U.S. health care system
3. providing background for health planning
4. developing board and staff collaboration.

It can be seen from this outline that the first and fourth elements deal with board/staff involvement and assume a consensus can be reached in setting objectives. The second and third impart technical knowledge and information relating to health planning and the health care system.

In the action planning module, an attempt is made to solve an actual agency or planning problem. This requires the building of a team, composed of consumers, providers, and staff, and entails an examination of their roles and relationships. The education consultants facilitate the development of, and provide assistance to, the team in identifying and working on a specific current problem; there is real engagement in and motivation for solving the problem. This action module is divided into three phases. Three full days are set aside for team building and problem identification. This is followed by six to eight weeks of effort to resolve the problem and a two-day feedback session. The objective of the action phase is team building, which results in ongoing collaboration for change at the conclusion of the demonstration. The consultants make it quite clear that the primary emphasis of the education project is to assist people in learning to work well together rather than to teach them the technical skills of planning.

Of the 15 health planning agencies in the region, eight completed the orientation module; four of these, along with three others, completed the action module. The seven completing the action module developed plans that mapped out how they would continue as a group. There is no follow-up report to determine whether this method of team building had a permanent effect or whether the teams incorporated nonattending board and staff.

Interactional Model

It should first be noted that the Columbia education model is a collaborative model of board education; it assumes that consumers and providers accept each other's values and can work together. The interactional model assumes value differences between consumers and providers; it focuses on developing those skills and techniques whereby consumers can, instead of accepting provider leadership and direction, take the initiative and exert their own influence in support of their concepts in board deliberations. The consumers' values and concepts may be similar to those of the providers, or they may be different. The point is that consumers, in their effort to achieve parity with providers, require education to enable them to achieve that equality. Thus, the interactional model refers to consumer education apart from that of the providers.

In a provocative paper, Bradley discusses his assumptions regarding the negative attitudes and feelings that must be overcome through health education. He believes that people must take charge of their own health and must change dangerous health environments in the workplace, negative aspects of the health care system, and their own passive acceptance of physician treatment.[21] Powerlessness and helplessness are "pervasive attitudes that affect everyone to some extent" and are "major obstacles to the development of health education."[22] He believes this powerlessness stems from childhood in which "young people are . . . put down, corrected, told they are unintelligent and incapable, given misinformation, discouraged from learning and assuming responsibility."[23] In time, many of these feelings are internalized, leading to attitudes of self-invalidation, limited expectations, powerlessness, isolation, fearfulness, and defensiveness. In turn, the person or group with such internalized feelings and attitudes develops distrust, a sense of isolation, and intergroup rivalry, factors that often make it very difficult for consumers, even those with similar goals and values, to act together.

One model to assist these individuals and groups in overcoming their sense of powerlessness has been developed by the New Jersey Department of the Public Advocate. Called the *Advocacy Project for Effective Health Planning*,[24] The project aims to develop a series of advocacy services:

- litigation
- public education through the media
- training of patient advocates
- systems monitoring
- monitoring health planning processes
- administrative and legislative lobbying
- mediation
- consumer organization strategies and skills development
- legislative research and representation

Two basic assumptions of the project are that (1) consumers should have a greater influence on health care services and (2) consumers should be able in time to gain control of health planning boards to redirect resources toward primary and preventive care. Its main goal "is to reduce and/or compensate for those structural barriers which are impediments to effective consumer involvement in the health care delivery and planning process."[25] The project is divided into three major components: (1) informational, educational, and research; (2) support; and (3) advocacy skills development.

In the informational component, the aim is to overcome the information disparity between consumers and providers by providing consumers with an independent source of research and technical assistance on a variety of planning and regulatory issues. Gaps in information will be identified and filled; a clearinghouse for information of all types will be established; statewide workshops will be held to discuss consumer roles in health care institutions and planning agencies and the constraints that prevent their being more active; and, finally, consumer activity in health planning will be monitored. Built into the Consumer Commission's concept of a national consumer network is the development of an information source vital to consumer decision making.[26] Other authorities on consumer participation in health planning have cited the need for an independent, autonomous consumer information source. Bradley, likewise, questions whether a consumer-oriented information resource could be developed through health planning agencies as suggested by the 1979 amendments because of the internal bias of health planners and the influence of the conservative agency philosophy on the health planner.[27]

The support component would supply services such as assistance in initiating litigation, requesting mediation, giving legislative testimony, drafting legislation and administrative regulations, monitoring the health planning and regulatory process, and coordinating with state agencies. This support service would thus back up consumer interests by carrying out activities that individual consumers on health planning agencies could not do for themselves. As such, the model calls for an advocate consumer agency that not only educates consumers and supplies them with information, but also takes an active role itself to ensure consumer concerns are not overlooked.

In the advocacy skill-building component, the model aims to assist consumers in overcoming their sense of powerlessness by teaching them skills to facilitate more active and effective participation in board activities. Through workshops jointly designed by the consultants and consumers, the following skills will be developed:

- problem solving and analytical techniques
- intervention strategies
- interactional skills
- policy analysis and regulatory review
- coalition building
- resource identification and mobilization
- patient advocacy

These are the types of skills that Forester believes are needed to overcome the structural and administrative disparities between consumers and providers. He emphasizes organizational skills in working with groups, developing leadership abilities, managing conflict, mobilizing support for special health issues, and building coalitions and alliances.[28] Development of such skills will also help counteract any effort by the planning agency to limit the active involvement of consumers in order to keep control of the agency's activities in the director's hands. Thus, this advocacy model is consistent with the recommendations of leading health consumer groups and authorities.

Formal Board Education Course

Under contract with the Health Resources Administration, the Educational Testing Service developed *A Course for Health Systems Agency Boards*.[29] This course was several years in the making and was tested on health planning agency board members before it was published as an official manual for use by planning agency personnel or consultants involved in educating health planning boards. It is a comprehensive course, requiring about 34 hours to complete, almost equivalent in length to a three-credit college level course. Basically, the course has four primary goals:

1. To help board members understand the nature, function, and process of the [health planning agency] and their responsibilities.
2. To help board members utilize the skills needed to function effectively on the board and to provide opportunities for board members to practice these skills to carry out board functions.
3. To help board members understand basic concepts of good board practice.
4. To help board members develop a self-directed program for continued growth of all members and indoctrination of new members.[30]

Each of these goals is then developed into discrete knowledge, skills, and activities modules needed to achieve them. Board members and staff should have at least the following knowledge:

- rationale for the enactment of the most recent health planning law
- mandates and functions of the planning agency
- milieu in which the agency operates
- structure, composition, and responsibilities of the agency
- functioning of the board

This knowledge provides board and staff with an in-depth understanding of the law and the operation of the agency as required by federal regulations.

The course focuses on the personal and technical skills required of staff and board members. Among those emphasized are the abilities to identify a problem; to determine the information needed to make decisions; to make decisions; to communicate with each other, agency staff, and outside agencies; and to use time efficiently. Given the heavy responsibilities thrust upon agencies, the efficient use of agency and board time becomes an especially meaningful skill. It should be noted the course spends considerable time on the systems method of planning. This is especially important because it helps to orient board members to the concept of linking goals, objectives, and services to each other and therefore viewing the health care system as an integrated whole rather than as a collection of isolated, discrete health components.

The third goal focuses on the board itself. In this module, the board as a human resource, its organization and structure, its relationship with staff and the executive director, and its everyday operation are highlighted.

Attention is given to such matters as bylaws, the openness of meetings called for in PL 93-641, assignment of board members to committees and positions of leadership, and frequency and purpose of meetings.

The final module is designed to encourage the board to go through a process of continuing self-education. Members are trained to use the course manual for orientation of new board members, although staff or consultants could lead such sessions.

It is important to note that the course can be broken into modules that can be taught separately or in any combination that is considered necessary for board/staff learning. Individual modules can be used as refresher courses. The flexibility and completeness of this citizen training course make it an especially valuable addition to the development of citizen/staff education modules. However, its focus on developing technical skills and collaborative, interactional techniques limits its use to planning agencies that stress the concordance model of decision making.

Other Board/Staff Training Methods

As noted earlier, there are two other means for educating staff and board. One is the informal, ad hoc method of using agency staff, sometimes with consultants, to orient new staff and board. In this case, staff would provide information and background on the subject under discussion, such as alternative methods of determining goal priorities or the conditions under which a computerized axial tomography (CAT) scanner would be needed by a health facility. Although these are only bits of knowledge and information, their accumulation over time adds greatly to each person's knowledge base and capacity to make informed decisions. Because it is used immediately in evaluating a situation and making a decision, the information is more likely to be remembered and used in future situations of a similar nature.

New board members have also gained information through slide show presentations on major health trends as well as on their own roles and responsibilities. In view of the fact that so many new board members and staff have little information about the health planning law and what it requires, such informal education sessions can give them a feeling of what is expected of them. While these sessions are formal presentations, they are considered ad hoc and informal because they are not part of the agency's planned work schedule. They take place as they are needed. Nonetheless, they are highly important and effective in educating board and staff.

A second method is the use of the health planning centers as an education and information resource. It was previously noted that these centers have been funded by the Department of Health and Human Services (HHS) to provide technical assistance and information to health planning agencies, including their boards. Until their mission was redirected in 1979, the centers provided numerous one- to three-day conferences on a vast range of subjects to assist agencies with the technical aspects of health planning, board governance, health regulations, and research findings. Courses quite similar to the Educational Testing Service course were developed on such topics as project review, legal aspects of agency operation, and methodologies for planning, as well as specific subjects such as mental health, disease prevention, and acute and primary care.

Because these sessions tended to be highly technical, they were often geared more for the professionals of the staff than for board members. The time required to attend the sessions and the frequency with which they were held—at least monthly in the first two years—was more time-consuming than most board members could afford from their own demanding schedules. Further, because the subject matter was not always germane to a specific agency's technical problems, their relevance for those attending varied widely. Center staff, however, tried to make up for this by providing individualized consultations to deal with specific agency issues and requests. Through the centers, the agencies tended to achieve a higher level of expertise and technical competence than would have occurred without them.

The real issue in all the education models for staff/board training is the relevance of the subject matter for both consumer and provider board members. A recent study on consumer/provider information needs sheds some light on this matter.[31] It showed that consumers and providers generally agreed on their major educational needs. They both felt a real difference between the need for information on "general concepts and background information" related to health planning and that for information on "special topics and current issues." There was a much higher level of interest in the special topics than in the general areas of interest. Among the special topics cited were

a. alternatives to institutionalization of the elderly and the mentally disabled
b. factors affecting the cost of health care
c. emergency medical services
d. physician extender personnel
e. primary health care centers and satellite clinics
f. factors influencing physician location
g. Professional Standards Review Organizations (PSROs)

Among the special topics, the major differences were that providers gave a higher priority to b, f, and g than did the consumers. Since they directly affect provider practice, this is not surprising. With respect to the general interest topics, both showed interest in

a. strategies of community health planning
b. measuring the health status of a community
c. defining and analyzing a health care system
d. a review of major health legislation
e. sources of data and other information
f. evaluative procedures for measuring the impact of health planning and health care services
g. guidelines in interpreting health statistics
h. history, structure, functions, and purposes of health planning
i. definitions of health planning terms and acronyms

Of these topics, there was agreement between consumers and providers on topics a, b, d, e, and g. Providers tended to favor c and f, while consumers were more interested in h and i.

These findings regarding the educational needs of one health planning agency board indicate more agreement between consumers and providers with respect to those needs than had been realized. Further, the fact that both tend to be more concerned with special interest topics than with general topics dealing with the method, process, and background of health planning shows that both want to be involved in substantive rather than process issues of planning. The differences appear to revolve around the providers' greater interest in more technical aspects of planning (evaluation and analysis of a health care system) and "bread and butter" issues that affect their practice (PSROs, cost structure, physician location), while consumers want to know more about the basic aspects of planning (history and the meaning of terms). Consumers are saying that they can be more fully involved if they have the same basic information as providers and planners. While this is only one study of board educational need, it reveals both the common and the separate needs of consumer and provider board members.

These various education models have basic differences in their philosophy and intended outcomes. Therefore, before a planning agency decides to undertake an educational effort it must determine which of the two decision-making models, concordance/consensus or conflict, best describes its board's milieu. This assessment indicates which type of education model would most benefit its board members. When values are shared, an education model that stresses technical and collaborative skills should be used. When consumers and providers are divided on a number of dimensions, an education model that stresses advocate interactional skills should be considered.

Staff Role

Staff members play an important role in board activities. Though the staff roles are somewhat dependent upon the relationship of the staff to the board, staff attitudes play a formidable role in board participation and effectiveness. Much of the board's behavior depends on the tone set by the staff and its concept of citizen participation.

If the staff has a genuine respect for citizen input, the participation process has the opportunity to grow and develop. If staff views the participation process as a nuisance and obstacle to staff-conceived plans and concepts, then a barrier is formed that has negative impact on the staff-board joint planning role. The staff, by its motivation, persistence, skill, and varying degrees of expertise, can undermine participation that at best involves a conglomeration of diverse backgrounds and interests.

Blum sees the staff and board as two power groups. The staff usually has the technology and skill, and the board has no one skill. According to Blum, it is a "futile gesture" to assume the two forces can be coequal. It is, after all, the staff that does the basic work.[32] Beck, too, says when referring to community boards that "it is important to note that when a community takes control of a service, the client and professionals are still not coequals because the bureaucratic structure remains . . . informal power still remains with the worker."[33] In other words, the staff can define the problem, determine the agenda, develop certain issues, and promote certain values.

In addition, the technical skills required by staff have not often been available except in larger cities.[34] Frequently, too, staff has had a specific health orientation, such as public health or health facilities, rather than the more useful, broader planning focus.[35] One of the biggest problems, according to the OSTI report has been the difficulty of attracting a qualified staff due to a shortage of trained personnel as well as a lack of funds to compensate them appropriately.[36]

If a staff lacks the technical skills, and if it is young and inexperienced, then another negative pattern may result. Instead of dominance and cooptation, a credibility gap ensues whereby the board has little faith in the leadership, expertise, or quality of the staff. This often occurs when the shift in expertise favors the board rather than the staff. It is, after all, not uncommon for board members not only to be skilled providers, but knowledgeable experienced consumers.

From the staff's perception, there are numerous board problems. One of the most undermining is lack of attendance.[37] Another problem involved in staff-board interactions is related to the training and educating of consumers and providers alike to their multiple responsibilities, including the relationship between planning and community needs, basic health information, and basic community information.

Most board members come with set attitudes regarding health status and health system needs. Providers have their special emphasis and interest. Consumers have their divergent views, whether sharing the values of the providers, antagonistic to the health system, or intimidated or awed by the health providers. Staff is faced with broadening the scope and outlook of the consumers and providers. Developing a rationale for planning takes time, and the obstacles are numerous, considering the poor attendance, lack of interest, board size, federal guideline difficulties, and staff credibility problems.

In a study of staff and board relations in New York City, Clark found that the "staff member influences both what a board member does and how he perceives board functioning. . . . In addition, the staff member seems to play a major role in creating the climate for questioning and discussing new, alternative approaches."[38] Staff thus controls in most instances the degree and manner in which board members involve themselves in planning decisions. With respect to the question, "Did staff member encourage new ideas for resolving the issue?" 34 percent of the board members said "No," 39 percent said "Yes," and the rest said "to some extent." With respect to the question, "Did staff help you clarify your thoughts about the issue?" 43 percent answered "Yes," 24 percent answered "No," and 34 percent answered "To some extent."[39] It can be seen from just these two questions that less than 50 percent of the 243 board members responding, over half of whom were consumers, felt that staff had fully encouraged them or helped to clarify their thoughts. This shows a differential in board members' perceptions about the helpfulness of staff toward their concerns. It implies that the staff, as well as the board, needs assistance in working together.

ISSUES IN TRAINING

The procedure that governs the flow of technical assistance availability and resources is a potentially major roadblock to full participation and cooperation of agencies in using such assistance. The key focus of this process rests with the agency's executive director, who serves as the funnel through which agency needs vis-à-vis training are expressed, and to whom the training body must refer before beginning a sequential program. This person, then, is strategically central to any decisions about training of staff, must pass on the agency "weaknesses" or some designation of need, and then approve the program and materials prepared to complete the training. It seems that often this is the very person whose schedule promotes delays in establishing education and training as an agency priority, owing to the numerous demands on his or her time and attention. The director, as receiver of the educational materials, may not have a viable mechanism for disseminating these materials to the staff, and the entire process of training can thereby be seriously hindered. Since this may become an obstacle to the fullest participation in regional training, more attention should be devoted to examining the role of the director in the training process in order to effect the best results in utilizing and implementing these resources.

Training programs are almost deficient in their evaluation and follow-up of the trainees. In order to evaluate these programs in a meaningful way, it is important that accurate records be kept of what is happening, such as notes about trainees' progress and training staff, curriculum outlines and program scheduling, lecture content, and attendance records. Failure to record what is occurring in the program will result in insufficient factual data or inaccurate information gleaned from personal perceptions. For instance, Cooper's study of six training programs noted at the outset of this chapter found that there was insufficient information available to assess the effectiveness of training in actual planning situations.[40] Thus, more research is required to evaluate actual activities in which trainees become involved after completing the training programs. Also, questions must be answered about where and in what capacity trainees were ultimately employed and how well they functioned in their roles. Such information should be related to the training experience, if appropriate.

Finally, the issue of consumer training requires further clarification and definition by legislators, training program administrators, training staff, and trainees in order to arrive at a meaningful assessment of the activity. What are they being trained for? To plan? To make decisions? To give advice? To provide a good public relations image? To advocate for particular interest groups? To gain a modicum of power and/or status? Until it is clear why the board is being trained, it is unlikely that many board members will have a strong interest in the training they are given, and each will put a personal perspective on the reason for training sessions and what can be derived from them.

TRAINING OF STAFF/BOARD RELATED TO PLANNING MODELS

The previous discussion has revealed that the complexities of the planning process and the intricacies of the political relationships involving the health planning agencies require some form of training for staff and board members. Changes have been taking place too rapidly in the health field

Table 11-4 Training of Agency Board and Staff by Types of Planning Models

	Planning Model			
Characteristics	Systems	Partnership	Alliance	Individual Action
Focus of training	Process of planning Identifying substantive issues in planning Comprehensive systems approach Interplay of technical work of staff with decision making of board Training for goal achievement	Process of developing policies Interplay of board-staff roles and functions in policy articulation and assignment for implementation Study of political, economic, and social factors involved in policy making Strategies of collaboration for implementation of policy	Process of problem solving of substantive issues regarding sectoral function of health Focus on strategies for setting policy, gathering allies and resources	Reality-oriented process of achieving specific programs Train staff/board to use limited staff resources and exploit resources of others to achieve objectives Strategies formulated to achieve goals
Who does training?	Primarily outside consultants with expertise in systems approach to planning and political strategies for implementation	Course organized by board/staff but segments taught by outside specialists, especially policy analysts and community organizers	Outside consultatnts with expertise in subject under study with staff as backup Specialists in program analysis, planning and strategies for implementation	Volunteer friend with special knowledge and loyalty to group gives ongoing assistance until problem is solved
When and how long is training given?	Given annually following the election of new board members; in weekly	Given annually following election of new board members in weekly sessions of 2 to	Given annually following election of new board members, weekly	Episodic training, indeterminate in length, informal course, geared

	meetings of 3 hours for 8 to 12 sessions Weekend retreats held in second or third quarters to train new staff/board members, as a refresher course for older members	3 hours for 8 to 10 meetings Weekend retreats held in second or third quarters to train new board members/staff, and refresher for key board members	sessions of 3 to 4 hours for 4 to 6 weeks Afterwards on an "as needed" basis	to problem and needs of group
Who gets trained?	Primary: whole board and staff Secondary: community health related groups, public health agencies, voluntary health institutions	Primary: board, executive committee and committee chairpersons; staff; administrators and unit heads Secondary: district/county board chairpersons	Primary: board/ staff and individual committees as needed Secondary: no other group unless requested	Primary: action oriented staff/ board at subarea level Secondary: specific committee/staff desiring assistance at central office level
Methods of training	Lectures, workshops with role playing and simulation	Lectures with discussion and clarification; small workshops with feedback techniques	Problem-solving workshops, case method with feedback and reenforcement techniques	Direct involvement in real problem of group
Education decision-making model used	Concordance/ agreement	Concordance/ agreement	Conflict/ negotiation	Conflict/ negotiation

to permit agencies to rest on their laurels once their staffs and board members have received such training. Many staff members come to the agencies without prior knowledge of health planning or awareness of the substantive issues in the field. They require training to understand issues related to the health field. Other staff members come into the agency from other health institutions. They require orientation to the operations of a health planning agency, the increasing complications of the health laws that affect the agency, and the intrarelationships and interrelationships involving the agency. For these same reasons, board members require training, education, and an orientation to the agency's mission, although there has been no uniformity in how this training is performed. Because a health planning agency potentially can conform to any of the four planning models discussed in this book, it is logical to assume that training should be geared to the planning model of the agency, i.e., the type of training must vary according to its structure, goals, and staffing patterns.

The various characteristics of training can be related to the four planning models used in this book (Table 11-4). The concepts and characteristics identified in the table are those of the author and subject to empirical verification.

Systems Model

Focus of Training

The foci of training in the systems model center on the substantive issues requiring solution. Training shows the participants how the systems approach can be utilized to come to grips with the major health and medical issues confronting them. In this way, the interrelationship of various issues and their solutions can be identified and should result in both a comprehensive approach and an in-depth analysis of the causes of the problems. Training also focuses on assisting staff and board members in the decision-making process to work more cooperatively on implementing the goals of the plan. Thus, the interplay of technical staff-board dynamics must be dealt with in training sessions so that one group does not overwhelm or retard the other from achieving the plan's objectives. Thus, training is as concerned with process as with substantive health issues, with the technical aspects of planning as with the political and social components.

The Trainers

It is unlikely that the range of expertise needed resides in any one person. A respected outside consultant firm with a multidisciplined staff is the most likely choice for engaging in this type of training. The normal competitiveness and minor frictions that exist within a planning agency usually are not conducive to the use of agency staff for such training. Involving agency staff as trainers may well exacerbate these tensions and become counterproductive to the agency's ongoing routine activities. Staff members are best suited for orienting new staff members to the functions and activities of the unit (e.g., data analysis, ambulatory planning, public relations) to which they have been assigned. If one consultant firm does not have all the expertise needed, then a primary contractor can be used, who, in turn, will hire the additional expertise required. These consultants should have proved ability in the systems approach to planning and a deep understanding of the politics of plan implementation. Too often, consultant firms are competent in one phase of planning and weak in other important aspects.

Duration and Timing of Training

Training should take place annually, preferably following the election of new board members in order to educate them rapidly to their tasks and the operations, methods, and goals of the agency. A prescribed course of topics should be given in three-hour weekly meetings for 8 to 12 sessions. These weekly sessions should impress upon new board members and staff the seriousness with which they are expected to take their roles as decision makers and technicians. The training should be largely completed within the first three months following the elections so full attention can be given to the normal business of the agency. These training sessions should be followed by two weekend retreats three months apart to offer intensive training to any new staff and/or board members who have joined the agency following the elections. In addition, they should serve as refresher courses for long-time staff members, a social opportunity for board and staff to become better acquainted, and a time for discussion of special problems that confront the agency. Finally, orientation sessions should be offered to new staff members. The difference between the focus of the orientation and education sessions is that the orientation focuses on the staff member's role in the specific unit to which he or she is assigned, whereas the annual education sessions provide the new staff member with an overview of agency operation and goals and the role of how his or her specific unit fits into the whole.

The Trainee

With respect to who is trained, there are three target populations. The first is the board, both at the central and subarea levels. If the agency opts for the plan to be developed at the central level, then the foci noted earlier are adopted. If the plan is actually developed in the subareas, then that focus is transferred to the subarea boards, and the central board is more concerned with plan coordination and implementation, setting areawide policy, and learning skills for mediating conflicts among the subareas for allocating scarce health resources. The second group is the staff. The focus for staff training has been outlined. In the third group are the hosts of medical institutions and community health groups that are linked to the central or subarea boards' planning activities. The agency staff, where possible, should be the primary trainer of these groups. It could provide special periodic seminars on selected topics of interest either to a single group or a general broad section of health bodies. The seminars could be on such topics as informing them about new federal or state laws that affect them, a special lecture on ambulatory care, or a brief series of seminars on the elderly and their health problems. In some cases, the agency takes the initiative in developing such educational seminars and in other situations responds to an institutional or community request. Such interaction should create positive public relations and develop a climate for securing the necessary cooperation of the health institutions in setting system goals and developing strategies for their implementation.

The Training Methods Used

There are many methods for training, but the most prevalent employs lectures and workshops involving the board and staff in actual examples of systems planning. Role playing, simulation techniques, and visuals followed by discussion are appropriate methods for smaller groups, such as board committees or specific units of staff. The small units are devoted to understanding and improving the dynamics of human relations among their members at the same time as they are engaged in substantive learning of special interest topics. The larger groups are more focused on resolving conflicts and seeking consensus in decision making while learning about the general planning process and their roles in it. The community training emphasizes lectures and question-and-answer methods. There is very little emphasis on reenforcement techniques to ensure the community groups understand and absorb the message of the lectures. The agency's interest in training community groups is to foster good will and to develop a positive image in the community.

The training manuals developed by Governments Services and Systems, Inc. of Philadelphia (GSS) on the systems approach to planning is an excellent training document to educate staff and board on the use of a common planning process. However, to train participants in the political and social interaction strategies required to implement the plan's goals requires simulation techniques. Such a technique is most appropriate for use in small groups where the individual's role and attitudes can be explored while he or she is learning how to plan and implement goals. The system planning model requires the most sophisticated and complex array of training methods and competent consultants because of its comprehensive vision and the changes in the health system necessitated by its plan and goals. These methods are consistent with the concordance/agreement decision-making model.

Partnership Planning Model

Focus of Training

The main focus of training in the partnership model is on training the board and staff in the art and science of developing health policy. This involves training the staff in the skills of research, theory, and the historical antecedents that create current need for policy changes. It requires the board members to learn the art of finding compromises in the decision-making process. As such, the focus of training is on the use of concepts developed in the social sciences, especially political science, economics, and sociology related to leadership training in small groups. The developing field of policy sciences is accented. Because this planning model is not concerned with implementation, no attention is given to this aspect of policy training. Its emphasis is on the concordance/agreement decision-making model.

The Trainers

Educators in policy sciences come from staff and outside consultants. The board members identify problems that require policy formulation. The staff then designs a curriculum on ways to diagnose and formulate policy alternatives. Outside consultants with a knowledge of policy science and experience in developing such policy for public bodies are brought in to explain how to diagnose an issue, using real life examples confronting the board and staff at the time. During the formulation of alternative solutions to the issue, community organization or other small group leadership consultants are used to assist the board and staff in coming to terms with their personal differences. The overall design and development of the curriculum is under the management of a board/staff training committee.

Timing and Duration of Training

As in the previous model, the most logical time to do the training is following the election of new board members or the arrival of a large number of new staff. Since there will be less attention to the technical, scientific, and methodological skills required in the systems approach to problem solving, the course can be shortened to eight to ten weeks of weekly three-hour sessions. Approximately at three-month intervals, a weekend retreat should be arranged to assist new board and staff in learning the policy science skills. More importantly, the retreats can be used to provide an opportunity for board and staff to become acquainted with each other as people in order to promote the collaboration required in achieving consensus on policy.

The Trainee

Policy making is primarily the function of the leaders of an organization and the executive or supervisory staff of the agency. As such the primary target group for the training consists of the officers of the agency board, the executive committee, other committee chairpersons not on the executive body, and agency administrators and unit supervisors. These are the groups who play the most important role in setting agency policy. Once trained, they use their newly developed skills in training their committee members or staff in the policy science methods. In this way, the effects of the formal training have a spin-off effect on all members of the board and agency staff. At the quarterly retreats, this leadership group invites board members and staff being groomed for future leadership or supervisory positions to join them. A secondary group to be trained consists of the district or county board chairpersons and officers, if time and funds permitted. The reason for this low priority under this model is that the central board develops areawide policy. The district boards serve primarily as a feedback mechanism to ascertain if the direction the central board is taking is largely acceptable to the constituents. These central board policies are criteria and guidelines that permit the district boards to monitor how well the health institution programs are being implemented within the districts. As such, the policies serve as sanctions, which are morally rather than legally binding on the district's health institutions. Refinements and flexible adaptations of the policy, not their determination, are the responsibilities of the districts. The central board sets policy, and the district boards monitor its implementation.

The Training Methods Used

The most effective means for training participants in the policy sciences is a combination of lectures on the elements involved in diagnosis with discussion and clarification. This is to be followed by small workshops in which the participants actually solve one or more health issues currently affecting the agency or the area. The policy science and human relations consultants then provide feedback to the participants on their use of skills and personal interaction with each other. Basic weaknesses found in the individual or the group's knowledge or performance are identified and given special consideration by the consultants.

The National Training Laboratory consultants and their methods are highly suitable for training the staff and board leaders in the dynamics of human relations, leadership, and the art of coming to decisions. Various professors from policy science graduate schools or consultant firms that specialize in developing policy can provide the technical and scientific skills needed in diagnosing problems and understanding the socioeconomic-political issues involved in the creation of policy alternatives.

Alliance Planning Model

Focus of Training

Planning under the alliance model is mainly concerned with a subcomponent of a sector in the health field. As such, the board and staff focus, for example, on devising the best method of insuring physicians and hospitals against malpractice suits as a subcomponent of the sector on health insurance and financing of health services. Because the various committees and functional units of the agency are concerned with their own special interests, the focus of this planning model is on the problem-solving process related to specific substantive issues that emerge. A further focus is on learning how to use different strategies for gaining resources and allies to implement the solutions planned. Large areawide development of policies or creation of comprehensive plans is not the interest of this planning model. Rather the maintenance of a stable, acceptable health system and making those adaptations required to have it perform more efficiently are the concerns of the decision makers. Because of its action orientation, emphasis would be on the conflict/negotiation decision-making model.

The Trainers

The primary skills needed are how to analyze and solve problems related to specific programs, and how to use strategies for implementing the solutions. As such, two types of consultants are needed. One teaches the board and staff the general skills and methods for solving specific problems, and the other is an expert in the program area in which the staff and board require assistance. The staff's role is to define the nature of the problem and secure the consultants needed.

Duration and Timing of Training

The training in the general principles and methods of problem solving and implementation takes place on an annual basis following the election of new board members. These sessions, of about three hours each, last four to six weeks. Thereafter, consultants are brought in on an "as needed" basis to work with the staff and board on current health problems as they emerge and require outside consultation; supervisors train new staff assigned to their units; new board members learn by observation and participation with those already trained.

The Trainee

The entire central board and staff are trained in the general methods and principles of problem solving. As required, specific board committees use consultants to assist them with individual problems that arise. District boards and committees are trained only if they request such assistance. No other group is trained.

The Training Methods Used

The major method of training involves workshops or laboratories in which participants learn how to use a problem-solving process on current agency program issues. The case method is used by committees and staff concerned with specific problems. Consultants help them to diagnose the problem and offer suggestions on how the solutions could be implemented. By using current problems as the case material, the consultants provide feedback and reenforcement to the efforts of the committees or staff who engage their services.

The most relevant problem-solving method for use in this model is the "disjointed incrementalist" concept developed by Lindblom.[41] The more formal rational planning processes that are widely taught and used by urban planners are not as relevant to this type of planning model. Community organization principles and concepts are also a feasible alternative because they focus on both a problem-solving process and ways of implementing them.

Individual Action Planning Model

Focus of Training

The major focus of training in the individual action planning model is on learning how to achieve very specific program objectives. It is completely oriented to reality since those involved must learn to solve a problem that immediately confronts them. Consequently, the training focuses on teaching staff and the board how to use limited resources to achieve their limited objectives. The emphasis should be on the conflict/negotiation decision-making model.

The Trainers

Most of the training takes place with the district or county-level boards or committees. These boards have little or no staff and little prospect of securing such paid staff from the central agency on an ongoing basis. Yet, it is expected that, over time, the district boards will have developed professional friends who have a commitment and loyalty to their goals and objectives. It is to these volunteer expert consultants the board or committees at the district level turn for help in solving their problems. Sources of such consultants would be community action agencies, graduate students who want to "be where the action is," professors who are community-oriented, or professionals from various public and private health agencies who devote part of their volunteer time to such groups. In large urban areas, there is usually an abundance of such volunteer talent, but it is more difficult to secure in rural areas unless a college or university is located nearby.

Duration and Timing of Training

Unlike the previous planning models, the individual planning model has no best time for offering training courses. Rather, the training is episodic, indeterminate in length, and informal. It lasts as long as the volunteer consultant and friend of the district body has the time to devote to it, or as long as the problem remains unsolved. Because district boards and their committees are involved in many health and medical issues simultaneously, the "training" can be expected to be a continuous process, although devoted to numerous and disparate issues that require attention.

The Trainee

The primary target population for training consists of the district boards and/or their committees. If staff exists at that level, then they, too, are a primary group for training.

The Training Methods Used

The trainer in this model is a consultant who is considered a friend of the group requesting assistance and, as such, is accepted as a peer of the group. The consultant happens to have some expertise needed by the board or committee at that time. Consequently, the consultant is asked to participate as an equal partner on the problem facing the group. What this means is that training takes place by doing, by participating with the volunteer consultant, and by analyzing his or her ideas in the same manner as those of the others in the group. Because of the consultant's professional expertise and training, his or her ideas may be given more weight than those of other members of the group, but they are just as readily rejected if they do not have merit in the eyes of the group as a way of solving the problem.

The basic concepts proposed by Friedmann in his provocative book on "transactive planning"[42] come closest to exemplifying the methods employed in this type of training. In this process, the application of knowledge is toward the outcome of securing action. Thinking and doing are inextricably intertwined in the group's aim at achieving its objective.

NOTES

1. John L. Cooper, "Training for Partnership?" (Ph.D. diss., Graduate Faculty of Political and Social Science of the New School for Social Research, 1974), p. 175.

2. Health Resources Administration, *Guidelines for Recruitment and Selection of Executive/ Professional Staff for Health Systems Agencies* (Hyattsville, Md.: Bureau of Health Planning, undated).

3. *Ibid.*, pp. 14–15.

4. Orkand Corporation, *Assessment of Representation and Parity for HSAs and SHPDAs*, Vol. 1, Contract no. HRA-230-76-0210 (Hyattsville, Md.: Bureau of Health Planning, Health Resources Administration, May 12, 1977).

5. *Ibid.*, Exhibit 11-10, p. II-21.

6. Health Resources Administration, *Board and Staff Composition of Health Planning Agencies: Project Summary*, no. HRA 78-609 (Hyattsville, Md.), p. 12.

7. Orkand, *Assessment of Representation,* p. II-101.

8. Douglas R. Brown, "Training Health Planners," *Hospitals* 46 (March 1972): 61–64.

9. *Ibid.*

10. Allan Steckler, Harry T. Phillips, and James N. Burdine, "The Concept of an Ideal HSA Board," *American Journal of Health Planning* 2, no. 1 (July 1977): 19–24.

11. John M. Bradley, "Volunteer Education: Key to Building an Effective Planning Process," *Health Law Project: Library Bulletin* IV, no. 5 (May 1979): 164–172.

12. Steckler et al., "Ideal HSA Board," p. 20.

13. Bradley, "Volunteer Education," p. 167.

14. "CIR Exposes HSA Purge of Health Activists," *CIR News* 9, no. 4 (November 1980): 6.

15. Edmund M. Burke, *A Participatory Approach to Urban Planning* (New York: Human Sciences Press, 1979), p. 59.

16. Samuel J. Bosch, Rolando Merino, and Ruth Zambrana, *Training of a Community Board to Increase the Effectiveness of a Health Center*, Public Health Reports, vol. 94, no. 3 (May-June, 1979): 277.

17. *Ibid.*, p. 279.

18. Terry E. Shannon, *Interim Report on Consumer Participation* (Hyattsville, Md.: Health Resources Administration, April, 1980), pp. 10–11.

19. Noreen M. Clark and Marcia Pickett-Heller, "Developing HSA Leadership: An Innovation in Board Education," *American Journal of Health Planning* 2, no. 1 (July 1977): 10.

20. *Ibid.*, p. 10.

21. John M. Bradley, "Health Education and the Community," mimeographed. Presentation at the Community Health Center Conference, University of Pittsburgh, December 8, 1979.

22. *Ibid.*, p. 2.

23. *Ibid.*, p. 3.

24. Marjorie Feinson, "Advocacy Project for Effective Health Planning," mimeographed (New Jersey Department of the Public Advocate, April, 1980).

25. *Ibid.*, p. 4.

26. Consumer Commission on the Accreditation of Health Services, "Development of a Consumer Health Network," *Consumer Health Perspectives* IV, nos. 4 and 5, July-October, 1977.

27. Bradley, "Health Education and the Community," p. 7.

28. John Forester, "Toward Democratic Health Planning: Political Power, Agenda Setting, and Planning Practice," mimeographed (Ithaca, N.Y.: Cornell University, Department of City and Regional Planning, April, 1980).

29. Educational Testing Service, *A Course for Health Systems Agency Boards*, Contract no. 30-75-0064 (Hyattsville, Md.: Health Resources Administration, undated).

30. *Ibid.*, p. 1.

31. Carol C. Riddick, Sam M. Cordes, and Charles O. Crawford,"Educational Needs as Perceived by Community Health Decision Makers," *Public Health Reports*, vol. 93, no. 5 (September-October, 1978).

32. Henrick Blum, *Planning for Health* (New York: Human Sciences Press, 1973), p. 404.

33. Bertram Beck, "Community Control: A Distraction, Not an Answer," *Social Work*, October, 1967, p. 16.

34. Donald Ardell, "Limitations and Priorities in CHP," *Inquiry* 10 (September 1973): 53.

35. Blum, *Planning for Health*, p. 408.

36. OSTI, "Organization for Social and Technical Innovations," *Final Report on Contract HSM 110-71-44*, April 1972, p. 7.

37. *Ibid.*, p. 9.

38. Noreen M. Clark, "Spanning the Boundary between Agency and Community: A Study of Health Planning Staff and Board Interaction," *American Journal of Health Planning* 3, no. 4 (October 1978): 42–45.

39. *Ibid.*

40. Cooper, "Training for Partnership?" p. 102.

41. Charles E. Lindblom, "The Science of Muddling Through," *Public Administration Review* 19 (Spring 1959): 78–88.

42. John Friedmann, *Retracking America: A Theory of Transactive Planning* (New York: Anchor Press-Doubleday, 1973).

Chapter 12

What Is Being Planned?

In the first generation of comprehensive plans completed by agencies funded under PL 93-641, eight issues were noted as critical:

1. health services for the poor
2. changing emphasis in health care delivery
3. training of health practitioners
4. identification of consumer priorities
5. rising medical costs
6. uneven distribution of medical care
7. uneven quality of care
8. overemphasis on treating illness

Five years have passed since these issues were identified, and all these issues have received some attention in the comprehensive health plans developed in the middle and late 1970s. Mainly because of federal and congressional initiatives, some improvement can be seen in all of them. The problems have by no means been solved, but an effort is being made to deal with them within the constraints of public and private fiscal allocations. A review of the literature, especially federally supported research findings and commission reports, indicates that some new initiatives were taken in the last half of the 1970s to deal directly with some of these issues. The focus on elimination of excess hospital beds, regionalization of health care services, and improved access to health care is related to the issues of the low level of services provided for the poor, high cost of care, and its uneven distribution. The recent emphasis on health education, disease prevention, holistic medicine, and home health care services is a reaction to the issue of the overconcentration on treating illness. In addition, the establishment of the mental health commission highlights the issues involved in this continuing problem. Given the changes that have occurred over the last five years, however, these same issues must be considered in a wider context.

MAJOR HEALTH PROBLEMS

Health Services for the Poor

The commonly held belief has been that most of the newly developed health services and facilities have been directed at the urban poor. Community mental health centers, family care centers, "ghetto medicine" outpatient services to the poor in New York City, lead poisoning, and "rat" eradication programs have all been designed to improve the health of the urban poor. To the extent that these and many other programs have been implemented, they have had some consequences. Yet, inadequate funds have so limited the scope of the programs that they have had little discernible effect on improving the health indicators that have been used to measure the health status of the residents over the last decade. In addition to the paucity of funds, the health care delivery system has not been altered to cater to the way the poor use these services, further reducing its effectiveness. In a provocative article on the failure of comprehensive health services aimed at urban Mexican-Americans, Cervantes notes how the services provided for these people were offered with little empathy, were inconsistent with the structure of their social and community organizations, and were aimed at a stereotypical "Chicano" who did not exist in reality.[1] He noted in contrast the diversity of medical services that Mexican-Americans utilize for different health needs. For example, the Catholic Church provided medical advice and services to middle-aged and older women; the pharmacy provided the patent drugs they used; the godmother was sought out for general medical advice, and the *bruja,* or witch doctor, was used when the patient felt the need of "spells" as a medical treatment. These are all sources of the health care delivery system used by Mexican-Americans for various types of health/medical problems. Yet, none of them is considered a traditional health service. Through this example, Cervantes was making the point that, while well-trained and skilled health and medical practitioners were needed as in the traditional model of medical care, it was essential for medical practitioners to have an understanding of the cultural and social organization of the people being served. In this way, more appropriate treatment can be provided to that population. Too often, health care delivery lacks this focus and in the process exhibits a callousness and disrespect to the population and its culture.

Statistics prepared by Rudov and Santangelo for the Department of Health and Human Services to compare the health status of minorities, especially the poor among the minorities, with that of whites and their respective utilization of health services reveal the following:[2]

- 32 percent of the lowest income, compared to 65 percent of the highest income, persons rated their health as excellent.
- 59 percent of whites, compared to 45 percent of nonwhites, visited a physician for pregnancy during the first trimester.
- During the ten years, 1965 to 1974, immunization rates for polio for nonwhites declined from 82 to 49 percent while the decline for whites was from 77 to 67 percent.
- A smaller proportion of nonwhites and low-income persons see a physician during the year.
- Short-stay nonfederal hospitalization rates are higher for low-income persons.
- A larger proportion of nonwhites and low-income persons report no regular source of care.
- Nonwhites are underrepresented in nursing homes and overrepresented in institutions for the mentally ill.

These are only a few of the statistics that show the inequity of services available to the poor and minorities. Because of the disparity, minorities have higher mortality rates in eight of the ten leading causes of death.[3] It is obvious that, if major shifts are to occur in health status indicators, there must be greater efforts to improve the health of the poor and minorities.

For children in low-income families, the statistics and findings are just as bleak, in spite of the enactment of such federal programs as Maternal and Child Health, Crippled Children's Services, Medicaid, and the Early and Periodic Screening, Diagnosis and Treatment (EPSDT) amendment to Medicaid:[4]

- 65 percent of black children living in families headed by females, compared to 19 percent in families headed by males, lived in poverty.
- Children in poor families have greater health problems and are less likely to receive primary and preventive health care than children from higher income families.
- Although 99 percent of all births take place in hospitals, five times as many black infants are born outside hospitals than are white infants.
- Death rates are higher for black than for white children. For example, 5.4 blacks, compared to 2.9 whites, per 10,000 children died from accidents, poisonings, and violence in 1976.

- Poor children are more likely than higher income children to be in poor health, have functional disabilities, and develop communicable diseases.
- Nine percent of poor children, compared to two percent from higher income families, are reported in fair or poor health.

Even though the EPSDT program was developed especially to overcome this disparity, only $150 million of a Medicaid budget of $10 billion were spent in 1977 to serve less than ten percent of the children eligible for this program.[5] Medicaid eligibility is required for poor children to receive services under this program. Yet, many states set their Medicaid eligibility level below the poverty line, coincidentally limiting the number of children who can participate in the EPSDT program; in the South, for example, only 24 percent of poor children receive Medicaid services. While there are other federal and state programs that offer services to children, this patchwork has a total capacity of 1.7 million children, with 40 percent already eligible for Medicaid. In essence, while there are a number of programs, their funding levels or eligibility requirements tend to permit services for only a small percentage of children at the most critical period of their lives. Thus, for minorities as well as children, receiving early and appropriate medical and preventive services is a major problem.

Shifts in Focus of Health Care

The health industry has often been characterized as a "cottage" industry, resistant to the changes required in our postindustrial society with its emphasis on computers, sophisticated technologies, and interdisciplinary teams of scientists, medical practitioners, and allied health professionals. Many claim that the solo practitioner is no longer able to serve patients properly because their conditions more frequently require a team approach. DeHoff believes that some form of group practice, whether a health maintenance organization (HMO), a foundation structure, a hospital-centered treatment complex, or a partnership of physicians, providing limited service in a group practice, will eventually supersede the solo practitioner who has so long dominated the practice of medicine.[6] In a 1972 survey of medical students, DeHoff found that 85 percent intended to enter group practice rather than engage in "solo" practice.

Tackling the issue from another perspective, Saward states that the American economy is close to reaching the limit with respect to the proportion of the Gross National Product that the nation is willing to devote to health services; also contending for large shares are such needs as housing, national defense, and education.[7] Consequently, the limited health dollars will have to be spent more efficiently; this will result in competition among different modes of health delivery in which the most efficient are likely to succeed. He believes that, on economic grounds, the delivery system will move away from solo practice and toward some form of group practice. These and other health analysts also recognize the potential disadvantages to this shift: the loosening of the patient-physician relationship, the loss of confidentiality through the indiscriminate use of patient information, and the diminishing autonomy of the medical practitioner. It is anticipated that practitioners most affected will resist the shift, creating tensions and delays that may dilute the full effects of the new modes of health delivery.

This trend toward group practice was given a major boost with the passage of PL 93-641. This act gives full recognition to the need for efficiency in the use of limited health resources through its emphases on group practice, integration and coordination of health services, health education, and the adoption of uniform cost accounting and reporting systems.[8] The end result of PL 93-641 will be to promote more effective and efficient health care for the entire population.

The changes that are taking place both in the organizational structure and in the services offered are still in their beginning stages, but powerful forces appear to be building toward additional initiatives. The movement toward group practices is expanding; they increased from 6,400 to 8,400 between the years 1969 and 1975.[9] More significant, however, is the fact that almost 75 percent of the new physicians have entered some form of group practice during this period of time, as predicted by DeHoff. In keeping with this trend is the fact that the number of HMOs has also increased dramatically between 1969 and 1978, from 37 to 203.[10] Whether either of these movements can replace the solo practice of medicine is unknown. There appear to be cost barriers beyond which persons will not pay to belong to an HMO, even though it provides a comprehensive array of services. Likewise, a large group practice can seriously dilute the patient-physician relationship, which presents a barrier to growth in both size and number of group practices.

With respect to the type of services offered, federal as well as private initiatives are clearly beginning to favor the growth of health promotion and education services. The focal point of this movement is in the Office of Health Information and Health Promotion of HHS, which has been promoting conferences in collaboration with national organizations in support of preventive type health services. McKeown points to three basic needs that must be met to keep individuals generally free from illness: "they must be adequately fed; they must be protected from a wide range of hazards in the environment; and they must not depart radically from the pattern of personal behavior under which man evolved, for example, by smoking, overeating, or sedentary living."[11] This leads to an emphasis on changing personal life styles and therefore a greater emphasis on health education and preventive measures.

Planners have also paid special attention to this interest in health promotion. The very first edition of the *American Journal of Health Planning* had as its focus holistic health.[12] Furthermore, the Surgeon General's report *Healthy People* is a catalog of health problems that can be solved only through health promotion and disease prevention.[13] Indeed, one must be impressed with the comprehensive health education and promotion program designed to reduce one of the highest rates of coronary heart disease in any area of the world, in North Karelia, Finland. A five-year program of health education resulted in a 31 percent reduction in the incidence of stroke, 21 percent reduction in the incidence of myocardial infarction, and a 20 percent reduction in the mortality rate from cardiovascular conditions.[14] Even health insurance companies are promoting this type of service. For example, Blue Cross and Blue Shield of Greater New York have distributed free copies of a special report written in layman's language, *Take Care of Yourself,* which is designed to help people determine when they can help themselves with preventive measures and when they should visit a physician.[15] It provides the kind of information that gives consumers a sense of self-confidence in their interactions with a physician and a willingness to accept greater responsibility for their personal health.

While there are many indications of a shift of concern with respect to both the delivery of health care services and consumers' involvement in their own care, it must be kept in mind that the dominant form of health care continues to be diagnostic-treatment services; the physician who works in a private office and uses the hospital for more sophisticated types of treatment and diagnosis remains the primary form of service. It is difficult to predict whether the new forces are temporary fads or the basis of a new emphasis of health and medical intervention for the future.

Rapid Rise of Costs of Care

Previous chapters have already alluded to rising costs as a major problem in medical care. The enactment of Titles XVIII and XIX of the Social Security Act simply accentuated the inflationary spiral that was already occurring in the field. Inflation has had an impact on (1) the escalation of costs on union and other third party payment contracts for medical care, (2) the deepening deficits confronting struggling municipal and voluntary hospitals, (3) the reduction in the quality and quantity of services available to the poor and lower middle classes, and (4) the shift toward utilization of less expensive medical care, such as paraprofessionals and, more recently, physician's assistants. Some of the causes of the inflationary trend to which health planners must address themselves are (1) the increasing use of expensive technologies; (2) the inefficiency of providing duplicate care for little used services such as maternity wards, open heart surgery, and cobalt treatments; (3) the rapid escalation of professional, technical, and supportive personnel costs; (4) the use of the more expensive inpatient treatment in the absence of less expensive ambulatory or nursing home care; and (5) the higher demands and greater expectations of patients. Health economists are especially concerned with the inflationary effects that an enactment of a national health insurance bill will have on medical care unless planning and corrective actions are taken in anticipation of its passage.

In a summary of research on ways of controlling the cost of health care, the National Center for Health Services Research studied hospital, consumer, and provider behavior to determine the best way to reduce costs.[16] While there were a number of potential opportunities, each had negative side-effects. For example, federal programs that guaranteed investors against a hospital's default on a loan also gave "management . . . no immediate incentive to make wise investment decisions."[17] The passage of a comprehensive national health insurance program will not have any adverse effect on inpatient costs, but it will substantially increase ambulatory costs because there are not enough physicians to handle the expected 30 to 75 percent increase in demand. Furthermore, the report notes that planners must consider the impact of cost containment on equity and quality of care, as well as its effect on the population's health status. Consequently, the report concludes, ". . . we still are not certain as to which button(s) to press or which *coordinated* initiatives to set in motion to contain costs and still secure an equitable and efficacious health care delivery system."[18]

Even the two most highly regarded strategies for controlling costs, HMOs and reduction of excess bed capacity, do not provide clear-cut solutions to this problem. For example, a study of three types of HMOs and a Blue Cross plan showed that only one of the HMOs had fewer patient admissions than Blue Cross[19] or fewer hospital days per 1,000 than Blue Cross.[20] While there are explanations for this, the fact that HMOs have no clear-cut advantage over traditional third party reimbursement raises questions about their cost effectiveness.

Similarly, reducing excess hospital beds is a complex and difficult strategy to achieve. Gottlieb identifies a number of constraints against hospital closings: constitutional prohibitions against government interference with contractual obligations or appropriation of property without fair compensation to the hospitals, physician resistance, the need to provide a means for payment of a hospital's debt, and the negative impact on the local community's economic structure.[21] He concludes that voluntary closure is the least expensive way to reduce capacity. In addition to these factors, Lewin identifies a number of societal characteristics that affect both the construction of new hospitals and community resistance to hospital closings. Among these are population shifts that either change the needed hospital capacity or require the development of hospitals for special groups, such as blacks or religious populations, and hospital sponsorships such as public or private.[22] Public hospitals are built mainly for the poor and private hospitals for the paying patient. These factors have encouraged the building of small hospitals, especially in urban communities, that cater to the needs of these special populations. The result is more hospital beds being built than are needed in the inner city and suburban areas of cities like Chicago and New York. This is what Lewin calls the "segmentation of hospital service areas" and, in many cases, a greater number of hospitals per capita than would occur in the absence of these societal factors. Thus, for both economic and social reasons, complex forces combine to fight against planning agencies or state regulatory agencies' efforts to eliminate excess hospital beds. Hospital and physician professional associations, aware of these inconclusive studies, believe that federal and state governments, in their efforts to cut hospital costs without dealing with the underlying causes of inflation, are using the hospitals as scapegoats for their own failure to achieve economic stability.[23]

Whatever the answer to controlling costs, it is apparent that the problem is so complex that no one solution will be effective. It appears that a reduction in health costs must also be accompanied by a reduction in the costs and inflation in the general economy.

Quality of Care

Closely linked to the maldistribution of medical care is the uneven quality of care that is delivered. A two-tier system of health care exists in which foreign born and educated physicians and the newly developing class of physician's assistants become the primary resources of medical care for the poor, while better trained and American-educated physicians gravitate toward lucrative private practices or prestigious positions in hospitals, medical schools, and research establishments. This is one dimension of the quality of care problem. The other dimension is related to the practice itself. According to Yordy, consumer dissatisfaction has been registered over excessive surgery, overuse of drugs as a form of treatment, and administrative failure to inform eligible clients of their rights to medical care under Medicaid.[24] There are those such as Ginzberg who maintain that, even with the passage of national health insurance, there will always be a differential between the care and treatment rendered to those completely dependent on such health insurance and those who can afford to pay premiums for a more personal and intensive level of treatment, nullifying to a limited extent the complete democratization of health care sought under national health insurance.[25] Health planners have an obligation to reduce the current disparity both in the supply and allocation of health personnel and the way treatment is rendered by medical practitioners to ensure a more even quality of care between the higher and lower income classes.

Part of the problem stems from the public's growing doubt that the large sums of money spent on medical research and care are justified by the minimal changes in health status indicators. As noted earlier, more attention is being given to changes in the environment and in life styles than to medical intervention. Further, there is a striking paucity of valid clinical knowledge about the efficacy and effectiveness of current medical care,[26] as well as insufficient information about the cost-benefit trade-offs. Ineffective methods may not only harm patients, but also waste scarce resources needed in research to uncover safer and more efficacious medical care. For example, a correlation has been found between the removal of healthy tissue during an appendectomy and the way in which the patient paid the physician or hospital. Welfare patients and those paying out-of-pocket had 40 percent healthy tissue removed, compared to 50 to 55 percent for those with commercial insurance or Blue Cross.[27] In other words, the better the insurance, the more likely the patient will have unnecessary surgery. This represents a perverse effect of comprehensive health insurance.

There is a wide variation in the incidence of serious complications or postoperative mortality for different hospitals. This difference could result in as much as 25 times more danger for a patient in one hospital than in another.[28] A study of maternal mortality shows that, in Michigan from 1950 to 1970, 60 to 80 percent of the deaths could have been prevented.[29] Finally, in selected areas of Washington, D.C., findings of a special study on children revealed that 12 percent of children in need of eyeglasses do not have them; that, of those who have them, 31 percent do not need them; that another 37 percent have an inadequate vision correction; and that 5 percent have glasses that make their vision worse.[30] All of these are examples of poor quality care. While a few affect the higher income family, most affect the poor.

Professional Standards Review Organizations (PSROs) and the National Health Services Corps (NHSC) have been assigned the major responsibility for both correcting poor quality care in medical institutions and providing care in medically underserved areas. It has been noted that PSROs are designed more for improving physicians' poor use of medical procedures (process standards) or identifying incompetent practitioners or dangerous equipment (input standards) than for improving the effect of practice on patients (output standards). Preliminary results indicate that PSROs are having an uneven impact. With respect to the NHSC program, it will be quite a while before a substantial number of medically underserved areas receive their first physician. There is already some question, however, about whether the students in the program are learning skills and developing the leadership capacities they will need when they become the only medical resource in the community.[31] Such communities need much more than medical assistance; they need help with health education, public health services, and environmental problems. NHSC professionals will be expected to help the community obtain more resources than they can personally supply. Are medical schools ready to add courses on community involvement, program planning, and public health intervention modalities and skills? Thus, the quality of care includes competence that comes from both medical knowledge and community leadership capacities. Failure to perform both types of functions will adversely affect the higher as well as the lower income members of a community.

Access to Care

Of the many issues involving the needs of the poor and elderly, the lack of access to medical care receives much attention. One of the problems encountered by health planners and policy analysts concerns the definition of the term. A staff paper developed by the National Academy of Medicine identifies at least 15 definitions already proposed. The following is the one it finally adopted:

> Access may be defined as the ability of a population or subgroup of the population to obtain essential health services in an appropriate manner. This ability is affected by economic, temporal, locational, architectural, cultural, racial, organizational, and informational factors which may be barriers or facilitators to obtaining health services.[32]

Each of these factors produces its own health indicators and data base. For example, the temporal factor could refer to the waiting time required to receive service, the number of days a person must wait for a scheduled appointment, or the length of time it takes to travel to a health facility.

Regardless of the factor focused on or the indicator used, it is agreed that the term is a complex one and, more importantly, that it affects the poor, elderly, rural, and inner city residents more than others. Some statistics taken from the National Academy report elucidate this point:[33]

- Although 87 percent of the population claimed to have a regular source of care, 24 to 31 million had no particular provider or regular entry into the medical care system.
- As of 1976, Spanish-speaking residents of the Southwest, urban blacks, and low-income groups were most likely not to have a regular source of care.
- Reasons cited for not having a regular source of care were not being sick, lack of insurance, or inability to afford a private physician or use of an emergency room.
- Lower income persons were more likely to use hospital outpatient departments, emergency rooms, public health centers, or neighborhood health centers.
- Three percent of the population stated that unavailability of a physician was the reason for not using medical care.
- In a large city like New York, travel time was cited as a barrier to using municipal hospital outpatient departments.
- It was found that moving health services closer to the centers of populations in need of medical care results in greater demand for these services.
- While Medicaid and Medicare have improved access to care for the elderly and poor, racial discrimination has affected the equal use of services between white and black persons, particularly in the South.
- Young adults, unemployed, and lower income families are much more likely than others to have no health care insurance.
- Even when people have insurance, 15 percent were found not to be covered for catastrophic illnesses and many more have little or no coverage for preventive health care services such as dental care, eyeglasses, or skilled nursing care in the home.
- Of those covered by health insurance, only three percent (6.5 million persons) belonged to prepaid group plans. The vast majority, 73 percent (151 million persons), had insurance that was based on fee for service.
- In 1976, higher income families visited a dentist twice as often as low-income families.

While progress has been made to improve access for the poor, these selected facts clearly illustrate the problems that remain to be solved if greater equity, one of the major goals of PL 93-641, is to be achieved.

The use of the regulatory strategy to achieve this equity may prove to be a two-edged sword. Even though most inner city poor depend on municipal hospital outpatient and emergency room departments for their health care, the cost containment philosophy of the act will result in the closing of the very hospitals that "will affect access, especially for the poor, the near-poor and central city and rural residents who may utilize such facilities."[34] This comes about because federal guidelines recommend less than 4 beds per 1,000 population and most of the excess beds are located in underutilized, antiquated, and inefficient medical institutions that serve these populations. Furthermore, it has previously been noted that the regulatory strategy is reactive in nature. It cannot be used to promote or force health providers to place new services where they are most needed but only to prevent providers from locating them where they desire. When negotiation and persuasion are possible between health planning agencies and health providers over certificates of need, this strategy might lead to more services for the poor. However, such trade-offs usually represent compromises between what the providers essentially want and what the planners believe is necessary.

With respect to physician location in rural areas, it seems that the use of physicians under obligation to the NHSC may be a positive strategy. For rural and other nonmetropolitan areas that are experiencing population increases, group practices work quite well as a way of attracting and maintaining physicians in these areas.[35]

Mental Health Services

In the last 20 years, there has been a dramatic change in the mental health field. Instead of largely custodial care in huge, impersonal institutions far from the communities where most of the patients lived, treatment is now provided to over 75 percent of patients in their own cities and towns. This dramatic change is known as deinstitutionalization. Since 15 percent of the American population have some form of mental disorder, over 30 million persons are affected.[36] The typical person treated is 25 to 44 years old. Only five percent of the elderly are counted in this number. Even the average length of stay has been radically reduced. The median length of stay is only 25.5 days in public mental hospitals, 8 days for acute care hospitals, and 14 days for private psychiatric hospitals. The role of the state mental hospital has thus been greatly reduced.

A number of factors account for this major change. Alternate care facilities for the aged, especially in nursing and community boarding homes, are more available and more often used. Under the impetus of the Community Mental Health Centers Act, the availability and use of outpatient and after-care facilities have increased. Psychoactive drugs have brought the more disturbing symptoms of many patients under control. The development of screening procedures has prevented inappropriate admissions of patients to state mental health facilities. Indeed, this treatment setting is now used primarily as a last resort, a major change from its previous role as the initial and primary source of treatment. As a result of these changes, a much larger role is taken by the acute care general hospitals and primary care outpatient medical facilities. They now treat almost 60 percent of all patients with a mental disorder. In fact, the specialty mental health sector treats only an estimated 20 percent of those with mental problems. The family physician, the local pharmacist, and the social worker come in contact with more persons with mental problems than do any other professionals, including those in the psychiatric services.

Included among those with mental disorders are an estimated nine million problem drinkers and an unknown number of heroin addicts. In spite of the increased availability of mental health services for drug addicts, alcoholics, and the mentally ill, there are still differences in the type of treatment facilities used by various population groups. Low-income persons use primarily public treatment services, such as community mental health center services, municipal and county hospital outpatient departments, and state and county inpatient services. Middle-income persons, many of whom now have insurance coverage for mental health services, use private treatment services, although they are more likely to use an inpatient service of a general acute care hospital rather than outpatient care in a psychiatrist's office. With respect to race, blacks used mental health services at a rate 30 percent higher than that of whites. They tended to use inpatient state and county public hospitals, community mental health centers, and outpatient psychiatric services at a higher rate than whites. Whites, on the other hand, tended to use inpatient private psychiatric and general acute care hospitals at a higher rate than blacks.

To provide treatment to this growing community-centered population, there has been a substantial increase in personnel. In just 13 years, the number of psychiatrists, psychologists, and social workers has doubled. Even more impressive is the substantial increase in the number of professionally trained mental health nurses, rising from just 20 in 1947 to 11,000 in 1976. From 1969 to 1977, the number of community mental health centers has grown from 205 to 649, a more than 300 percent increase. All of these changes provide fresh evidence of the dramatic changes that have taken place in mental health services. Yet, there are major unsolved problems. In fact, deinstitutionalization has developed its own problems.

While there has been less "warehousing" of patients in state mental hospitals, the warehousing custodial treatment is now becoming more common, especially for the elderly, who are placed in nursing homes where they receive far less professional treatment than they would have received at state institutions. This has occurred because there has not been a concomitant shift in funds from state to community services to take care of the many discharged patients. As a result, large populations of single room occupants have established themselves in large, older hotels no longer profitable for commercial trade. Little or no services are provided to those who live in such places, which are located mostly in urban areas. In some cities, such as New York, where the hotels are again becoming commercially valuable, these former mental patients are arbitrarily and, in many cases, violently evicted from the hotels, although they have no place to go. While the number of patients hospitalized at state institutions has been reduced, statistics indicate that the number of readmissions has greatly increased; the high number of discharges from these hospitals may indicate no more than a fast revolving door that holds the census down.

At least 20 percent of those with mental disorders, about seven million persons, received no care during any calendar year. In addition, distribution of services in the United States has been inequitable, with the greatest concentration of services in the Northeast and lower levels of care in the South and Rocky Mountain sections. Finally, since the majority of mental health services are offered in nonpsychiatric treatment settings, such as physicians' offices, there appears to be a major organizational and training problem in linking the mental health system to the general health system; physicians need training either in medical school or as continuing education to assist them in identifying, diagnosing, and making appropriate referrals of the many patients they see in their daily practice.

As with physical health, there is a need to shift the emphasis on diagnosis and treatment to an emphasis on prevention. It was found that of the 12 highest risk health behaviors, 10 were related to one or more of the mental disorders. Among these are smoking, alcohol use, drug use, driving, sexuality, risk management, family development, coping, stress management, and self-esteem.[37] Preventive services can potentially yield high dividends to those persons identified as high risk with respect to these 10 behavior situations. In sum, dealing with these life style issues calls for a more integrated health/mental health strategy, a far cry from the current division that separates these two forms of service.

GOALS AND OBJECTIVES OF HEALTH SYSTEMS PLANS

The Bureau of Health Planning has computerized the goals and objectives of all first-generation plans produced under PL 93-641, including the long-range and short-range implementation plans. Called AGPLAN (referring to the health planning agency's plans), this computerization has involved indexing the goals and objectives so that it is possible to extract the information in a variety of forms, e.g., all goals or objectives related to national standards, to the priorities stated in Section 1502 of PL 93-641, to services, to settings, or to system characteristics, such as availability or accessibility. It is the only data base that deals with basic health planning information on a national level. (See Appendix 12-A for a list of key words and samples of the types of information that can be extracted from the AGPLAN computer base.)

Most health plans deal with some or all of the basic health system components:

1. primary care
2. acute care
3. specialized acute care services (CAT scanner, open-heart surgery)
4. mental health
5. alcohol services
6. drug abuse
7. developmental disabilities
8. long-term care
9. home health care
10. emergency medical services
11. prevention services
12. health education
13. environmental services

Almost any medical or health service can be linked to one or more of these 13 components. In many plans, several of these components are grouped under one heading. For example, mental disorders may include mental health, alcoholism, drug abuse, and sometimes developmental disabilities. Specialized services are often found with acute care, and long-term care is often linked to home health care. Regardless of how the goals and objectives are actually formatted in health plans, the key words in AGPLAN can be used to retrieve any goal or objective that refers to any of the major medical service components.

The major deficiency of the system is its failure to include the most recent health plans. It has been well recognized that there were many deficiencies and inconsistencies in the first plans. Because of their limited data base, many health planning agencies were unable to quantify their goals in their first plans. Thus, the information in the remainder of this section can at best provide a guide to the thinking and health issues of the agencies in the years 1977 through 1979 when the first generation of plans were produced. Since then, agencies have become more specific and more comprehensive in their analysis of areawide health systems, and more goals and objectives have been quantified. Compared to the plans produced under predecessor health planning agencies, these plans represent a quantum jump in both quality and scope.

A ten percent sample of all long- and short-range health plans indexed by AGPLAN was used to seek information on the following questions:

1. What percentage of goals and objectives were stated in quantifiable form?
2. Which medical components received the most attention in these health plans?
3. On which characteristics of the medical system did the health plans focus?
4. What type of goals and objectives were most prevalent?
5. What percentage of goals and objectives were accorded high priority status in the plans?

Quantification of Goals and Objectives

Table 12-1 demonstrates that there are more qualitative goals and objectives than quantitative ones. This is to be expected in view of the lack of data for many of the functional medical components. Because these are first-generation plans, it could be expected that all of the functional components would have more qualitative than quantitative statements. Surprisingly, however, mental health and alcohol/drug abuse had 50 percent or more quantitative statements. This is especially surprising for the mental health component, because it is generally thought to have much "softer" data than the more precisely measured elements of acute care, HMOs, and emergency medical service components.

In almost all cases more objectives were quantified than goals. For example, 23 acute care objectives were quantified to 12 acute care goals. These findings are expected because goals are often perceived as more generic, timeless achievements that represent the optimum feasible potentials while objectives are time-bound. There should be a way to determine when objectives have been achieved, and that usually calls for some sort of measurement or indicator. For example, an emergency medical service goal states:

> An adequate supply of trained personnel to meet the emergency medical services needs of the NY-Penn area should be made available to the community.

Table 12-1 Ratio of Quantitative to Qualitative Goal/Objective
Statements by Selected Medical Service Components

Service Component by Goals/Objectives	Quantitative and Qualitative Statements					
	Quantitative		Qualitative		Total	
	No.	%	No.	%	No.	%
Mental health*						
Goals	120	34	230	66	349	100
Objectives	295	84	55	16	350	100
Total	415	59	285	41	699	100
Alcohol/drug abuse*						
Goals	45	27	121	73	166	100
Objectives	104	84	20	16	124	100
Total	149	51	141	49	290	100
Primary care						
Goals	40	35	73	65	113	100
Objectives	94	58	69	42	163	100
Total	134	49	142	51	276	100
Acute care						
Goals	12	29	29	71	41	100
Objectives	23	56	18	44	41	100
Total	35	43	47	57	82	100
HMOs						
Goals	5	33	10	67	15	100
Objectives	3	15	17	85	20	100
Total	8	23	27	77	35	100
Health education						
Goals and objectives	70	22	246	78	316	100
Emergency medical services						
Goals and objectives	42	22	153	78	195	100

*Data for the mental health and alcohol/drug abuse components were taken from "Program Information Note 80-1" by Reagan Gray-Kettering, Claudia Kirk, and Milt Schoeman, Bureau of Health Planning, Feb. 20, 1980.

This goal sets no date when the "adequate supply" should be achieved nor does it state what an adequate personnel supply is. It is a general statement of need. However, its objective states the following:

> To develop, by 1981, an adequate supply of EMS-trained first responders (firemen, policemen, and others who are often first to arrive at the scene of an emergency) so that an individual with EMS training can be expected to be among the first to respond to 95 percent of all emergencies.

This objective is far more specific than the goal; it indicates who should be trained (firemen, policemen, and others), when that training should be completed (1981), and what is a sufficient number of trained first responders (personnel trained in emergency medical services are the first to respond to 95 percent of all emergencies). The only information lacking to make this a complete measurable objective is the number of persons who would be considered "adequate" to meet 95 percent of all emergencies. One can infer that the data to determine that number do not exist, that experience will provide a firm estimate based on actual utilization. Many goals and objectives call for studies and collections of data in order to provide a firmer basis for quantified goal and objective statements.

Priority and Type of Goals and Objectives

Approximately 40 percent of all the goals and objectives were considered to be high priorities for the health planning agencies (Table 12-2). This is an unusually high percentage, since these are first-generation statements that often lacked sufficient data for the rational determination of priorities. Secondly, the potential political repercussions of identifying priorities when all the health providers consider their own medical components high priority make the citing of even a few priority statements a potentially divisive force in a health service area. The fact that so many were identified indicates the seriousness with which most health planning agencies take the federal guidelines that call for a determination of priorities. It is not surprising that primary care (59 percent), HMO (53 percent), and the number of acute care medical beds (50 percent) all were considered very

Table 12-2 Type and Priority of Goals and Objectives by Selected Medical Components

Service Components	Priority of Statements		Type of Statements		
	High (%)	Low (%)	Status (%)	System (%)	Others (%)
CAT scanner	24 (39)	37 (61)			
Acute medical beds	29 (50)	29 (50)			
Emergency medical services	75 (38)	121 (62)	25 (16)	131 (84)	
Health education	97 (33)	199 (67)	72 (34)	127 (60)	11 (6)
HMOs	18 (53)	16 (47)	3 (12)	23 (88)	
Acute care	82 (29)	154 (71)	22 (14)	131 (86)	
Primary care	68 (59)	47 (41)	0	115 (100)	
Total	393 (39)	603 (61)	122 (18)	527 (80)	11 (2)

high-priority areas. More surprising is the fact that acute care services, which account for about 40 percent of the health care expenditures, had the lowest percentage of high-priority statements (29 percent). Health education might have been expected to have the lowest percentage of high-priority statements. The reduced emphasis on acute care may be explained by the fact that significant acute care components, such as CAT scanners and acute care medical beds, were disaggregated and dealt with separately.

With respect to the type of statements that were found in these health plans, 18 percent were status goal/objective statements that dealt mostly with mortality, morbidity, or disability. Positive status statements were drafted for the health education component, such as improving the degree of immunization among school children or raising the percentage of persons living in areas with fluoridated water. Two medical components, CAT scanner and acute care medical beds, do not lend themselves to health status statements; primary care also has no health status statements. Some primary care goals or objectives might be expected to deal with reduction of morbidity through early diagnosis, screening, or detection. However, all the statements in AGPLAN deal with various facets of the primary care system rather than with the impact improvement of the system will make on the health status of people. Finally, as anticipated, health education had the most statements concerned with the health status of the population (34 percent). Given the fact that health education speaks to the issues of a healthful environment, a positive life style, and prevention of disease through screening, detection, and providing information, this heavy emphasis on health status would be expected.

Content of Goals and Objectives

Just what are the main concerns of the goal/objective statements? Although each of the medical components covered a large number of issues, for this analysis only the five or six most important were selected from each medical component (Table 12-3). Some of the substantive areas were combined into a single category because of the difficulty in determining in which one a statement belonged. In some cases, a statement belonged to more than one category.

The content areas that received the most attention are coordination/comprehensive health system (345 statements), availability/accessibility (414), information giving/health education (272), and prevention (245). Federal guidelines asked health planning agencies to give special attention to availability, accessibility, and cost of medical care. The planning agencies responded to the request with respect to the first two, but to a much

Table 12-3   Most Frequently Noted Types of Substantive
Statements by Selected Medical Components

Substantive Statements	Medical Components							
	Health Educa-tion	HMO	Acute Care	Primary Care	Mental Health	Alco-hol/ Drug Abuse	Emer-gency Medical Ser-vices	Total
Assessments/ studies	24	6	4	34	0	0	22	110
Information giving	41	0	3	24	134	55	15	272
Availability/ accessibility	72	12	56	143	30	35	66	414
Prevention	73	4	0	32	67	42	31	245
Coordination/ comprehensive health system	25	5	0	14	62* 183	34* 85	33	345
Continuity	0	0	0	0	115	22	0	137

*Data from the mental health and alcohol/drug abuse components were already separated. Because of the large number of statements related to these two areas, it was considered best to show them in their disaggregated form.

lesser degree with respect to the third. Much of this has to do with the fact that planners have had very little exposure to financial issues in their graduate education; also, cost data usually are closely guarded by the health providers. In more recent years, the heavy emphasis on cost containment has led to renewed interest in this system characteristic. Cost issues may well be the top priorities in the most recent health plans.

In spite of the generally low priority given to health education and prevention in the federal guidelines, strong emphasis was nevertheless given to them by the citizen health planning boards. This is probably an indication that consumers especially want to know more about the medical system and how to prevent illnesses by taking responsibility for their own health. This emphasis is consistent with the large amounts of information that have been disseminated in the 1970s through television, newspapers, and magazines. The inclusion of such goal/objective statements is merely a reflection therefore of what is already occurring in the larger society.

In health education, although an emphasis on disease prevention and even the need for education services would be expected, the provision of health education information is accorded only third place in the frequency of statements recorded. However, the emphasis on the need for more health education services implies that, once these services are in place, more information would be available for dissemination to the public.

Availability/accessibility of HMOs, acute care and primary care services, and emergency medical services were the most frequently mentioned needs for these medical components. In contrast, coordination and development of a comprehensive mental health system, along with information giving, were considered the main system issues in mental health services. The Community Mental Health Centers Act gives high priority to the development of such a system. At the same time, since the public needs service while this system is still in its uncoordinated and fragmented state, the planning agencies have emphasized continuity of mental health care.

The main surprise of this analysis is the low emphasis given to assessments and studies of the various medical components. Such studies are usually needed before quantifiable statements can be made or the priority of goal/objective statements determined.

In sum, in most situations, the data support the anticipated outcome of the priorities, concerns, and needs of the health service areas as represented by the health plans. The main surprise is the attention given to the nonmedical determinants of health care, as expressed in the health education component. In spite of the problems that usually attend the development of long- and short-range health plans and the pressure brought to bear by the federal government through its guidelines, most health planning boards displayed their independence by focusing on the needs of their own health service areas. However, the very development of these plans reflects the authority, power, and priority of Congress and the federal government with respect to comprehensive health planning. The fact that health plans now exist for nearly every geographical area of the United States contrasts sharply with the total failure of planning agencies to develop such plans under the Comprehensive Health Planning Act of 1966.

MAJOR HEALTH PLANNING OBJECTIVES FOR REGION II

A study of 13 health planning agencies' first-generation plans for Region II (New York, New Jersey, Puerto Rico, and the Virgin Islands) was completed by the author in 1978.[38] The purpose of the study was to discover the high-priority goals and objectives for the region in order to assist the HHS regional office in planning for its future resource needs. Initial analysis revealed that few planning agencies had set priorities among their goals and objectives. Consequently, it was not possible to rank medical needs based on the priorities in the plans; it was possible, however, to identify the frequency with which certain types of services were mentioned. In addition, since planning agencies tended to identify goals most important to them among the first statements in each of the plan's health system components, priorities could be inferred. This method provided a crude guide to the most important medical areas and substantive issues in each planning agency.

Major Objectives for Region II

For the region, mental health received the most attention in the 13 health plans, followed by primary care, acute/specialized care, long-term care/home health, and health education (Table 12-4). The least number of objectives were cited for environmental health, emergency medical services, and disease prevention. Overall, there appears to be a strong emphasis on community-based rather than institutionalized services. This is to be expected in view of the major emphasis given to both cost containment and developing quality services that can be rendered at lower costs, such as primary care and home health care.

Given this large number of objectives, an examination of their content reveals the ten most important for the region (Table 12-5). Of these ten objectives, only two deal with the cost containment emphasis of PL 93-641, reducing the number of acute care beds and the length of stay. All others add services and therefore will increase the cost of medical services. Of the other eight objectives, five call for increasing the availability of services (adding physicians, long-term care beds, home health services,

---

Table 12-4   Health Care Field by Number of Objectives Cited for Region II

Health Care Field	Number Objectives Cited	Rank
Mental health	226	1
Primary care	130	2
Acute care/specialized services	128	3
Long-term/home health care	120	4
Health education	106	5
Environment	75	6
Emergency medical services	61	7
Prevention	55	8

Source: Herbert H. Hyman, "Most Important Regional and State HSP/AIP Objectives," mimeographed (New York, N.Y.: DHHS Region II Division of Health Resources Development, Public Health Service, October 1978).

Table 12-5 Most Frequently Cited Regional Objectives in Health Plans

Objectives	No. of Health Plans Mentioning This Objective
1. Increase the physician:population ratio.	12
2. Reduce number of hospital beds.	12
3. Develop regionalized plans for specialized services.	10
4. Increase number of long-term care beds.	8
5. Increase home health services, especially for elderly.	8
6. Increase number of community mental health centers.	8
7. Reduce length of stay or bed days.	7
8. Increase primary care services to medically indigent.	6
9. Coordinate long-term care services with others.	6
10. Coordinate mental health with other services.	6

Number of health planning agencies in region = 13.

Source: Herbert H. Hyman, "Most Important Regional and State HSP/AIP Objectives," mimeographed (New York, N.Y.: DHHS Region II Division of Health Resources Development, Public Health Service, October 1978).

community mental health services, and primary care services for the poor) and three are concerned with improving the efficiency of services (coordinating long-term care and mental health services, and developing plans to regionalize high-cost special services, such as CAT scanners).

The question is whether the short-range objectives, those that will be implemented in the current year, are consistent with the long-range objectives. Table 12-6 shows these objectives for five health care fields. Basically, they are consistent with those noted in Table 12-5, but there are exceptions. They tend to focus on the preliminary steps to implementation and thus place greater emphasis on surveying existing services, developing methodologies to assess need, planning services, and establishing the mechanisms required to implement the objectives. As each planning year passes, there should be a closer consistency between long- and short-range objectives.

An examination of these 23 short-range objectives reveals their emphasis on the more discrete types of services or actions, such as developing a coordinating committee for a specific county, adding a 24-hour mental

Table 12-6 Short-Range Objectives Most Frequently Cited for
Selected Health Care Fields in Region II Health
Planning Agencies

Objectives	No. Times Mentioned

Health Education

1. Provide health education in subregions. — 4
2. Emphasize nutrition, disease prevention, and patients' rights in health education courses. — 3
3. Coordinate health education efforts in subregions and develop planning committees for regional health education. — 2
4. Evaluate health education courses to determine if they meet state standards. — 2

Mental Health (DA/A1/DD)

1. Increase number of community mental health centers. — 7
2. Add special mental health services, such as community residences, consultation/education, and 24-hour crisis service. — 7
3. Assess and undertake surveys such as inventorying mental health services, quality of care, and reducing waiting time. — 5
4. Add nonhospital detoxification beds. — 5

Primary Care

1. Increase physicians to an established ratio (1:2200-1:3500) with special emphasis on underserved areas. — 9
2. Assess primary care need for specific programs, such as an HMO in a rural area, reducing medically underserved areas; assess ways of providing primary care for the poor. — 5
3. Reduce insurance barriers to primary care services. — 4
4. Add new primary care services as women-infants-children programs to children, and immunize school enterers. — 4
5. Increase dental services in underserved areas. — 3

Acute Care/Specialized Services

1. Develop regional plans for specialized services. — 10
2. Reduce excessive services such as medical/surgical, obstetric, and pediatric beds and hospitals with too few cardiac surgery cases, newborn babies, or less than a 90 percent occupancy rate. — 7
3. Assess need for acute beds. — 3
4. Coordinate services with the establishment of councils, such as a specialized service committee or hospital coordinating council. — 2
5. Study reimbursement policies and hospital discharge planning. — 2

Long-Term/Home Health Care

1. Expand variety of services, such as social adult day care, basic home health care services in all agencies, increasing number — 10

Table 12-6 Continued

of home health care visits and adding two levels of care in long-term facilities.	
2. Add 1200 long-term care beds in region.	8
3. Coordinate services, such as county screening programs, developing long-term care/home health care coordinating council, and linking long-term care with mental health.	5
4. Develop plans for home health care services, a pilot geriatric hospital, and establishing long-term care service areas.	3
5. Eliminate financial barriers to care.	2

Source: Herbert H. Hyman, "Most Important Regional and State HSP/AIP Objectives," mimeographed (New York, N.Y.: DHHS Region II Division of Health Resources Development, Public Health Service, October 1978).

---

health crisis service, or developing an adult geriatric day care service. This is to be expected, in as much as the emphasis is on implementation. Major findings for the region are as follows:

- Nine of the short-range objectives will increase services in the region.
- Two would reduce costs.
- Three would result in improved coordination of services.
- Four would assess the need for additional services.
- Two would add new services.
- Two would reduce financial barriers to service.

It can be seen from these findings that the implementation of short-range objectives increases the costs of medical care, since only 2 of the 23 objectives directly reduce costs of care. There is also an increase in the efficiency in the use of existing services, however, through improved coordination and assessment of current services. While the short-run costs of efficiency through coordination may well raise initial costs of care, it is hoped that, in the long run, the costs to the system will be reduced.

Most of the objectives attempt to deal with both major purposes of PL 93-641, the reduction of costs and the improvement of accessibility and availability of services. This is evidenced by the short-range objectives that focus on improved coordination, use of less restrictive settings (such as HMOs and physician's assistants), and regionalization of services. Other objectives, although they would increase the cost of services, make services more accessible to the poor and reduce financial barriers to their use, especially primary care services. The findings suggest that the planning agencies in Region II are more concerned with adding new services than with reducing costs. In spite of the exhortations of PL 93-641 and the federal guidelines, local citizen planning bodies appear to go their own way, although they always stay within the broad guidelines of federal and state policy.

Both the national and regional goal statements reveal the richness and diversity of the health care field. While federal guidelines are intended to ensure that all health service regions have a basic set of medical care services, each area has generally selected its own goals and objectives to meet its own population's needs. Even the crude first-generation health system plans provide an insight into the direction the system is taking. The details may be obscure and the analytical assessment may be found wanting, yet the blueprint has been made for what a health system should be like. Whether these first-generation goal/objective statements ever bear fruit depends on a host of political, cultural, social, and economic factors. That some goals will be accomplished is a foregone conclusion, but whether they will be the most important cannot be predicted at this time. All that is known is that the health planning system has reached its adolescence and is striving to attain maturity.

Comparison of Health Plans' Objectives with Major Health Issues

Health planning agencies are giving attention to all major health care issues, although not all agencies are giving equal attention to every issue. For example, health services for the poor is an implied issue in almost every system goal. HMOs, increase in the number of primary care physicians, and the wider use of physician's assistants are only some of the more obvious ways that planning agencies are attempting to meet the needs of the poor. These same strategies are also prominent in efforts to change the emphasis of the health care delivery system. Regionalization of high-cost medical technologies and specialized services, such as the CAT scanner or open heart surgical suites, and sharing of support services are other methods used to increase cooperation within the health care system.

It has already been noted that both the national and the Region II surveys have indicated unusual interest in goals related to health education and disease prevention. These are two of the main dimensions in the consumer movement toward personal responsibility for health, which in the long run would reduce medical expenditures. In addition, all health plans and their goals focus directly on strategies for constraining rising medical costs. Some strategies involve cost-efficiency measures, such as use of ambulatory surgery, physician's assistants, or HMOs; others are direct regulatory efforts to reduce costs by denying medical programs that are not needed or too costly compared to alternatives.

Medical issues dealing with uneven quality and uneven distribution of medical care are also treated in the health plans. However, establishing PSROs, reducing the dual levels of care (one for the poor and a second for all others), or ensuring that medically underserved areas receive a minimal level of medical care are not given as much attention as the previously mentioned health issues. Part of the reason is that health economists, physicians, or health planners do not agree on standards for defining quality. Also, reliance upon the NHSC and physician's assistants to fill the gap in medically underserved areas is viewed only as a temporary measure. No one yet knows how to motivate physicians to work in areas that guarantee long hours for minimal financial rewards and limited status and prestige. Since the more desirable urban and suburban practice areas are now saturated with physicians, some physicians have begun to move into the outer rural areas or the inner urban areas, but not in sufficient numbers to overcome the major deficiencies that continue to exist.

The health plans have a curious mixture of expressed concerns regarding treatment. Many of the introductions to the health plans and the sections that deal with health status strongly advocate changing the balance from treatment to more concern for disease prevention and health promotion. Yet, the body of each plan hardly touches the subject, especially in considering goals and objectives that promote this alternative to treatment. Part of the reason stems from the emphasis in the federal guidelines on cost containment and on those components of the medical system responsible for the rapid rise in medical costs, e.g., acute care hospitals and long-term care nursing homes. Yet, the bias of health care providers and their consumer allies toward mental health, emergency medical services, drug abuse, and specialized services tends to crowd out interest in alternatives to treatment. Consequently, while disease prevention, health education, health promotion, and environmentally caused illnesses, are often mentioned, little emphasis is given to these in the action strategies of the health plans.

Mental health planners have been planning community mental health systems since the mid-1960s. They believe mental health planning parallels health planning. Where health planners have involved mental health planners in the development of their health systems plans, the mental health component, which usually includes alcoholism and drug abuse, has been developed as one of the most comprehensive units of the health plan. The national and Region II surveys indicate that for the most part mental health has been given the proper attention. The major concerns of mental health planners have been filling in the gaps of the comprehensive community mental health service systems, ensuring continuity of care, fostering coordination, and informing the public of the availability of mental health services. The most recent amendments to the Community Mental Health Centers Act will further this movement toward an integrated health/mental health plan.

In sum, the first generation of health plans has displayed an awareness of the major problems affecting health and the deficiencies within the medical system. Taking into account competing interests and scarce resources, the citizen governing bodies have felt it necessary to focus initially on the most pressing of the medically oriented treatment issues, leaving other health concerns on the "back burner" until they have dealt with the matters of rising costs, lack of primary care services, and the poor's difficulty in gaining access to medical care.

HEALTH PLANNING MODELS

A study of Region II agency applications does not include the characteristics or the dynamics of the models to permit an analysis of empirical relationships between plan characteristics and planning models. While the paradigm is hypothetical, the relationship of its various characteristics or elements is based on the author's knowledge and experiences (Table 12-7). Nevertheless, an empirical study is required to test the model in order to make necessary modifications or to reject it if it proves too far removed from reality. The author's conception of a comprehensive health plan is based on the idea that an agency surveys the entire range of health and health-related factors that affect the health of a population. Based on that survey and an identification of the problems requiring attention, the agency board and staff make decisions on the parts of the system requiring change. They attempt to deal with the causes of the problem insofar as this is possible rather than just the symptoms. Thus, while the final plan is not comprehensive in what it attempts to improve, it is comprehensive in making a diagnosis of the operation of the system and its impact on people. This is in contrast to a health planning agency reacting to situations that force it to make a study of individual issues and to offer recommendations without any attention to their impact on other situations in the health field; in this reactive process, planning is arbitrary and ad hoc, and it often treats only the symptoms of the problem.

Systems Model

The systems model calls for the development of a comprehensive health plan that takes into account all three major sectors of health: personal health care, environmental health, and socioeconomic health-related conditions. In this model, an examination is made of the available health status and system indicators and specific studies are carried out. Based on these, health goals, policies, objectives, priorities, and alternative plans of action are designed and a plan of action proposed to implement the final plan.

Table 12-7 Relationship of Plan Elements to Planning Models

Plan Elements	Planning Models			
	Systems	Partnership	Alliance	Individual Action
Comprehensiveness of plan	Very comprehensive	Some arbitrary comprehensiveness	Occasional comprehensiveness	Almost no comprehensiveness
Emphasis of plan	On personal health care/ environmental health and socioeconomic. All steps in plan process completed	Main focus on personal health care & narrow aspect of environmental health plan diagnosis/goals & policies; no implementation	Focus mainly on one part of personal health plan at a time includes policies/implementation related to area studied	Mainly on a subarea of personal health care program plan & implementation
Input-Delivery System-Output-Outcome Focus	Focus on delivery system & outcome	Focus on input/ delivery system	Focus on input/ delivery system	Focus on input/ delivery system
Evaluation	Use of health status/system indicators to evaluate outcome	No evaluation	No evaluation	No evaluation
Emphasis on cause/symptoms of health issues	Prevention & treatment of illness/delivery system emphasized	Some focus on prevention; mostly on improving delivery system or treating illness	Focus on symptoms of illness/ delivery system	Focus on symptoms of illness/delivery system
Agency initiative	Initiates study/ action	Some initiation; mainly reacts	Some initiation; mainly reacts	Mainly reacts
Type of change sought in health system	Structural changes	Maintenance of system with changes as needed	Maintenance of system	Both acceptance of system & "demo" structural changes

The agency then takes steps to carry out the plan. The primary emphasis of the plan is on the delivery system and how it affects the outcome, or the personal health status of the region's population. Health indicators are used to measure what impact the plan has on the health of the region. Only peripheral attention is given to output indicators because these are perceived mainly as means to the end of improved personal health. For example, whether the surgical team produces a lower level of necessary operations or the number of persons receiving health treatments is increased is secondary to whether they produce a positive impact on the health status indicators that measure the population's health.

The plan should focus on the causes of health problems, regardless of where they are located. The high infant mortality rates of minority groups may be due to poor nutrition or a pregnant woman's failure to receive medical attention until the very end of her pregnancy. However, a deeper analysis may show that caring for several young children with no help; an inadequate welfare budget; living in a drafty, vermin-infested apartment; and breathing the black smoke issuing from apartment buildings around an expectant mother are the more relevant causes of her difficulties. These socioeconomic conditions in turn reflect themselves in such health indicators as high infant mortality or morbidity rates among minority groups. It may be necessary to deal with all causes of the problem simultaneously in order to make an appreciable impact on a high infant mortality indicator. In treating the causes, the focus is primarily on preventing the illness while taking short-term steps to treat people with the symptoms.

In order to deal with the causes of problems, the plan should map out an implementation strategy whereby the health planning agency takes initiatives in both studying and taking action to implement the plan's objectives. It is anticipated that most of the changes sought would result in structural changes both in the health system and the nonhealth systems such as welfare, education, and employment that impact on the population's health.

Most long- and short-range health plans are intended to reach this level of comprehensiveness and detail. However, the first generation of health plans are skewed in favor of medical treatment and show less concern for nonhealth forces that affect health. Environment, socioeconomic, and cultural factors are often recognized in the health plans as causes of numerous diseases, but little is done to deal with them. Most plans are oriented toward symptoms rather than causes.

Partnership Model

In the partnership model, the plan is general in nature, with an arbitrary selection of health issues to which the agency addresses itself. There is no systematic analysis of all the factors that affect the population's health. The primary focus is on those elements of the delivery system that have an impact on personal health care, such as ambulatory care, hospitals, or long-term health care facilities. Some attention is generally paid to those environmental issues such as air or water pollution on which the public demands the agency's response. Almost no attention is given to socioeconomic health-related factors. The plan itself is incomplete. The agency defines the problems of those health issues it studies and offers policies and goal recommendations. However, it may or may not suggest a plan of action or specific program actions required to resolve the problems. These are left to the discretion of the individual and independent health institutions to carry out with encouragement from the agency. The plan focuses mainly on the inputs to improve the delivery system such as personnel needs, addition of ambulatory services, or introduction of new technologies to improve health care treatment. The agency generally does not provide evaluations of these changes and may not even monitor the parts of its goals and policies that are implemented by health institutions. Any evaluation that takes place is done by the implementing institutions themselves and may not be made available to the agency.

Because the health issues studied by the agency are arbitrarily selected, often in response to public demand or health crisis, the partnership model planning agency may emphasize prevention of illness, but more likely it will focus on improving the delivery system that treats persons who already are ill. Consequently, the agency reacts to demands made upon it rather than initiates actions for study and implementation. Neither does the agency offer structural changes in the health system, but more likely suggests modifications in the existing system to which the health providers can readily adapt.

The diagnosis and policy recommendations offered by Cervantes with respect to improving services to urban Mexican-Americans is an example of a policy plan that reacts to a negative health situation and asks for adaptations in that system to accommodate the needs of an urban minority group.[39] In this respect, he sums up his recommendations with emphasis on "C-care": congenial, courteous, convenient, complete, consistent, and compassionate. Similarly, Clark's recommendation for "medical regionalization," in which community health institutions, especially hospitals, are linked to university medical schools, focuses on personal health care, the need for prevention, and the involvement of the consumer.[40] The emphasis of his plan is on an improvement in the health delivery system and the inputs required to improve it. It is assumed that these improvements will produce positive effects on health status indicators. All the problems he defines are related to personal health care and deficiencies in the health delivery system. He accepts the existing health care system but cites the need for its integration and modifications of services.

Alliance Model

The plan that is produced in the alliance model is very similar to the partnership model plan; differences are only minor. The primary differences are in the degree of comprehensiveness and the focus of the planning process. The alliance model planning agency is mainly concerned with only one component of the personal health care system, such as ambulatory care, special health problems of the elderly, or drug abuse. It considers only one health issue at a time. However, with respect to that issue, it not only identifies goals and policies, but also aggressively initiates an action plan. This is possible because the actors involved are generally health providers who recognize the nature of the problem and are in a position to take action with respect to it. The only other difference from the partnership model is that the agency is seldom concerned with prevention and causes of illness. Instead, it focuses on treating the symptoms of illness or on improving the health delivery system itself. It accepts the existing health system but may offer slight adaptive changes to it. Basically, the overall emphasis is on the maintenance of the medical system.

Daniels' study of the "Mid-Southside Health Planning Organization" of Chicago exemplifies this type of plan.[41] Its major interest is on one segment of personal health care, providing ambulatory care to a minority group. The goal was to translate a number of basic principles such as universal eligibility, ease of accessibility, and continuity of care into reality through the development of an HMO. The health provider and the community health-oriented organizations collaborated to design the plan and submitted a proposal for its implementation, which was eventually accepted by the Office of Economic Opportunity. In this case, the alliance took the initiative in the planning, and the health planning agency of Chicago at first reacted negatively to the subarea's initiative. It wanted to control the grant that would result from the proposal, but later embraced it after political pressure was exerted by the subarea body. The plan aimed at providing an integrated delivery system to replace highly fragmented and unreliable health services then available to the residents. This study illustrates how an alliance can convert a need into an action plan.

Individual Action Model

The individual action model is primarily concerned with project type planning in which a very narrow segment of the medical system, such as the improvement of a surgical unit of a community hospital, is demanded by residents of one part of the region through their representatives on the planning agency. As such, the project plan is a reaction to a medical need with an emphasis on improving the delivery system, particularly increasing personnel or facilities for a small segment of the region. Only occasionally does a participative model plan represent a structural change in the system, and this only occurs on a "demonstration" basis. There is, thus, very little emphasis on changing the system; instead, there is a concern with its maintenance and achieving equity in the allocation of medical services to minority or other disadvantaged groups. Most planning agency studies for a specific geographical area, population, or health facility are representative of this type of planning, provided the study goes beyond recommendations into plan implementation.

NOTES

1. Robert A. Cervantes, "The Failure of Comprehensive Services to Serve the Urban Chicanos," *Health Services Reports* 87 (December 1972): 932–40.

2. Melvin H. Rudov and Nancy Santangelo, *Health Status of Minorities and Low-Income Groups,* No. HRA 79-627 (U.S.DHEW: Health Resources Administration, Office of Health Resources Opportunity, 1979).

3. *Ibid.,* Table 7, p. 47.

4. U.S.DHEW, "Children and Youth: Health Status and Use of Health Services," in *Health: United States—1978* (Hyattsville, Md.: Office of the Assistant Secretary for Health, December 1978).

5. U.S.DHEW, *EPSD&T: The Possible Dream,* No. 77-24973 (Washington, D.C.: Health Care Financing Administration, 1977).

6. John B. DeHoff, "Health Care Delivery Systems: What's Here, What's Coming," *Maryland State Medical Journal,* October 1972, pp. 44–48.

7. Ernest W. Saward, "The Organization of Medical Care," *Scientific American,* September 1973, pp. 169–175.

8. U.S. Congress, *Conference Report on National Health Planning and Resources Development Act of 1974,* 93rd Congress, December 19, 1974, pp. 4–5.

9. U.S.DHEW, *Health: United States—1978,* Tables 125 and 128.

10. U.S. Comptroller General, *Report to the Congress: Health Maintenance Organizations Can Help Control Health Care Costs,* PAD 80-17 (U. S. General Accounting Office, May 6, 1980), Table 2, p. 11.

11. U.S.DHEW, *Promoting Health: Issues and Strategies* (Washington, D.C.: Office of Health Information and Health Promotion, 1979), p. 3.

12. American Association of Comprehensive Health Planning, *American Journal of Health Planning,* no. 1 (July 1976).

13. U.S.DHEW, *Healthy People: The Surgeon General's Report on Health Promotion and Disease Prevention,* no. 017-001-00416-2 (Washington, D.C.: U.S. Government Printing Office, 1979).

14. U.S.DHEW, *Promoting Health,* p. 8.

15. Donald M. Vickery and James F. Fries, *Take Care of Yourself: A Consumer's Guide to Medical Care* (Reading, Mass.: Addison-Wesley Publishing Company, 1977).

16. U.S.DHEW, *Controlling the Cost of Health Care*, Policy Research Series (National Center for Health Services Research, May 1977).

17. *Ibid.*, p. 4.

18. *Ibid.*, p. 17.

19. Andrew A. Sorensen, Richard P. Wersinger, et al., "Commentary: A Note on the Comparison of the Hospital Cost Experience of Three Competing HMOs," *Inquiry* 16 (Summer 1979): 167–171.

20. J. William Gavett and David B. Smith, "A Comparison of the Hospital Cost Experience of Three Competing HMOs," *Inquiry* 15 (December 1978): 327–335.

21. Symond R. Gottlieb, "Reducing Excess Hospital Capacity Is a Tough But Necessary Job," *Hospitals, Journal of the American Hospital Association* 52 (December 1978): 63–68.

22. Health Resources Administration, *Societal Factors and Excess Hospital Beds—An Exploratory Study*, (under contract to Lewin and Associates, Inc.), vol. 2, June 1979.

23. "Health Leaders Join in Attacking Hospital Cost Control Proposal," *American Medical News*, March 23, 1979.

24. Karl D. Yordy, "National Planning for Health: An Emerging Reality," *Bulletin of New York Academy of Medicine* 48 (January 1972): 32–38.

25. Eli Ginzberg, *Men, Money and Medicine;* Rene Dubos, *Men, Medicine and Environment* (New York: Praeger Publishers, Inc., 1969).

26. U.S.DHEW, *Health: United States—1978*, Chapter VI.

27. *Ibid.*, Chapter VI.

28. *Ibid.*

29. *Ibid.*

30. *Ibid.*

31. Donald L. Madison and Budd N. Shenkin, *Preparing to Serve—NHSC Scholarships and Medical Education*, Public Health Reports 95, no. 1 (January-February 1980): 3–8.

32. Carolyn R. Kohn, *Access to Health Care* (National Academy of Medicine: Institute of Medicine, Division of Health Services, May, 1980), pp. 2–5.

33. *Ibid.*, Chapter 4.

34. *Ibid.*, p. 5–3.

35. Philip G. Cotterill and Barry S. Eisenberg, "Improving Access to Medical Care in Underserved Areas: The Role of Group Practice," *Inquiry* 17 (Summer 1979): 141–153.

36. Information for this section is taken mainly from U.S.DHEW, *Forward Plan for Health: FY 1978–1982* (Washington, D.C.: Public Health Service, August 1976), pp. 80–82; "Mental Disorders," in U.S.DHEW, *Health: United States—1978*, Chapter IV.

37. Gerald L. Klerman, *Dealing with Alcohol and Drug Abuse and Mental Illness*, Public Health Reports, vol. 93 (November-December 1978): 626.

38. Herbert H. Hyman, "Most Important Regional and State HSP/AIP Objectives" mimeographed (New York, N.Y.: DHHS Region II Division of Health Resources Development, Public Health Service, October 1978).

39. Cervantes, "Failure of Comprehensive Services."

40. Harry T. Clark, Jr., "Planning a More Effective Health Care System," *Inquiry* supplement (March 1973): 40–45.

41. Robert S. Daniels, James W. Wagner, and Lloyd A. Ferguson, "An Example of Subregional Health Planning: A Further Report," *Inquiry* 9 (September 1972): 57–62.

Appendix 12-A

AGPLAN Key Words

AGPLAN KEY WORDS RELATED TO SECTION 1501

The following phrases represent the key words used to extract goals and objectives programmed into the computer as part of the AGPLAN project. All goals or objectives that contain any reference to "Med/Sur bed supply" can be elicited by punching in this key phrase. The same is true for goals or objectives related to primary care, medically underserved areas, etc. An example of this process is shown at the end of this appendix.

- Med/Sur bed supply
- Med/Sur bed occupancy
- OB inpatient services
- Neonatal care units
- Ped bed supply
- Ped bed occupancy
- Open heart surgery
- Cardiac cath
- Radiation therapy
- CAT scan
- End-stage renal dialysis (ESRD)

1. Primary care
   Individual health protective services
   Detection services
   Ambulatory care
2. Medically underserved
   Physician shortage
3. Rural areas
   Isolated areas
4. Economically depressed
   Poor
   Impoverished
   Low-income
5. Multiinstitutional systems
   Coordination and consolidation of institutional health services
   Referral patterns
   Regionalized tertiary services

6. EMS
7. Medical group practices
    Medical partnerships
    Multispecialty groups
    Prepaid group practice
8. HMO
    Prepaid health plans
9. Physician's assistants
    Physician extenders
    Paramedics
10. Nurse clinicians
    Nurse practitioners
    Nurse midwives
11. Shared services
    Sharing medical records
    Purchase of drugs
    Hospital management
12. Quality of care
    Quality for medical care in hospital
    In-service education
    Tissue review
    Medical review
    Peer review
    Utilization review
13. PSRO
14. Comprehensive health services
    Consolidated health services
    Integrated health services
15. Geo integrated services
16. Disease prevention
    Nutrition
    Environment
    Occupational safety
    Food protection
    Radiation safety
    Biomedical and consumer product safety
    Sanitation
    Fluoridation
    Screening
    Immunization
    Dental prophylaxis

17. Uniform cost accounting
    Financial accounts
    Cost centers
    Operational costs
18. Reimbursement system
    Rate review
    Rate regulation
    Third party payments
    Health insurance
19. Utilization reporting system
    Professional activity study
    Uniform hospital discharge
    Data sets
    Medical audit program
20. Management procedures
    Hospital administration
    Management information systems
21. Health Education
    Health promotion
22. Minority
23. Handicapped
24. Women
    Geriatrics
    Senior citizens
    Aging

The following are two examples showing the relationship between goals and the use of AGPLAN's key words to extract them from the computer.

Example 3:
Goal: Promote the development of comprehensive community health
  education programs.
The goal does not need further enhancement as it already contains key word descriptor (Health education).

Goal: The incidence of venereal disease should be stabilized by 1990 and
  eventually reduced. (Health education)
Recommended action: . . . through health education in the schools and the community, improved case finding, and better treatment, the incidence of untreated cases, and thus ultimately of VD will decrease. This goal should be enhanced to include the key word descriptor (Health education).

Example 5:
Goal: Increase the financial and geographic accessibility of dental care and dental hygiene services by 1985. (Health education) (Rural areas) (Medical group practices) (Disease prevention)

Recommended action: Promotion of school *health education,* establishment of satellite dental clinics in *isolated areas, prepaid financial arrangements* and *nutrition* education. [Emphasis added.]

Chapter 13

The Planning Process in Action: The Systems Approach

A case study of New York City's health Planning District E can be used to illustrate the systems approach to health planning. District E is located on the upper west side of Manhattan, adjacent to the Hudson River. It is one of the 33 health planning districts into which the New York City health planning agency has been subdivided. District E encompasses two community planning districts, 9 and 12, and some 300,000 persons reside in the area (Figure 13-1).

The case illustration uses a systems approach to planning patterned after the *National Health Planning Guidelines* and Palmer's "An Advanced Health Planning System" model.[1] The facts, data, and references to groups are true where such information is available; for the most part, however, they are based on simulated data on what is known about the district. The systems approach is used because of the emphasis it is given in the National Health Planning and Resources Development Act of 1974. Under this legislation, each health planning agency is mandated to develop long- and short-range plans. In this illustration, only a long-range plan will be developed. The steps in the planning process are shown in Table 13-1.

Table 13-1 Basic Steps in Systems Planning Process

Basic Steps	Phase	Title
Base case	I	Introduction; collect data
	II	Predict consequences of present programs
Goals/objectives	III	Analyze desired outcomes
	IV	Set goals and objectives
Long-range recommended actions	V	Identify alternative actions
Resource requirements	VI	Estimate resources needed
	VII	Evaluate and select priority plan

Figure 13-1   Location of District E in Manhattan

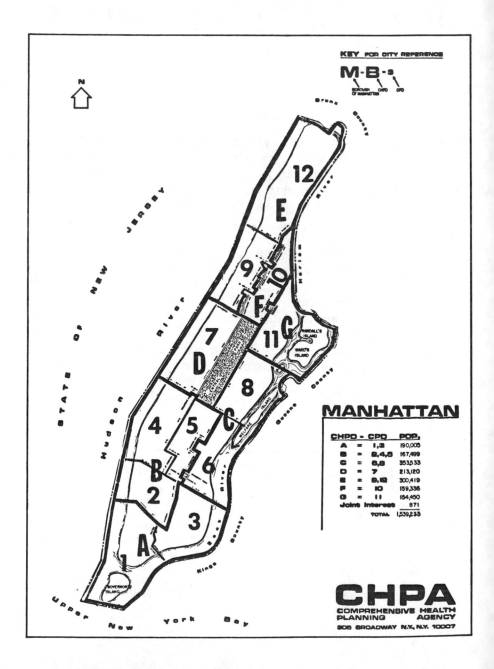

BASE CASE

The base case includes the collection of data that are relevant to the district's health needs and resources, a demographic description, and the estimation of potential gaps between need and service. The base case describes what has occurred, what currently exists, and what is likely to happen if nothing is done to change the health system in the future. In this case study, the forecasts are made for the year 1985, and the current year in which the plan is being developed is 1980. Health indicators are used as surrogate measures to state objectives of desired health system outcomes, especially of what happens to people using health services. Indicators are defined by the planning guidelines as

> quantifiable measures chosen to reflect the health status of the population or to represent how well the health system is perform- ing. Direct indicators (such as infant mortality or disability days, and cost per patient day . . .) measure the level and/or change in community health and in health systems performance. Indirect indicators (such as percent of the area population with incomes below the poverty level . . .) indicate social or environmental conditions which have been attributed to affecting the health of the area's residents.[2]

Three basic components of health are involved in the analysis of the health system. These are the health status of persons who use or are likely to use health services; the health system, which is primarily concerned with the functioning of the health delivery system itself, such as hospitals, clinics, mobile units, and personnel needed to operate these; and the health-related environment, which refers to the housing, income levels, transportation system, education, and other basic services that have a major impact on the health of people and the operation of the health system. Traditionally, little emphasis has been placed on the health-related environment, and it is not likely that, in spite of its impact on the health of people, much more attention will be paid to it in terms of actual health plans developed in the near future under the systems approach. The importance of including this component in a diagnosis of the district, even if in a peripheral manner, is to alert the governing board to its potential influence in solving problems that cannot be affected by health care inter- ventions only. As can be seen in this case illustration, awareness of the impact of the environment is noted in the base case, but is not taken greatly into account in the actual formulation of the district's health plan.

Introduction: Conceptual Framework

The long-range plan has five broad goals:

1. to restrain health care cost increases
2. to promote a healthful environment
3. to reduce gaps and inefficiencies in the health system
4. to improve the health of the community's residents
5. to emphasize prevention and early treatment of disease.

It is necessary to understand how the health care system must be reorganized in order to reach these goals. The New Jersey State Health Plan offers an excellent conceptualization that clearly demonstrates the differences between the present and proposed health systems.[3] Figure 13-2 depicts the proposed system as a pyramid in which preventive and primary care services are emphasized at the community level. These are the services most used by the population. General hospital inpatient services, long-term nursing care, mental health services, and other such secondary care services that require a larger population base than is available at the community level are offered at the subregional level. At the top of the pyramid, specialized services are offered at the regional or state levels. Such services might include burn units, blood banks, trauma centers, and renal transplant centers. Figure 13-3 shows the full range of services that should normally be offered at each of the three levels; this reorganization of services takes into account five major trends that have been occurring in the health care field:

1. Growth in the national economy is limiting the capacity of the health care system to grow.[4]
2. Acute care hospitals can no longer operate as autonomous units of service. Sharing and integration of services are being demanded to conserve scarce resources.
3. Through various forms of regulation, Congress and the executive branch of government are increasing restrictions on the use and expansion of medical services.
4. A growing interrelationship between health providers and the general public is making each more sensitive and responsive to the needs and demands of the other.
5. The organization and role of health professionals is changing as consumers put more stress on taking charge of their personal health needs and are accepting less costly, but appropriate services such as ambulatory surgery and physician's assistants.

Figure 13-2 A Model for Organizing the Health Care System

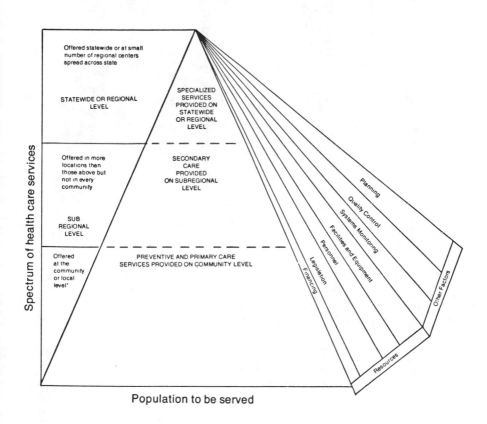

*Some of these services, because of factors associated with their efficient delivery, should be planned and administered at the subregional level but offered with easy access to everyone.

Source: Adapted from the New Jersey State Health Plan: 1978–1982, Vol. 1 (Trenton, N.J.: New Jersey State Department of Health), Section 3, p. 10.

Figure 13-3 The Health Care System of the Future

Services which should be offered Statewide or at a small number of regional centers spread across the State.

**STATEWIDE
OR
REGIONAL
LEVEL**

SPECIALIZED SERVICES OFFERED ON A STATEWIDE OR REGIONAL BASIS

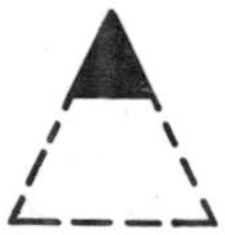

1. Burn Units and Centers
2. Blood Banking
3. Organ Banking
4. Cardiac Surgical Centers
5. Level II and Level III Perinatal Centers
6. Renal Transplant Centers and Histocompatibility Laboratories
7. Complex Neurosurgery Services
8. Trauma Centers
9. Rehabilitation Center Services
10. CAT Scanners
11. Megavoltage Radiation Oncology Units

EXAMPLES OF BENEFITS

Closure and consolidation of excess capacity will result in:

1. Lowering costs
2. Increasing efficiency by improved utilization
3. Improving quality by insuring volumes necessary to maintain staff proficiency
4. Reducing lengths of stay (LOS) because of increased demands on services—thereby encouraging referral below
5. Discouraging unnecessary admissions

EXAMPLES OF NEEDED CHANGES

1. Adequate support services after patient leaves this setting:
   a. Home health services
   b. Outpatient rehabilitation services
   c. Expanded ambulatory care opportunities
2. Improved utilization review
3. Implementation of Federal Guidelines, State Planning and Licensure Regulations

Figure 13-3 Continued

SUBREGIONAL LEVEL

Services offered in more locations than the specialized services noted above but not offered in every community.

SECONDARY CARE PROVIDED ON SUBREGIONAL LEVEL

1. General hospital inpatient services including
   a. Medical-Surgical Services
   b. Obstetrics—Level I
   c. Pediatrics
   d. Psychiatric
   e. Intensive Care Unit
   f. Coronary Care Unit
   g. Diagnostic Radiology (excluding the CAT Scanner)
   h. Emergency Department Services
   i. Physical Medicine and Rehabilitation
2. Long-Term Nursing Care
   a. Skilled Nursing Care
   b. Intermediate Nursing Care
   c. Boarding Care
3. Behavioral Health Services
   a. Drug Abuse, Alcohol, and Mental Health
   b. Mental Retardation/Developmental Disabilities
4. Renal Dialysis Services
5. Emergency Transport Services—Advanced Life Support Services
6. Home Health Services (Planning and Administration)
7. Health Maintenance Organizations

EXAMPLES OF BENEFITS

1. Increased utilization resulting in cost savings and encouraging a reduction in LOS
2. Improved alternatives to inpatient care through increased opportunities for ambulatory care
3. Elimination of costly excess capacity through regionalization
4. Increased accessibility throughout the system

EXAMPLES OF NEEDED CHANGES

1. Expanded alternatives to inpatient care—Examples:
   a. Home Health, Outpatient Rehabilitation
   b. Increased ambulatory services at community level
   c. Third party financing of ambulatory care
2. Improved transportation networks from below
3. Emergency transport to level above
4. Implementation of Federal Guidelines, State Planning and Licensing Regulations
5. Utilization Review

Figure 13-3   Continued

8. Burn Programs
9. Specialized Dental Care
10. Ambulatory Surgery
11. Homemaker Services (Planning and Administration)

6. Improved Scheduling of Elective Admissions
7. Preadmission Testing

COMMUNITY PREVENTIVE AND PRIMARY CARE SERVICES

EXAMPLES OF BENEFITS

Prevention and Health Promotion Services

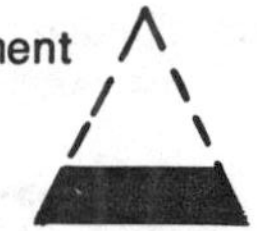

1. Child Growth and Development Surveillance
2. Family Planning
3. Immunizations
4. Hearing, Speech and Vision Screening and Follow-Up
5. Nutritional Status Screening
6. Cervical Cancer Screening and Referral
7. Hypertension Diagnosis and Medical Management
8. Periodic Physical Examinations
9. Personal and Family Health Education
10. School Health Programs
11. Walk-In Mental Health Centers
12. Environmental Health Programs (e.g., air and water control, fluoridation of waters)

1. Prevention of disease
2. Early diagnosis and treatment of problems
3. Viable alternatives to institutionalization
4. Cost savings

EXAMPLES OF NEEDED CHANGES

1. Organized transport systems to services at this level and above
2. Third party coverage for ambulatory care and preventive services
3. Additional financing for improved public health programs
4. Efficient employment of paraprofessionals

Services offered at the community or local level*

*Some of these services, because of factors related to their efficient delivery, should be planned and administered at the subregional level but offered with easy access by everyone.

Figure 13-3 Continued

COMMUNITY PREVENTIVE AND PRIMARY CARE SERVICES	EXAMPLES OF BENEFITS

13. Occupational Health Programs
14. Lead-Paint Screening and Follow-Up
15. Screenings and Referrals for Other Specific Diseases
16. Crisis Intervention—e.g., Suicide Prevention

Acute Ambulatory Care

1. Medical
   a. Eye Care
   b. Emergency First Aid
   c. Injections
   d. Nutrition Counseling and Education
   e. Office Visits
   f. Physical Therapy
   g. Pre-Natal and Post-Natal Care
   h. Prescription Drugs
   i. Speech Therapy
2. Dental Health—Extractions and Restorations
3. Mental Health—Diagnosis and Treatment

Source: Adapted from the New Jersey State Health Plan: 1978–1982, Vol. 1 (Trenton, N.J.: New Jersey State Department of Health), Section 3, pp. 11–13.

These trends collectively foster a more efficient health care system that emphasizes prevention, early diagnosis, and primary care, all of which are offered at the community level. At the same time, efficient use of high-cost medical services will become even more essential as resources are either limited or transferred to other health care uses. Regionalization of specialized services, elimination of excess acute care beds, and use of less costly medical interventions already have been introduced to improve efficiency. Regulatory measures, such as PSROs, appropriateness review, certificate of need, and prospective rate reimbursement have also been aimed at reducing medical costs.

In contrast to the triangle-shaped model of the proposed health care systems model (Figure 13-2), the current medical model can be depicted in the shape of a diamond with the largest expenditures for subregional highly specialized and acute care hospital services while minimal services are offered at the community level and the regional/state levels (Figure 13-4). Detailed examples of how the medical model currently functions are given in Figure 13-5.

Demography

Of the 300,000 people residing in District E, 62 percent live in Community Planning District (CPD) 12, and 38 percent in CPD 9. The population in the district has declined by 9 percent since 1960, which compares with a similar decrease in the population in the City of New York in the same period. During this period, the decline in the white population has been almost 18 percent, compared to an increase in minority population of 5 percent. The white population, nevertheless, continues to be the dominant group, with 67 percent of the total population in the district. A comparison of the two CPDs shows a vastly different white-nonwhite balance in each. CPD 12 has 81 percent whites while CPD 9 has only 43 percent. Thus, not only is the population in the district declining, but a major exchange is also taking place among the races from white to minority groups; the preponderance of the whites live in CPD 12 and of the minority groups in CPD 9.

The two CPDs also show differences with respect to age. Seventeen percent of the CPD 12 population are 65 and over compared to 11 percent for CPD 9. At the other end of the age distribution, there is no difference among those under 15 years old, who make up 18 percent of the population in both districts. Nor is there a significant difference in sex distribution— 53 percent females and 47 percent males in both CPDs.

Using a cohort survival population projection, further population changes through 1980 have been forecast. These show a district population

Figure 13-4 The Existing Organization of Health Services—A Medical Model

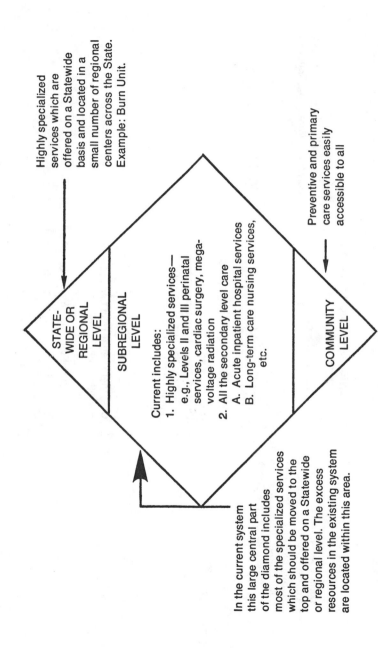

Highly specialized services which are offered on a Statewide basis and located in a small number of regional centers across the State. Example: Burn Unit.

STATE-WIDE OR REGIONAL LEVEL

SUBREGIONAL LEVEL

Current includes:
1. Highly specialized services—e.g., Levels II and III perinatal services, cardiac surgery, megavoltage radiation
2. All the secondary level care
   A. Acute inpatient hospital services
   B. Long-term care nursing services, etc.

Preventive and primary care services easily accessible to all

COMMUNITY LEVEL

In the current system this large central part of the diamond includes most of the specialized services which should be moved to the top and offered on a Statewide or regional level. The excess resources in the existing system are located within this area.

Source: Adapted from the New Jersey State Health Plan: 1978–1982, Vol. 1 (Trenton, N.J.: New Jersey State Department of Health), Section 3, p. 15.

Figure 13-5   The Existing System*

Highly specialized services which
are currently offered on a *Statewide*
or *Regional Basis* (located in a
small number of regional centers
spread across the State)

STATEWIDE OR REGIONAL LEVEL

Examples of existing services
currently offered on a *Statewide*
or *Regional* basis:
Burn units

Problems with the Existing Organization

There are not enough highly specialized
medical services regionalized at this
level. As a result there are excess
resources at the subregional level
resulting in:

A. Underutilization of expensive inpatient
    services
B. Cost inefficiency resulting in the waste
    of millions of dollars
C. Increased Lengths of Stay
D. Low Patient Volume and Unnecessary Risks
    to Patients
E. Unnecessary Admissions
F. Increased Indigency

*Darkened areas refer to the portion of the diamond (the shape of the existing system) being discussed.

Figure 13-5 Continued

SUBREGIONAL LEVEL

Services currently offered on a
Subregional Basis

Examples of existing services currently
offered on a Subregional Basis:

1. General hospital acute inpatient
   services
   a. Medical-surgical
   b. Obstetrical-Level I perinatal
      care
   c. Pediatric
   d. Psychiatric
2. Highly specialized tertiary services
   a. Level II and III perinatal
   b. Cardiac surgery and cardiac
      diagnostics
   c. Radiation therapy
   d. Renal disease services
   e. Hemophilia service
   f. Computerized axial tomography
   g. Trauma services

Figure 13-5 Continued

3. Long-term care services
   a. Skilled nursing care
   b. Intermediate nursing care
   c. Boarding homes
4. Chemical dependency services
5. Home health services
6. Mental health services
7. Ambulatory surgery
8. Developmental disabilities services
9. Rehabilitation services
10. Health maintenance organizations
11. Other ambulatory care services

Problems with the Existing Organization

1. Excess resources at this level—e.g., approximately 3,000 excess hospital beds statewide. (See below)
2. Underutilization of existing services:
   a. Obstetrical services
   b. Cardiac services
   c. Megavoltage radiation services
   d. Pediatric services
   e. Medical-surgical beds
3. Overutilization of:
   a. Hospital emergency rooms
   b. Hospitals as entry level into system
4. Increased Lengths of Stay

Figure 13-5 Continued

5. Many of the services—particularly the expensive tertiary services—are not serving a wide enough service area and need to be regionalized.

6. Results
   a. High unit cost results from the underutilization of inpatient beds and services.
   b. Lowered quality of care and increased risks to patients because many of the specialized services are not generating adequate patient volumes to insure staff proficiency.
   c. Inadequate alternatives to inpatient care.
   d. Increased indigency.

Figure 13-5 Continued

COMMUNITY LEVEL

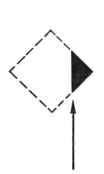

Services offered at the
*community or local
level*

Problems with the Existing Organization

1. Large unmet need for:
   a. Preventive and health promotion
      services
   b. Primary care services
   c. Acute ambulatory care services
2. Some services currently offered at
   this level should be planned at
   levels above—e.g., emergency medical
   services
3. Inadequate third party financing
   of preventive, primary care, and
   acute ambulatory services
4. Inadequate alternatives
   to inpatient care

Examples of the general types of
services currently offered at
community level
1. Public health programs
2. Preventive services
3. Primary care services
4. Emergency medical services

Source: Adapted from the New Jersey State Health Plan: 1978–1982, Vol. 1 (Trenton, N.J.: New Jersey State Department of Health),
Section 3, pp. 16-19.

of 314,000, a gain of 4 percent over the 1970 population. However, the gains come mainly among the under-14 population in CPD 12 with a 28 percent increase, and in the over-65 populations in both CPD 9 and 12 where increases of 16 percent and 10 percent respectively are predicted. In contrast, the adult working population (15 to 64 years) either shows a modest increase (4 percent in CPD 9), or an actual loss (3 percent in CPD 12). This forecast continues the trend that started in the 1960s when the white population of CPD 12 began leaving the area, and the younger minority population with small children began moving into CPD 9. A significant increase of 19 percent is expected in the over-65 population of CPD 9, but that still represents only 30 percent of the aged in the district. Seventy percent of the over-65 population will continue to reside in CPD 12.

Socioeconomic Status of District

The socioeconomic index was proposed as a way of measuring the health-related environmental factors of the district and how the CPDs compared with each other. The index is composed of three factors: education, median income, and overcrowding. The three factors used in the scale were chosen because data related to them are easily obtainable from the 1970 census. A 12-point scale, ranging from a plus six to a minus six, which is referred to as the SES Rating Scale, was developed. This scale was then divided into five levels of environmental well-being: upper if the rating was 4 to 6; upper middle, 1 to 3; middle, 0; lower middle, −1 to −3; and lower, −4 to −6. The standard against which the CPDs were measured was the Manhattan borough of New York City, chosen because the residents and conditions of the district were most influenced by the activities of the borough of Manhattan rather than the city as a whole. The three indicators chosen for comparison were median family income, percentage of the population over 18 years old with four years of high school, and percentage of overcrowded household units (over 1.5 persons per room). The central value of the borough was used as the norm and a rating of plus two to minus two could be given, depending on how the CPDs compared to the borough. For example, the standard of the median family income for Manhattan was $8,983 in 1970. On the basis of the scale shown in Table 13-2, CPD 12 would receive a 0 rating and CPD 9, a −1 rating on the income factor. In like manner, the other two factors were measured against the Manhattan standard. The scores of each of these three factors were then totaled. The final total of the factors represented the location of the CPDs on the SES Rating Scale. The maximum positive score a CPD could receive was six (a rating of two on each of the three factors), and

Table 13-2   Ratings of CPDs 9 and 12 on Income Scale

If income is	The rating is	CPD 12	CPD 9
<$4,492	−2 (50% less than standard)		
$4,492 to $8,534	−1 (from 6% to 50% of standard)		$7,717
$8,534 to $9,432	0 (from 5% less to 5% more than standard)	$8,879	
$9,432 to $13,474	+1 (between 6% to 50% over standard)		
>$13,474	+2 (more than 50% above standard)		

that would represent an "upper-upper" level of environmental well-being.

On the basis of this index, the two CPDs had the profiles shown in Table 13-3. Based on the rating, CPD 12 has a middle SES rating; CPD 9, a lower middle SES rating. The implications of this rating should alert the planners and the district governing board to the potential greater negative impact of environmental factors on the health of the residents of CPD 9.

Health Status Indicators

The wellness of the population in the district is measured by health status indicators. These are taken from the Department of Health's Vital Statistics for 1980 and compared with the Manhattan borough measures.

Table 13-3   SES Ratings of CPDs 9 and 12 by Income, Education, and Overcrowding

Factor	CPD 12 Value	Rating	CPD 9 Value	Rating	Manhattan (Standard)
Education	50.4%	−1	48.2%	−1	57.11%
Income	$8,879	0	$7,717	−1	$8,983
Overcrowding	2.64%	+1	3.65%	0	3.63%
Total SES rating		0 (middle)		−2 (lower middle)	

With respect to deaths caused by accidents, suicides, homicides, and drug dependence, the district had a lower rate by 10 percent (for accidental death) to 35 percent (for homicidal death) than the borough of Manhattan. With respect to some selected morbidity rates, the district had lower rates per 100,000 population on venereal disease, hepatitis, lead poisoning, measles, and tuberculosis than the borough of Manhattan. For example, it had a 60 percent lower hepatitis rate than did Manhattan; 60 percent lower rate of measles; and 25 percent lower rate of lead poisoning. In a population health survey carried out by the health department, it was found that in every age cohort a significantly high percentage of persons surveyed in the district, compared to those in New York City as a whole, reported they were in excellent health (Table 13-4). The survey also indicated that for all age categories, except the 5 to 14 years cohort, the residents of CPD 9 reported higher rates of excellent health than did those in CPD 12. When this finding is compared to the SES Rating Index, which shows CPD 9 to have a lower index than CPD 12, it raises the question of whether a correlation exists in this district between environmental factors and a person's sense of well-being. One would have anticipated a lower rate of reported excellent health for CPD 9 than 12 on the basis of the SES Rating Index.

Likewise, when the population's health status in the CPDs was compared to that in New York City on the basis of income, it was found that, in every income grouping, the CPD residents reported a higher rate of excellent health than did those of New York City (Table 13-5). The data also show that, in four of the six income categories, a greater percentage of CPD 9 residents reported excellent health than did those in CPD 12. In CPD 12 and New York City, the pattern holds true that, as income rises, there are higher percentages of persons reporting excellent health. This is not true for CPD 9, however.

Table 13-4 Comparison of Population's Health Status by Location and Age (in percentages)

Reported Excellent Health	Age				
	0-4	5-14	15-44	45-64	65 plus
CPD 9	74	31	58	33	32
CPD 12	56	52	49	27	15
New York City	41	36	39	21	11

Table 13-5   Health of CPDs 9 and 12 by Annual Income Levels

Reported Excellent Health	Income*					
	$0-29	$30-49	$50-69	$70-99	$100-149	$150 plus
CPD 9	63	47	26	74	40	70
CPD 12	19	21	34	58	57	59
New York City	18	20	25	31	38	42

*Expressed in hundreds. All entries are in percentages.

The general health status indicators for the district compared to Manhattan or New York City suggest that the district is generally healthier, by both objective reporting of morbidity and mortality rates and by the residents' own self-perceptions of their health, than the rest of New York City.

Health System Indicators

The health system indicators generally measure how well the health delivery system is functioning in providing the services needed by the residents of the community. The two general categories for comparison are availability of hospital beds per 1,000 population and availability of ambulatory medical services.

Hospital Beds

The district is fortunate in having seven hospitals that provide general and specialized care. They provide a total of 3,100 beds or about 10 beds per 1,000 population, which is more than double the 4.5 national average and about twice New York City's average of 5.2 beds per 1,000 population. Counted among these hospitals are two large general medical centers, St. Luke's with a bed complement of 705 and Columbia-Presbyterian Hospital with 1,488 beds. The other hospitals are satellite community or specialized hospitals. While on the surface there would appear to be more than sufficient beds to meet local population needs, it is unknown how many of these hospital beds really serve the district population. Columbia-Presbyterian Hospital accepts patients from the entire metropolitan area and nation, while St. Luke's receives patients from all over Manhattan. Jewish Memorial Hospital, with 200 beds, serves numerous residents from the borough of the Bronx. Thus, without a patient origin survey, it is not possible to know how many of the beds are actually available for service to the district's population and whether there are sufficient beds to meet the population's needs.

Ambulatory Care Services

Ambulatory health facilities include outpatient or emergency room services of a hospital, a district health center, a physician's private office, or group practice services. Based on the population health survey, it was found that residents of the district made 5.6 visits per person annually. This compares favorably with 5.4 visits for the City of New York in the same period. The question is whether there are sufficient resources to meet the 1.7 million ambulatory visits required for the district's 300,000 population. An examination of various records reveals that there were 2,200,000 private physician office visits, 790,000 hospital/outpatient and emergency room visits, and 205,000 group practice visits. The 3.2 million visits represent what is potentially available in ambulatory care services located in the district. This is about 1.5 million more visits than are needed by the residents of the district itself. While there are no hard facts, it can be estimated that the surplus is taken up by residents of other districts, boroughs, or the metropolitan area.

It is known that less than 50 percent of the visits to Columbia-Presbyterian, St. Luke's, and Jewish Memorial outpatient/emergency room facilities are made by residents from the district. Although 520 physicians practice in the district, many have nonresident patients who are attracted by the physicians' affiliations with such prestigious hospitals as Columbia-Presbyterian and St. Luke's. Thus, while on the surface there appear to be sufficient ambulatory resources available, it is not certain whether they do in fact meet the needs of the district's population, especially those minority, low-income residents who reside in CPD 9. The forecast to 1985 reveals that the hospitals in the district have submitted applications for expanding their outpatient/emergency room facilities to serve an additional 250,000 patients annually. One can conclude that there should be sufficient ambulatory facilities to meet the population's needs after this expansion.

The planning agency's borough planning team reported the above facts and their finding to the district's citizen board. On the basis of the health status and system indicators, the board concurred that the general health needs of the district were being fairly well met. However, the board members, with the assistance of the health planners, decided to consider whether there might be some specific health issues that required closer examination. In this deeper analysis of the health system and the health status of the population, some 30 new health indicators were examined by the planning team meeting with the district's citizen board.

Using the Delbecq[5] nominal method in which each member of the district board was asked to identify two health problems or issues that affected the member personally or the member's constituency, the 15 members present identified 23 separate issues. The planners converted their ideas, with the members' consent, into two categories of health indicators:

- health status indicators
  1. percentage of children under 14 years old reported as abused
  2. percentage of children under 14 years old affected by lead poisoning
  3. frequency of lung cancer per 1,000 in adults, 18 years old and over
  4. number of children 13 to 19 years old per 1,000 with serious dental problems
  5. percentage of total population with a balanced diet
  6. population with hypertension per 1,000 by age, sex, and ethnicity
  7. disability due to chronic pulmonary dysfunction per 1,000
  8. children up to 3 months old visiting a physician for routine non-illness related matters, visits per 1,000 children
  9. inoculations of children per 1,000, 12 years old and under
  10. narcotic drug abuse per 1,000 by age cohorts, 14 years old and over
  11. number of admissions to psychiatric hospitals or units per 1,000 population
  12. number of persons per 1,000 visiting physician for a perceived illness
  13. percentage of population having chest x-rays in last calendar year
  14. persons with chronic mental illness per 1,000, 65 years old and over

- health system indicators
  15. number of radiologists per 1,000 population
  16. number of laboratory technicians per 1,000 population
  17. number of private, noninstitutional physicians practicing with offices in the district per 10,000 population
  18. number of institutional and patient advocates per 1,000 patients receiving care at an inpatient or group practice ambulatory care facility
  19. average length of waiting time per clinic visit
  20. number of physical therapist contact hours available per 1,000 permanently disabled persons
  21. number of drug-related outpatient visits per 1,000 persons with drug-related problems

22. ratio of direct to indirect support services available in all hospitals serving the district
23. number of psychiatric beds available for all age groups per 10,000 population.

The planners presented ten additional health problem issues. Of these, the committee agreed to accept seven for further study:

- health status indicators
    1. physical development disorders per 100 children, 7 years old and under
    2. reduction in the average length of hospital stay in a general hospital from the current 13.2 days

- health system indicators
    3. ratio of resources available to serve children with physical development disorders per 1,000 children, 7 years old and under.
    4. percentage of district residents with a "medical home" (i.e., their own family doctor or clinic where they are registered and accepted for treatment of medical services as needed)
    5. percentage of population, 14 years old and over, aware of correct entry point for medical problem

- related health indicators
    6. number of children per 1,000, 6 to 18 years old, involved in court system
    7. air pollution (particulate matter) μg/cu mm.

The committee asked the staff to study these 30 health indicators and report at the next meeting on the actual or estimated levels of the indicators in comparison to the borough of Manhattan, New York City, and the United States. In addition, they wanted to know what the likely forecast of these indicators would be for the district by 1985 if no other services than those already available or actually planned were introduced. The planning team indicated that data were not collected on a routine basis for most of these indicators. It would require a special effort on their part to get what data they could and establish estimates for the others through talks with experts in the fields related to the various health indicators. Therefore, they asked that the 30 indicators be put on a priority list, and they would first attempt to obtain data related to those with the highest priority. The committee set up such a list using a five-point scale. The members individually rated each indicator, awarding a five for the highest priority and a one for the lowest. When the scores were added up, each indicator had a total score based on the collective judgments of the committee. The staff agreed to examine the indicators, starting with the highest priorities. They believed they could research at least 20 of the 30 indicators by the next meeting. All agreed that, if time permitted during this planning cycle, they would also consider the low priority indicators. If this could not be done, they would be given the highest priority for study in the next planning cycle.

On the basis of their study of data, interviews with health experts, and statistical manipulation of tangential data, the planning team secured data or "good" estimates on 22 of the 30 indicators. An examination of Table 13-6 shows that on seven of the indicators (numbers 3, 6, 10, 11, 14, 20, and 21), the district had poorer measures than the borough of Manhattan. The planners noted that these required special attention. In addition, the planners pointed out that on eight of the indicators (numbers 1, 2, 4, 7, 8, 9, 17, and 20) the forecast for 1985 indicated that the problem would become worse if no intervention other than that already planned occurred. They further noted that it was unclear on some indicators in which direction an improvement was being made. For example, with respect to indicator 20, is having fewer psychiatric beds considered an improvement or a worsening of the indicator? A reduction might signify that fewer persons were mentally ill and fewer beds were consequently needed. Or it might mean that more persons were being treated in the community than in the hospital because of earlier detection when ambulatory treatment was possible.

The planners then made a presentation of each indicator, describing what it meant, its potential amenability to solution based on the knowledge available, and the clarity of direction constituting improvement in the indicator. The planners also noted on which indicators the data were somewhat valid, which were based on expert opinion, and which were subjective "guesstimates" based on their own hunches and study of material. They explained that while these differences in accuracy between current and future data were open to challenge, they would develop information systems to collect reliable data for any indicator that was eventually selected for inclusion in the final plan. Since the planning cycle was to be repeated on an annual basis, the accuracy of the data was secondary to the general direction of the indicator in the future and the importance placed upon it by the committee.

However, the planners' own study of the indicators revealed that not all were equally important as future objectives. They, therefore, asked the committee to choose which of the 22 indicators they believed were the most important for the in-depth study and analysis required if specific objectives and intervention alternatives were to be selected. They suggested that two criteria be used for ranking the importance of the indica-

Table 13-6   Health Indicators by Jurisdiction*

	Jurisdiction				
Indicator	District E	Borough	NYC	USA	District Forecast: 1985
A Health Status					
1. Child abuse/100 children	4.2	5.0	4.5	3.2	4.8
2. Chronic respiratory disability per 1,000 adults	E U 70 50	E U 75 55	E U 65 45	E U 64 40	E U 75 58
3. Lead poisoning 6 μg/100 ml of blood	4%	3%	3%	2%	2%
4. Percentage of population with adequate diet	66%	64%	70%	58%	62%
5. Frequency lung cancer deaths/ 1,000 population	1.26	1.26	1.26	.9	2.0
6. Percentage of children under 3 mos. inoculated	74%	81%	72%	62%	80%
7. Alcoholic deaths cirrhosis/100,000	13	15	16	11	16
8. Breast cancer operations/ 100,000 women	50	87	87	85	55
9. Hypertension/ 1,000 population by race	W B 21 34	W B 25 36	W B 22 33	W B 20 33	W B 25 39
10. Percentage of women 45 and over receiving annual Pap test	15%	40%	40%	30%	17%
11. Percentage of population with annual physical check-up	50%	70%	59%	45%	75%
12. Percentage of mental illness 65 and over	12%	12%	11%	8%	10%
B Health System					
13. Avg. length of hospital stay (days)	9.0	9.5	8.5	8.0	8.5

Table 13-6   Continued

			Jurisdiction		
Indicator	*District E*	*Borough*	*NYC*	*USA*	*District Forecast: 1985*
14. Percent need by permanently disabled for physical therapy service available	35%	62%	45%	25%	42%
15. Radiologists/ 10,000 population	6.1	12.2	9.8	4.3	8.0
16. Lab technicians/ 10,000 population	12.5	10.4	8.5	6.0	13.0
17. Waiting time for outpatient/ emergency room clinic visits (hours)	5	6	4	3	6
18. Air quality (particulate matter)	105	125	95	—	75
19. Institutional patient advocates/ 1,000 patients	2.5	2.0	1.5	1.0	5.0
20. Psychiatric beds/ 10,000 population	1.7	2.0	.83	2.0	1.5
21. Percentage receiving care of every 1,000 children with developmental disorders	1.1	1.5	1.15	1.0	1.2
22. Percentage of population with "medical home"	35%	35%	38%	NA	NA

*All data are made up and used for illustrative purposes only.
Key: E—Employed; U—Unemployed; W—White; B—Black.

tors—amenability to change and clarity of direction for improvement in the indicator.

On each criterion, the individual committee members were given a ten-point scale and asked to rate where on the scale (10 for high and 1 for low) they would place the indicator, first with respect to amenability and then with respect to clarity of direction. These separate ratings were added. The totals of all members were then added to come up with a group total for each indicator. In other words, the 22 indicators were ranked according to the subjective numerical ratings of the 15 committee members.

While this particular ranking was done in a committee meeting as a whole, the group could have subdivided itself into two or more task forces and gone through the same process. In that event, the committee would have first had to agree on the criteria upon which they would be ranking the indicators. The benefit of task forces would be a greater opportunity for in-depth analysis and discussion of the indicators and the application of the criteria, before the actual individual ratings. Or the indicators could have been divided into health status indicators to be studied by one task force, and health systems indicators by the other.

Once this ranking was completed, the planners noted that a second ranking would be required by the committee. They indicated that, even apart from the criteria of amenability to action and clarity of direction, not all of the 22 indicators were equally important. For example, would they rate an indicator that was already above the borough's or New York City's standard, such as number 16, number of laboratory technicians per 10,000 population, as a more important indicator requiring special intervention than number 3, lead poisoning of children, which had a 33 percent higher rate than the borough or the city as a whole? Consequently, the committee agreed to place each indicator in one of three categories, high, medium, or low priority with scores of 3, 2, and 1, respectively. Each committee member then multiplied the sum of the two criteria ratings by the general importance of the indicator for an overall score.

After all scores for each indicator were added, the indicators were ranked from highest to lowest, and it was agreed to study only those in the upper half. The 11 indicators finally chosen were

1. percentage of population with adequate diets
2. percentage of women with annual Pap tests, 45 years old and over
3. child abuse per 100 children
4. alcoholic death from cirrhosis of the liver per 100,000
5. hypertension per 1,000 population by race
6. chronic mental illness per 1,000, 65 years old and over
7. chronic respiratory disability per 1,000 adults, employed and unemployed
8. length of waiting time for outpatient and emergency room clinic visits
9. ratio of services available to need for physical therapy of permanently disabled

10. number of institutional patient advocates per 1,000 patients, both bedridden and ambulatory
11. percentage of children under three months old receiving inoculations.

An alternative format for determining health system needs, and one that is used for most health plans, is to examine each of the functional components of the medical care system separately. These include such components as primary care, specialized services, mental health, acute care services, and long-term care. Each of these medical components is subjected to study to determine if there are any problems associated primarily with availability, accessibility, or costs of service and secondarily with quality, continuity, and acceptability. This planning model tends to treat each medical component as an autonomous subsystem with little or no attention paid to its relationship to other subsystems or the health status of high-risk population groups. In short, eight to ten of these functional miniplans constitute the basic health plan, which is generally referred to as resource planning. The primary aim of resource planning is to develop a comprehensive, efficient medical system that is consistent with the medical model depicted in Figure 13-5.

Summary of Base Case

At this point, the base case is completed. The district committee was informed of the general demographic and socioeconomic status of the district and its subareas, CPDs 9 and 12. It also was alerted to the general health status and health system indicators and how the district compared with the borough, which the committee chose to use as its standard of comparison. It also considered some of the health-related indicators. The general finding of this preliminary study was that the district on all *general* indicators exceeded the borough's standard. However, this did not mean that everyone in the district received medical attention that was up to those standards. For example, the demographic data and socioeconomic index noted that CPD 9 had a lower index rating than CPD 12; at the same time, CPD 9 had both a younger and a larger minority population than did CPD 12. This would require the planners and the committee to pay special attention to this subarea of the district. On the other hand, CPD 12 had a much larger elderly population, which was concentrated in certain sections and would also require special attention. In spite of the differences between the two CPDs, the residents of CPD 9 perceived themselves as having a higher level of excellent health than those in CPD 12.

Given this overall favorable health picture compared to the borough of Manhattan, the committee decided to concentrate on specific health problems that lent themselves to deeper analysis and study. Through a series of meetings and examination of an initial list of 30 health problems, the committee narrowed down its concern to 11 which it felt merited attention for intervention in the next fiscal year. These 11 health problems were expressed in terms of quantifiable indicators on which forecasts were made of the probable direction the indicators would take without any planned intervention.

DETERMINING GOALS AND OBJECTIVES

Goals and objectives are determined in two phases. The first deals with the analysis of desired outcomes, and the second, based on these, deals with the actual setting of goals and objectives.

The committee has already identified the 11 health issues on which it desired to focus in the coming year. The planners suggested that further study of the constraints and intervention alternatives would give the committee data to use to identify goals and set specific objectives.

Analysis of Desired Outcomes

The following is a summarized description of the constraints the committee would have to take into account in setting goals. The staff collected the data and presented the findings.

Constraints

1. Percentage of Population with Adequate Diets. Three main constraints were identified: (a) there is difficulty in defining "an adequate diet" so data can be collected and changes in the indicator measured, (b) there is insufficient staff working in the nutrition field to meet the present needs of the population, and (c) the public is indifferent to the whole subject of nutrition and balanced diets.

A further study of the resources available revealed that the percentage of persons who were considered to have an adequate nutritional diet was 45 percent rather than the initial measure of 66 percent. A minor change of 1 percent was predicted to occur by 1985 if nothing more is done than the continuation of current programs. The middle-income classes were believed to be those most amenable to nutrition education. The 45 percent estimated to be financially able to buy nutritious foods were members of this group. There are doubts whether many of the remaining 55 percent could be influenced to change their dietary habits.

2. Number of Persons per 100,000 Who Died of Breast, Uterine, and Lung Cancer. The narrower emphasis on the preventive aspect of women taking Pap tests was changed to a consideration of the three most important causes of death by cancer in men and women. It was felt that a concerted attack on uterine cancer alone was too limited to affect a major proportion of the population.

The main constraints were (a) an increasingly elderly population with a higher incidence of cancer, (b) lack of cooperation among existing health facilities, (c) lack of adequate detection services in both the district and borough of Manhattan, (d) lack of funds to pay for increased services, and (e) lack of awareness generally among district residents regarding cancer and the importance of early detection.

A further study has shown that the programs operating and planned will serve only 20 percent of the population at risk. The change in the indicator shows the current and forecast 1985 levels for lung cancer to be 94 and 102 deaths per 1,000, respectively; for breast cancer, 81 and 78 deaths per 1,000; and for uterine cancer, 47 and 47 per 1,000. The cure rate is presently 33 percent, but the American Cancer Society believes that, with early detection, the cure rate can be increased to 50 percent.

3. Child Abuse and Neglect per 100 Children. The major constraints were (a) the lack of funds directed at the problem, (b) the psychological resistance to reporting incidences of child abuse and neglect by professionals and the general public of the problem, (c) a general cutback in health services, (d) a lack of trained personnel to deal with the problem once it is discovered, and (e) a lack of cooperation among existing services and agencies related to the problem.

Because of the staff cutbacks and the constraints noted, only about 20 percent of the population who were brought to the attention of the authorities were being served.

4. Deaths from Alcohol per 100,000 Population. This indicator was broadened to include all deaths due to alcohol abuse, rather than restrict it to those caused by cirrhosis of the liver.

The major constraints were (a) failure of Medicaid and Medicare health insurance to cover alcoholism as an included insurance treatment cost, (b) local prejudices against alcoholics, and (c) detecting and treating the causes of the disease rather than just the symptoms.

5. Hypertension per 100 Persons by Race. The major constraints were (a) apathy on the part of the professional community toward dealing with the disease, (b) lack of facilities (clinics and concerned personnel), and (c) classification of hypertension as a condition and not a disease.

The main problem is the failure of professionals to treat the condition in its incipient stages rather than encouraging the patient to begin treatment when its serious symptoms begin to develop, which results in life-long suffering.

6. Chronic and Severe Mental Illness per 1,000 Population 65 Years and Older. The major constraints were (a) a negative attitude by the public that there will always be elderly mentally ill, (b) an indifference to meeting the needs of the aged and mentally ill because of that negative attitude, and (c) the limited financial capacity of elderly with fixed incomes to obtain treatment for themselves.

Given these constraints, it was estimated that only about 10 percent of the elderly in need of service received it. They are generally perceived as persons who have lived out their lives and so are given a lower priority by public and private officials in the allocation of resources compared to other adults and the young.

7. Chronic Respiratory Disability per 1,000 Adults, Employed and Unemployed. The main constraints were (a) governmental resistance to taking effective antipollution measures, (b) continued intensive cigarette smoking advertising campaigns, (c) resistance on the part of smokers to give up the habit, and (d) indifference by legislators to respiratory diseases.

There is little that can be done unless the public, as represented by community leaders, political leaders, and government officials, takes a more active role in reducing the more severe causes of chronic respiratory diseases, automobile and factory pollution, and cigarette smoking. Further study revealed that the rate of the indicator should be changed from a rate per 1,000 to a rate per 10,000.

8. Length of Waiting Time for Outpatient/Emergency Room Clinic Visits. The main constraints were (a) inadequate facilities to meet the needs of the existing community; (b) overbooking of appointments to ensure adequate work for employees, causing an uneven flow of patients and periodic excessive waiting time; and (c) lack of a directory of health services, causing an excessive number of referrals to assist patients in finding a correct portal of entry.

The base case indicated that there are potentially sufficient clinic resources to meet need. However, it was unknown to what extent those resources catered to district population needs compared to those of non-district residents. The constraints also imply that services are provided with the convenience of the staff in mind rather than the patient.

9. Ratio of Services Available to Need for Physical Therapy of Permanently Disabled. The main constraints were (a) a cutback in funding for this type of treatment, (b) limited medical coverage by insurance programs, and (c) reduction in eligibility levels for Medicaid, thereby reducing the number eligible for services under this program.

The major resources for the disabled are spent on persons holding jobs, with the elderly a poor second in the receipt of such services.

10. Number of Institutional Patient Advocates per 1,000 Patients, Both Bedridden and Ambulatory. The main constraints were (a) the overcrowded conditions in hospitals and the general feeling of alienation felt by the patient, (b) reduction in Medicaid eligibility levels, (c) lack of trained personnel to serve as patient advocates, and (d) lack of cooperation by existing institutions to meet needs of patients.

While advocates are required for all patients, they are most needed to assist patients of low-income groups who attend clinics and are placed on ward services in hospitals.

11. Percentage of Children under Three Months Old Receiving Inoculations. The committee reconsidered this indicator and concluded that, with the proliferation of family planning clinics and after-baby care services, the fairly high percentage of those already covered would be maintained with the services currently available and planned. It was agreed to review the situation during the next annual planning cycle to determine if further intervention was required.

Indicator Levels

In addition to describing the constraints, the staff presented its data on the level and type of services currently available in the district. The planners asked the committee to review these data with the aim of arriving at realistic goals for 1985. As an aid in decision-making the staff suggested that the committee use a graphic method based on indicator levels. A distinction was made among current, predicted forecast indicators without intervention, and desired indicator level with intervention.

The current indicator level is the value the indicator has in the current year. For the study of District E, this is 1980.

The predicted forecast indicator without intervention refers to the value the indicator will have in a future specified year if no special actions are taken by health planners or agencies. The future year in this study is 1985.

The desired indicator level with intervention is the value that will be reached with planned long-range actions. This is similar to the goal levels, which is an expression of optimal feasible improvement that can be achieved given the constraints of scientific knowledge and political, economic, and social factors. The long-range objective represents a partial or complete fulfillment of the goal within a stated time period. For this case illustration, that time period is five years.

In Figure 13-6, the hypothetical example shows percentage of population with a medical home to be 35 percent for the current indicator level and 70 percent for the predicted forecast without intervention. This increase assumes the passage of some form of national health insurance or the liberalization of health insurance benefits, particularly to the low-income population, which is the group most likely not to have a medical home. Episodic visits to various outpatient/emergency room clinics for service does not constitute a medical home unless the patients perceive that as the place where they receive their primary health care. With intervention, it was believed that the desired level could be increased to 90 percent of the population. Consequently, the indicator gap, the difference between the desired level or goal and the forecast level without intervention, is 20 percent. This is the gap that requires planning and program intervention. The objective is the level that can be achieved through program intervention in an attempt to close the gap between the desired and forecast indicator levels. If by 1982, the program interventions can close the gap by 10 percent and an additional 10 percent between 1982 and 1985, then the objectives are to increase the percentage of the population with a medical home by 10 percent for 1982 and by another 10 percent by 1985. Thus, objectives can be viewed as the intermediate steps toward achievement of the desired indicator level or goal. On the basis of actual experi-

Figure 13-6   Hypothetical Outcomes for Indicator: Population with a Medical Home

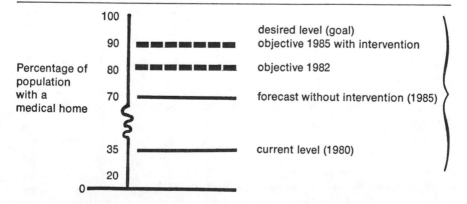

ence, either the objectives or the goal might be changed either upward or downward.

Setting of Goals and Objectives

The committee understood from this illustration that it had to arrive at goals that had some feasibility. The goals or desired indicator levels are predictions of what the committee would like to see occur. They are based on projections of staff; on studies of possible new technologies being planned, but not yet perfected; and on a knowledge of cultural, social, and economic trends of the district that may have a bearing on the population. For example, the repair of the West Side Highway has detoured heavy traffic into the local streets of the district, increasing the level of automobile pollution. Since this is likely to change only in the 1980s, it can be expected that the indicator, respiratory disability of adults, will not show a marked improvement without intervention. Taking such factors into account, the committee, with assistance from the staff, set the objectives to be achieved by 1985 (Table 13-7).

The desired level in most cases is an ideal goal of what is technically feasible under positive circumstances of interest, financial availability, and administrative effectiveness. The objectives represent the committee's view of how much of that desired level can be achieved, given the reality constraints and the positive trends that may change some of the negative constraints into positive forces. Thus, the committee felt it could

Table 13-7   Indicators and Health Issues for District E

Indicator Levels	*Health Issues Requiring Intervention**									
	1 %	2 per 1,000	3 per 100	4 per 100,000	5 %	6 %	7 per 10,000	8 hours	9 %	10 per 1,000
Current level – 1980	45	75	4.2	13	10	12	600	3	80	2.5
Forecast without intervention for 1985	46	78	4.8	16	12	10	650	4	82	3
Desired level with intervention	50	70	2.0	10	25	8	530	1	85	5
1985 objective	48	70	3.5	10	20	9	530	2	85	5

*Health issues identified earlier in this chapter.

actually achieve its desired levels or goals with respect to indicator issues 2, 4, 7, and 10. On all other objectives, the committee felt confident that its objectives would result in improved health care for the residents and a more effective delivery system even where it believed its goals could not be fully attained.

Health Status Goals and Objectives

G1: Increase the percentage of persons with an adequate diet in District E from 45 to 50 percent.

Obj. 1.1: Increase the percentage of persons with an adequate diet from 45 to 48 percent by 1985. Special attention is to be given to low-income families and families headed by a female in CPD 9 and the elderly in CPD 12.

G2: Decrease the cancer mortality rate for breast, uterine, and lung cancer for persons in District E from 75 to 70 per 100,000 persons.

Obj. 2.1: Reduce the mortality rate of lung cancer from 94 to 70 per 100,000 persons by 1985.

Obj. 2.2: Reduce the mortality rate of breast cancer from 81 to 61 per 100,000 persons by 1985.

Obj. 2.3: Reduce the mortality rate of uterine cancer from 47 to 35 per 100,000 by 1985.

G3: Reduce the rate of child abuse and neglect from 4.2 children per 100 children to 2 in District E.

Obj. 3.1: Reduce the rate of child abuse and neglect from 4.2 to 3.5 per 100 children by 1985. Special attention should be given to families with children aged 10 and under.

G4: Reduce the mortality rate due to alcoholism from 13 to 10 per 100,000 persons.

Obj. 4.1: Reduce the mortality rate due to alcoholism from 13 to 10 per 100,000 by 1985 in District E, with special emphasis on persons 18 to 35 years old.

G5: Increase the percentage of blacks under treatment for hypertension from 10 to 25 percent of the population in District E.

Obj. 5.1: Increase the percentage of blacks under treatment for hypertension from 10 to 20 percent by 1985, with special emphasis given to those living in CPD 9.

G6: Decrease the percentage of persons 65 and over with severe mental illness from 12 to 8 percent of the elderly population in District E.

Obj. 6.1: Reduce the percentage of the elderly population with severe mental illness from 12 to 9 percent of persons 65 and over by 1985, with special emphasis to those residing in CPD 12.

G7:   Reduce the rate of persons with chronic respiratory disability from 600 to 530 per 10,000 population in District E.

Obj. 7.1: Reduce the rate of respiratory disability for unemployed from 580 to 530 by 1985 and for employed adults from 750 to 700 by 1985 in District E.

Health System Goals and Objectives

G8:   Reduce the waiting time for outpatient and emergency room visits from three hours to one hour.

Obj. 8.1: Reduce the waiting time for outpatient and emergency room visits from three hours to two hours by 1985 for persons residing in CPD 9.

G9:   Increase the percentage of permanently disabled persons receiving physical therapy from 80 to 85 percent in District E.

Obj. 9.1: Increase the percentage of permanently disabled persons receiving physical therapy treatment from 80 to 85 percent in District E by 1985.

G10: Increase the number of patient advocates from 2.5 to 5 per 1,000 patients, including in- and outpatients in District E.

Obj.10.1: Increase the number of patient advocates from 2.5 to 5 per 1,000 inpatients by 1985 in District E.

Long-Range Recommended Actions and Resource Requirements

In order to make informed decisions, the staff, working with the agency's plan development committee, devised a worksheet for each of the ten health indicators that contained data related to health services available, target population, goal and objective levels, and recommended actions and their estimated costs. The committee and staff also planned to solicit proposals from the relevant public and private health agencies that expressed interest in and had some expertise with the problems under consideration. The basic data compiled for the worksheets for the indicator, mental illness of elderly are shown in Exhibit 13-1.

Exhibit 13-1   Summary Worksheet for Mental Illness of Elderly

A. Objectives to be reached
    1. Name of indicator: Mental illness of persons
                                 65 years old and over (percent)
    2. Current measure: 12 percent
       Desired goal: 8 percent
       Objective 1985:   9 percent

B. Resources available to meet objectives currently in operation

Health Care	Community Education	Others
a. 1980–1985		
—Washington Heights Community Mental Health Center	None	None
—Nursing Homes		
—State Hospital		

C. Demographic Data

	1975	1980	1985
1. Population at risk age 65 plus:	4860	5140	5456
2. Number receiving service:	540	570	744

    3. Ethnicity:
    4. Income below $4,500:   All groups
                                  Over ½ of elderly live on less
                                  than $3,000 per year
    5. Sex: Females outnumber males 6:4

6. Percentage of persons reached by service:	11	11	14

D. Constraints to improving the health indicator
    1. Negative attitude of public toward elderly in general
    2. Elderly on fixed income unable to afford private treatment.

E. Estimate of how well programs mentioned in "B" are working
    1. Current programs are limited. It is estimated they serve about 10 percent of mentally ill 65 years old and over.

F. New program being recommended to meet objective
    1. Name of program

Exhibit 13-1 Continued

>   a. Health promotion: Mental Health Task Force on
>   Services to Aged—education service for nursing homes
> 2. Brief description of program: purpose of program is to
>   educate and train nursing home staff to deal better with
>   problems of the mentally ill elderly and to instruct staff on
>   methods for reorienting patients with chronic brain syn-
>   drome (senility).
> 3. Cost of program
>   a. Medium cost:
>   b. Source of funds: New York City Department of Health
>   c. Agency for implementation: voluntary hospitals in
>   District E
> 4. Constraints of program
>   a. Not all nursing homes will want to participate.
>   b. Nursing home staff may be ambivalent to program.
>   c. Patients in nursing homes may reject service.
> 5. Expected impact of program on objectives:
> 1985
No impact
>
> 6. Impact on other indicators or objectives. (Put number of
>   indicator after appropriate prediction.)
>
> | | 1985 |
> |---------------------|------|
> | a. High: | 2,6 |
> | b. Medium: | 1,5 |
> | c. Low: | |
> | d. No impact: | |
> | e. Negative impact: | |

The objectives and recommended program interventions are listed in the following, with a summary of their cost and target populations. This information was based on more extensive data collected for each indicator.

Indicator 1:   Percent of population with an adequate diet

Objective: Raise percent with adequate diet from 45 to 48 percent by 1985.

Target population: 43,000 of all ages and ethnicity

Programs: 1. Expansion of the Bureau of Nutrition's existing program for educating the public.

Cost: Medium at $85,000 from city tax levy funds
Impact: Low

2. Educate public to presence and use of the Women, Infants and Children federally funded program and the Title VII "Meals on Wheels" program for the elderly.
Cost: Substantial to high at $200,000 to $250,000 annually from federal funds.
Impact: High

Indicator 2:   Mortality Rates from Breast, Lung, and Uterine Cancer per 100,000 Population

Objective: Reduce mortality rates of lung cancer from 94 to 70 by 1985; breast cancer from 81 to 61 by 1985; and uterine cancer from 47 to 35 by 1985.

Target population: 48,884 males 45 and older and 88,770 females 35 and over.

Programs: 3. Develop and distribute a directory of existing detection services during a "Cancer Awareness Week."
Cost: Medium at $100,000 per year from New York City Department of Health
Impact: Medium

4. Cancer education in the district's schools.
Cost: Medium at $100,000 per year from New York City Board of Education
Impact: Medium

Indicator 3:   Child Abuse and Neglect per 100 Children

Objective: Reduce the incidence of child abuse from 4.2 to 3.5 per 100 children by 1985.

Target population: 2,110 children, 0-4 years of age.

Programs: 5. Bilingual publicity and education campaign on child abuse.
Cost: Substantial—$150,000 per year from state and federal funds.
Impact: High

6. Expansion and improvement of the child abuse and neglect service unit at St. Luke's Hospital.
Cost: Very high—$430,000 per year from Federal Community Mental Health Act.
Impact: High

Indicator 4:   Percent of Alcohol Abuse.

Objective: Reduce percentage of those suffering from alcoholism from 13 to 10 per 100,000 persons by 1985.

Target population: 51,000 black men and white women, aged 45 to 64 and white men, 65 and over

Programs: 7. Training of staff at Community Mental Health Center to treat alcohol abusers.
Cost: Medium to substantial—$50,000 to $200,000 from federal government's Alcoholic Abuse Act
Impact: High

8. Public health education in schools, churches, and community facilities regarding alcohol abuse
Cost: Medium at $20,000 from Alcoholic Abuse Act
Impact: Low

Indicator 5:   Percentage of persons under treatment for hypertension

Objective: Increase percentage of blacks under treatment from 10 to 20 percent by 1985 and whites from 20 to 30 percent by 1985.

Target population: 60,000 blacks and 48,000 whites, 15 to 64 years old.

Programs: 9. Health education through public displays
Cost: Substantial at $150,000 from New York City Department of Health per year
Impact: Medium

10. Diagnosis/treatment for 25 percent of target populations
Cost: Very High at $22 million with 50 percent from Medicaid, 10 percent from New York City Department of Health and 40 percent out-of-pocket
Impact: High

Indicator 6:   Chronic Mental Illness of 65 Years Old and Over per 100 Persons

Objective: Reduce percentage of elderly with mental illness from 12 to 8 percent by 1985

Target population: 5,140 elderly with mental illness

Programs: 11. Educate and train nursing homes' staff in treatment of mentally ill.
Cost: Medium at $30,000 from Medicaid funds
Impact: Medium

12. Neighborhood ambulatory day care and home support services through expanded neighborhood mental health centers
Cost: Very high at $400,000 per seven centers by 1985, from Federal Community Mental Health Act and Medicaid funds
Impact: High

Indicator 7:	Rate of Respiratory Disability of Employed and Unemployed Persons per 10,000 Adults
Objective:	Reduce the incidence of respiratory disability from the anticipated level of 580 by 1985 to 530 for unemployed adults and for employed adults from 750 to 700.
Target population:	50,000 adults, 15 to 64 years of age
Programs:	13. Establish one store front family health center in CPD 9 and 12.

Cost: Substantial to high at $150,000 to $350,000 by 1985 from Health and Hospital Corporation and tax levy funds from New York City.
Impact: Medium

14. Antismoking campaign.
Cost: $60,000 from U.S. Office of Health Promotion
Impact: Low

Indicator 8:	Average length of waiting time for outpatient/emergency room clinics in the district
Objective:	Reduce waiting time for clinic visits from 3 to 2 hours by 1985.
Target population:	54,331 persons who use such clinics in the district
Programs:	15. Development of a triage system in district clinics

Cost: Medium at $60,000 for public/voluntary hospitals
Impact: High

16. Train public in medical self-help in emergency situations
Cost: Medium at $100,000 from city/voluntary hospitals
Impact: Medium

Indicator 9:	Percentage of patients with total disability receiving physical therapy treatment
Objective:	Increase percent of people served from 80 to 85 by 1985
Target population:	800 persons with total disability and in need of physical therapy
Programs:	17. Home visit treatment by bilingual physical therapists

Cost: Substantial at $120,000 from Medicaid/Medicare funds
Impact: High

18. Develop a physical therapy pick-up and home care service

Cost: Very high at $300,000 from Medicaid/Medicare funds

Impact: High

Indicator 10:   Number of Advocates per 1,000 Patient Population

Objective: Increase number of advocates from 2.5 to 5 per 1,000 patient population by 1985.

Target population: Patient population of 210,000 which is expected to be reduced to 150,000 by 1985.

Programs:

19. Development of a centralized patient advocate center to coordinate patient problems and make medical referrals
    Cost: High at $250,000 to $275,000 from federal and state funds
    Impact: High

20. Develop a comprehensive directory of health services and distribute to all patients attending hospital clinics and inpatient services
    Cost: Low at $20,000 to $25,000 from New York City Department of Health
    Impact: Low

A review of these programs indicates the following:

- The programs will have a generally high impact in achieving at a medium or higher level the objectives of the ten health indicators.
- Many of the programs are aimed at health education of substantial segments of the adult population. This implies that there will be a duplication of effort or an oversaturation of health education focus in alerting the population to the services available to them. The assumption of most of these programs is that adequate resources are available, but are simply going unused or are being used in an inefficient manner.
- The emphasis of the programs is on the prevention, early detection, and maintenance of a person's independence as far as possible.
- Only six of the programs are for personal care services, with an emphasis on developing services not now available to the district's population.
- The cost of these programs is substantial, at an average of $150,000 per program, except for the estimated $22 million for the hypertension treatment program.
- The costs of the programs would be borne largely by existing federal grant programs, especially Medicaid, Medicare, and community men-

tal health funds. City tax levy dollars would be relied on to a lesser degree.

- Most of the goals for 1985 will not be achieved by the program interventions because of the numerous constraints inhibiting their success.

The committee sought initially, through health promotion programs, to teach the district's population how to prevent illness and where to go to get early treatment. The committee believed that the cumulative effect of health education activities would change the public's orientation from seeking assistance only in time of dire need to prevention and early detection and treatment. The committee was building upon what is known in the health field rather than counting on new medical breakthroughs that might have a substantial impact on a particular disease. While much medical research was taking place in the two major district hospitals—Columbia-Presbyterian and St. Luke's—anything that developed from it would be perceived as a bonus by the district committee.

Table 13-8 summarizes the large array of data that have been discussed. Three of the indicators, 2, 5, and 7, were logically subdivided into their component parts. Thus, cancer (2) was divided into cancer of the lungs, breast, and uterus and treated separately for analysis. The table also vividly illustrates the impact of the programs on indicators other than the ones for which they were specifically designed. Thus, on the first indicator—percentage of population with an adequate diet—seven other actions have a spillover impact on it in addition to those designed to achieve the committee's goal. Some members of the committee were concerned that oversaturation could generate negative public opinion toward the program originally designed for a particular indicator.

The staff pointed out that this concern and other insights the committee members had drawn would assist them in developing alternative plan designs.

SELECTION OF PLAN DESIGN

In the absence of unlimited resources, the committee had to select its priorities among the objectives and select the actions that could best achieve them. Before designing these plans, the staff reviewed the entire range of alternative actions, their costs, and forecasts of indicator levels, and modified these where new insight or knowledge made it appropriate.

Table 13-8 Relationship of Actions to Indicators

					Summary of Task Force Actions													
Indicators for objectives					1	2a	2b	2c	3	4	5a	5b	6	7a	7b	8	9	10
Desired level					50%	70	61	35	2.0	10	18	18	8%	530	700	1	85%	5
Current level					45%	94	81	47	4.2	13	24	34	12%	500	700	3	80%	2.5
Predicted 1985/present action					46%	102	78	47	4.8	16	25	39	10%	580	750	4	82%	3
Provisional 1985 objective					48%	70	61	35	3.5	10	20	30	9%	530	700	2	85%	5
	Source				IMPACTS													
Action	Funds	Agency	Feasibility	Cost	1	2a	2b	2c	3	4	5a	5b	6	7a	7b	8	9	10
1	C	V	H	M												H		
2	C/F	V	M	M												M		
3	C	P	H	S	H					L	M	M		L	L			L
4	C	P	M	S	H				M	L	M	M	L	L	L		L	
5	S, F	C	M	S	L				H									
6	S, F	V	H	VH					H	M						M		
7	F	PR	H	M-S					H	H						M		
8	F	PR	H	M	L				L	L			H					
9	C	PR	M	S									L				H	
10	PR/C/S/F	PR	H	VH									L				H	
11	C/S/F	C	M	M	H					L	L	L						
12	F	C	L	S-H	M													
13	C	C	H	M	M													
14	F	C	H	M	M													

Table 13-8 Continued

No.										
15	C/PR	PR	L	M	L	L	L	H	M	L
16	C/PR	V	M	VH	M	L	L	M	M	L
17	C/S/F	C	M	M	M	M	M	M	M	
18	C/S/F	P	M	S-VH	M	M	L	L	L	M	M
19	S/F	C	L	H	L				M	H
20	C	C,V	H	M		M	L		M	L

C–City   PR–Priv.   H–High
S–State   P–Public   M–Med.
F–Fed.   V–Volun.   L–Low

Low: 0-$25,000
Medium: $25-$100,000
Substantial: $100-$199,000
High: $200-$299,000
Very High: $300,000 & up

Impact
L–Low
M–Medium
H–High

After reviewing the staff's modifications, the committee met with the staff to consider the design of a final plan. The staff suggested that the committee consider a number of criteria in designing plan alternatives. One suggested criterion was feasibility for implementation. The planner defined feasibility as the capacity of an agency to translate an action into reality by developing a staff, creating an administrative structure, obtaining a suitable location, securing the necessary knowledge to carry out the service, and obtaining community and public acceptance. Any major hindrance or obstacle to achieving these requirements would constitute a serious feasibility problem and would greatly reduce the capacity of the action to achieve its objective. The committee agreed to accept feasibility as the first criterion and, in addition, added seven other criteria various members wanted considered. Each of these eight criteria was defined:

1. feasibility—the capacity to translate an action into reality.
2. cost—the availability of funds within the fiscal year for implementing the action.
3. cumulative action impact on objectives—the secondary impact actions designed for a specific objective have in helping to implement other objectives, thus producing a multiplier and reenforcement effect in achievement of the objective.
4. quantitative impact on mortality rates—selection of only those programs that have a direct influence on lowering the mortality rates of the indicators related to various types of disease, such as cancer and hypertension.
5. direct effect on personal health status—the selection of those indicators and their related actions that have an impact on the personal health status of the district residents
6. direct effect on health systems—the selection of those indicators and their related actions that tend to improve selected components of the health system
7. prevention of illness and maintenance of health—identifying and selecting those indicators that focus primarily on prevention of poor health and maintaining the health of residents at an optimal level
8. urgency of the program to meet current objectives—selecting only those actions that will have a major impact in the short run on improving conditions that are in or may be approaching a crisis stage.

The committee and staff examined the eight criteria and came to the following conclusions. First, they felt that cost was as important a factor in program implementation as were the other feasibility components and agreed to combine these two criteria. They could find little distinction between the criteria relating to personal health status and prevention, and decided to combine them. They rejected the criterion dealing with mortality because they reasoned that (a) their primary orientation was on prevention and health maintenance rather than mortality; (b) through this orientation, one outcome of a successful program would be a reduction of mortality rates; and (c) the technical knowledge for radically reducing mortality rates of the major causes of death was not available. They also rejected the criterion dealing with health systems because only two of the ten indicators had this as their focus. The committee considered it irresponsible to propose a plan that focused on only a few programs. Consequently, the final four criteria to be used in designating alternative plans were (1) feasibility, including the cost component; (2) cumulative action impact on objectives; (3) direct effect on personal health status, which would include the concept of prevention of illness and health maintenance; and (4) urgency of the action in meeting current objectives.

One of the committee members pointed out that, just as the original indicators were of unequal value, so too were the final ten indicators. Some were more important than others. The staff agreed with this point of view, but noted that through the original ranking there was fair agreement that these remaining ten indicators all had fairly high significance for the committee. The real question the staff noted was whether they differed in the degree to which the goal levels would be reached by 1985. For example, it was noted that several objectives would reach the "desired goal" set up by the committee, such as 2, 4, and 9. Others would reach the goal only partially, such as 6 and 8. The staff, therefore, recommended a weighting based on the percentage of the gap that would be closed between the forecast level without intervention for 1985 and the desired goal. Thus, for example, if 100 percent of the goal would be achieved by the objectives for indicator 10—number of institutional advocates per 10,000 patients— it would be given a weight of one. On the other hand, for indicator 1, only 50 percent of the gap between the 1985 forecast level of 46 percent and the desired goal of 50 percent would be reached by the objectives' level of 48 percent.

$$(W) \text{ Weight} = \frac{(G) \text{ difference between goal level} - (O) \text{ objective level}}{(G) \text{ gap between goal level} - (F) \text{ forecast level without intervention}}$$

$$W = \frac{G-O}{G-F}$$

$$W = \frac{.02}{.04}$$

$$= 50\% \text{ for indicator } 1$$

The judgments already made on the impact the various actions would have on the ten indicators are shown in Table 13-8. By giving scores of 3 for high impact (H), 2 for medium impact (M), 1 for low impact (L), 0 for no impact (blank space) and −1 for a negative impact (N), it is possible to obtain the cumulative unweighted score of the actions on each of the indicators (Table 13-9). It is also possible to obtain the cumulative effect one action has on the different indicators it influences. By multiplying the weights given for the degree of the gap closed, it is then possible to treat all the indicators and the action impacts on them as though they were of equal value.

The effects on the indicators of weighting are shown in Tables 13-10 and 13-11. An analysis of the results of weighting shows that there is considerable shifting in the rankings of the indicators. For example, with weighting, 1 fell from the first to the third rank while 4 climbed from second to first rank; 6 fell from third ranking to a seventh ranking with weighting. Weighting thus has a tendency to equalize the objectives in their relationship to each other. The tables also illustrate a shuffling of ranks due to the action impact on the various indicators. The change in ranking of the actions was not evident among the first four or the last five, but came primarily in the middle rankings where slight shifts take place. Thus, proposal 15 fell from an eighth ranking to an eleventh ranking with weighting. On the other hand, proposal 5 climbed from a ninth ranking to a fifth ranking with weighting.

Assisted by the staff, the committee selected four criteria, or organizing principles, to develop alternative plan designs. The impact of the various patterns of actions in achieving the plan's objectives was then assessed. In addition, the committee evaluated the costs of each set of actions in

Table 13-9 Ranking of Indicators

Rank	Unweighted	Weighted
1	1	4
2	4	2
3	6	1
4	3	9
5	2	5a
6/7	5a	10
6/7	5b	6
8	8	7
9	9	3
10	10	8
11	7	5b

Table 13-10 Impact of Actions on Indicators: Unweighted

Summary of Task Force Actions

Indicators for objectives	1	2a	2b	2c	3	4	5a	5b	6	7a	7b	8	9	10
Desired level	50%	70	61	35	2.0	10	18	18	8%	530	700	1	85%	5
Current level	45%	94	81	47	4.2	13	24	34	12%	500	700	3	80%	2.5
Predicted 1985/present action	46%	102	78	47	4.8	16	25	39	10%	580	750	4	82%	3
Provisional 1985 objective	48%	70	61	35	3.5	10	20	30	9%	530	700	2	85%	5

Action	Source Funds	Agency	Feasibility	Cost	Unweighted Scores	IMPACTS 1	2a	2b	2c	3	4	5a	5b	6	7a	7b	8	9	10
1	C	V	H	L	3												3		
2	C/F	V	M	M	2												2		
3	C	P	H	M	10	3					1	2	2		1	1			1
4	C	P	M	M	10					1	1	2	2		1	1			1
5	S,F	C	M	M	6	1				3	2								
6	S,F	V	H	H	8					3	2						2	1	
7	F	PR	H	L	8					3	3			3			−1		
8	F	PR	H	L	4	1				1	1			1					
9	C	PR	M	H	4									1				3	
10	PR/C/S/F	PR	H	M	4									1				3	
11	C/S/F	C	M	M	6						1	1	1						
12	F	C	L	M	2		2	2	2										
13	C	C	H	M	6		2	2	2										
14	F	C	H	M	6		2	2	2										
15	C/PR	PR	L	H	7		2	2			1	1		3			−1		
16	C/PR	V	M	L	11		2	2			1	1		2					1

Table 13-10 Continued

17	C/S/F	C	M	H	14	2	2	2						2	2		
18	C/S/F	P	M	H	19	2	2	2	1	1	1	1		2	2	2	
19	S/F	C	L	M	4	1					1			1	1		3
20	C	C,V	H	L	1								1	1	1	1	1
Total Unweighted Scores					17	10	10	12	14	10	11	12	6	8	9	12	2

C–City   PR–Priv.   3–high impact
S–State   P–Public   2–medium impact
F–Fed.   V–Volun.   1–low impact
                             −1–negative impact

Table 13-11 Impact of Actions on Indicators: Weighted

Summary of Task Force Actions

						Indicator 1	2a	2b	2c	3	4	5a	5b	6	7a	7b	8	9	10
Indicators for objectives						1	2a	2b	2c	3	4	5a	5b	6	7a	7b	8	9	10
Desired level						50%	70	61	35	2.0	10	18	18	8%	530	700	1	85%	5
Current level						45%	94	81	47	4.2	13	24	34	12%	500	700	3	80%	2.5
Predicted 1985/present action						46%	102	78	47	4.8	16	25	39	10%	580	750	4	82%	3
Provisional 1985 objective						48%	70	61	35	3.5	10	20	30	9%	530	700	2	85%	5

| | Source | | | | Weighted | IMPACTS | | | | | | | | | | | | | |
Action	Funds	Agency	Feasibility	Cost	Scores	.5	1.0	1.0	1.0	.5	1.0	.7	.4	.5	1.0	1.0	.7	1.0	1.0
1	C	V	H	L	2.1												2.1		
2	C/F	V	M	M	0.7												0.7		
3	C	P	H	M	5.70	1.5					1.0	1.4						1.0	
4	C	P	M	M	7.70	1.5					1.0	1.4	.8		1.0	1.0			1.0
5	S,F	C	M	M	6.00	.5				1.5	2.0		.8		1.0	1.0			
6	S,F	V	H	H	5.90					1.5	2.0				1.0	1.0	1.4	1.0	
7	F	PR	H	L	5.30					1.5	3.0			1.5			.7		
8	F	PR	H	L	2.50	.5				.5	1.0			.5					
9	C	PR	M	H	3.50					.5	1.0			.5					
10	PR/C/S/F	PR	H	M	3.50									.5					3.0
11	C/S/F	C	M	M	3.60	1.5					1.0	.7	.4	.5					3.0
12	F	C	L	M	1.00	1.0					1.0								
13	C	C	H	M	6.00		2	2	2										
14	F	C	H	M	6.00		2	2	2										
15	C/PR	PR	L	H	4.40	.5					1.0	.7	.4	1.5				.7	
16	C/PR	V	M	L	9.10		2	2	2	2	1.0	.7	.4	1.0			.7	1.0	

Table 13-11 Continued

17	C/S/F	C	M	H	12.20		2	2			1.4	.8		2.0	2.0		
18	C/S/F	P	M	H	15.50	1.0	2	2	2	.5	1.0	.7	.4	.5	2.0	2.0	1.4
19	S/F	C	L	M	3.30	.5				.5					.7	.7	3.0
20	C	C,V	H	L	0.80									.5		.7	1.0
Total Weighted Scores					8.5	10	10	10	6.0	14.0	7.0	4.0	6.5	6.0	6.0	8.4	7.0	7.0

C–City
S–State
F–Fed.

P–Public
PR Priv.
V–Volun.

Weightings

3–High Impact
2–Medium Impact
1–Low Impact
−1–Negative Impact

relation to the benefits produced. Once this analysis was completed, the committee could determine which plan would produce the greatest benefits at the lowest costs. The following are the alternative plans that evolve from the application of the four organizing principles to the 20 actions previously described:

PLAN 1

Organizing Principle:	Urgency—Selection only of those actions that will have a major impact in the short run on improving health conditions that are in or may be approaching a crisis state.

Component Action Nos.	Description
3	Cancer directory
5	Bilingual education on child abuse
6	St. Luke's child abuse center
7	Train Community Mental Health Center staff on alcohol abuse
8	Community education on alcoholism
9	Community education on hypertension
10	Hypertension treatment services
12	Mental health centers for elderly
14	Antismoking campaign
16	Self-help training for emergencies

PLAN 2

Organizing Principle:	Feasibility—the capacity to translate an action into reality within the five-year period.

Component Action Nos.	Description
2	Women, Infants, and Children, and Meals on Wheels programs
4	Cancer education in schools
7	Train Community Mental Health Center staff on alcohol abuse
8	Community education on alcoholism
11	Train nursing home staff to care for elderly
14	Antismoking campaign
20	Directory of health services

PLAN 3

Organizing Principle:	Personal health—selection of those actions that have an impact on personal health status, prevention of poor health, or maintenance of health at an optimal level.

Component Action Nos.	Description
1	Nutrition education
2	Women, Infants, and Children, and Meals on Wheels programs
4	Cancer education in schools
6	St. Luke's child abuse center
7	Train Community Mental Health Center staff on alcohol abuse
8	Community education on alcoholism
10	Hypertension treatment services
12	Mental health centers for elderly
14	Antismoking campaign
16	Self-help training for emergencies

PLAN 4

Organizing Principle:	Cumulative action impact—selection of those actions with a secondary impact on other objectives, producing a multiplier effect in the achievement of the objective

Component Action Nos.	Description
3	Cancer directory
4	Cancer education in schools
7	Train Community Mental Health Center staff on alcohol abuse
14	Antismoking campaign
15	Triage system in outpatient clinics
16	Self-help training for emergencies
17	Train bilingual physical therapists
18	Mobile vans for physically disabled

An examination of the four plan designs reveals the following:

- Only two actions, numbers 7 and 14, are affected by all four organizing principles, while 4, 8, and 16 are affected by three.

- Three actions, 13, 19, and 20, are not affected by any of the organizing principles.
- Organizing principles of urgency and personal health are affected by ten actions, while feasibility is affected by 7 and cumulative impact by 8.
- Except for seven actions affected by the urgency principle that are also found among those affected by the personal health principle, the pattern of actions affected by the organizing principles tends to be unique. Thus, only Plans 1 and 3 have significant overlapping actions.

These findings indicate that almost all the actions are affected by one or more of the organizing principles and that the four plans are indeed distinct plan designs. In order to provide further guidance to the committee in the selection of a final plan, it was next necessary to determine the impact of the alternative plan designs on the achievement of the objectives. The percentage of an action's impact in achieving an objective is based on the following values:

High impact = 60–100 percent achievement of an objective
Medium impact = 35– 59 percent achievement of an objective
Low impact =   0– 34 percent achievement of an objective

The committee had already established the level of impact each action had on the various objectives (Tables 13-10 and 13-11). To illustrate, Plan 2 shows that actions 2, 4, 7, 8, 11, 14, and 20 were derived from the organizing principle of feasibility. An examination of Table 13-10 shows, that for objective 3, only two of the seven actions of plan 2, numbers 7 and 8, impact on it. Action 7 has a high impact and action 8 a low impact on objective 3. Together, they project a 75 percent achievement of objective 3, based on 60 percent for the high impact of action 7 and 15 percent for action 8. In like manner, the expected percentage of achievement for each objective in relation to the alternative plans was derived. These values are shown in Table 13-12.

Table 13-12 shows that Plan 4, based on the cumulative action impact principle, has the greatest impact, both weighted and unweighted, in achieving the objectives. It reveals that 84 percent of all the weighted objectives would be achieved with 7 of the 14 being accomplished by 100 percent or more. Only 8 of the 20 actions would be used to accomplish this. At the other extreme, Plan 2 would result in the lowest rate of achievement, 34 percent. This plan is based on the feasibility principle.

When the costs of the plans are taken into account, Plan 2 costs the least at $480,000–$955,000, while Plan 3 costs the most at $23.3–$23.8 million

Table 13-12 Degree of Achievement of Objectives for Alternative Plans (Weighted and Unweighted)

Objective	Weight Assigned	Percent of Objective Achieved Plans				Weighted Percent of Objective Achieved Plans			
		1	2	3	4	1	2	3	4
1 Population with an adequate diet	.5	125	135	110	170	62.5	67.5	55	85
2a Reduce mortality rate of lung cancer	1.0	105	35	70	140	105	35	70	140
2b Reduce mortality rate of breast cancer	1.0	105	35	70	140	105	35	70	140
2c Reduce mortality rate of uterine cancer	1.0	105	35	70	140	105	35	70	140
3 Child abuse per 100 children	.5	195	75	135	75	97.5	37.5	67.5	37.5
4 Rate of alcohol abuse/100,000	1.0	200	105	140	135	200	105	140	135
5a Increase hypertension treatment; % of blacks	.7	50	50	50	150	35	35	35	105
5b Increase hypertension treatment; % of whites	.4	50	50	50	150	20	20	20	60
6 Reduce mental illness of elderly	.5	105	90	125	170	52.5	45	62.5	85
7a Reduce respiratory disability of unemployed	1.0	15	15	15	100	15	15	15	100

Table 13-12 Continued

Objective	Weight Assigned	Percent of Objective Achieved				Weighted Percent of Objective Achieved			
		Plans				Plans			
		1	2	3	4	1	2	3	4
7b Reduce respiratory disability of employed	1.0	15	15	15	100	15	15	15	100
8 Reduce outpatient clinic waiting time	.7	20	0	115	0	14	0	80.5	0
9 Increase % of disabled with physical therapy	1.0	135	0	75	0	135	0	75	0
10 Increase advocates per 1,000 patient pop.	1.0	15	30	15	45	15	30	15	45
Average objective achieved		81%	47%	75%	108%	68%	34%	57%	84%
No. objectives 100% achieved out of 14		8	2	5	10	4	1	1	7
No. actions involved in each plan out of 20		10	7	10	8	10	7	10	8
Annual increase in costs		$23.4–$23.6 million	$480,000–$955,000	$23.3–$23.8 million	$850,000–$1,050,000				

dollars annually. There is thus a wide discrepancy in the range of costs. However, an examination of the actions shows clearly that all the plans would be fairly similar in cost if the $22 million required to implement the hypertension treatment action were omitted. Though their costs vary significantly, Plans 1 and 4 produce the greatest benefits. Yet, even at an annual cost of $22 million, the hypertension treatment action of Plan 1 would only achieve 35 percent of its weighted objective by 1985.

If the actions of the two plans were grouped according to their major functions of education, training, and service, the differences and similarities between them would be clearly illuminated:

Plan 1	*Plan 4*
Education Actions	
Cancer directory	Cancer directory
St. Luke's child abuse center	Cancer education in schools
Community education on alcohol abuse	Antismoking campaign
Community education on hyper-tension	
Antismoking campaign	
Training Actions	
Community Mental Health Center staff on alcohol abuse	Community Mental Health Center staff on alcohol abuse
Self-help for emergencies	Self-help for emergencies
	Bilingual physical therapists
Service Actions	
St. Luke's child abuse center	Triage system in outpatient clinics
Hypertension treatment	Mobile vans for physically dis-abled
Mental health centers for elderly	

The primary differences between the two plans rest on two features: (1) Plan 1 provides a richer number of health education actions than Plan 4, and (2) Plan 1 has a different array of service actions that are also much more costly to operate than those of Plan 4. Table 13-12 reveals that the actions of Plan 4 already produce a higher rate of objective achievement than Plan 1 with respect to reductions in hypertension and mental illness among the elderly. It seemed clear to the committee that any trade-offs in designing a final plan would be based on Plan 4, which appeared to have the best balance of costs to benefits. The committee therefore decided to take the following actions to improve its benefits at the least cost.

1. It rejected the two high-cost service actions of Plan 1 because of their limited benefits, hypertension treatment and development of mental health centers for the elderly.
2. It decided to accept the St. Luke's child abuse service action of Plan 1 because it would significantly raise the percentage achievement of objective 3, reduction of child abuse, from 37.5 to 97.5 percent weighted.
3. To round out its education function, the committee added the actions on hypertension and child abuse education from Plan 1.

The result of these changes was the introduction of Plan 5, based on the best features of Plans 1 and 4. This final plan thus included the following 11 actions:

- education actions
  1. cancer directory
  2. cancer education in schools
  3. St. Luke's child abuse center
  4. community education on alcohol abuse
  5. antismoking campaign

- training actions
  6. Community Mental Health Center staff on alcohol abuse
  7. self-help for emergencies
  8. bilingual physical therapists

- service actions
  9. St. Luke's child abuse service
  10. triage system for outpatient clinics
  11. mobile vans for physically handicapped

The committee expected Plan 5 to achieve the following results:

1. It would raise the rate of achievement of the child abuse objective.
2. While reducing by almost $22.4 million annually the cost of two treatment actions, at a nominal cost it would improve health education on hypertension and alcohol abuse.
3. A wider scope of services would be offered under the combined plan than would have occurred under either Plans 1 or 4.
4. 11 of the 14 objectives would be 85 percent or more achieved, with 8 completely achieved by 1985. Only two, reducing waiting time and increasing the number of patient advocates, would be minimally achieved with Plan 5.

Plan 5 would thus be a major improvement over any of the other plans considered singly. The committee decided therefore to adopt Plan 5.

Funding of Plan

The committee structured the plan so that it could be developed in modules as funding became available over the five-year period. The committee was particularly mindful of the fact that cutbacks were being made at all levels of government. Four major sources are initially being considered to fund the plan. These are city, state, and federal governments and voluntary hospitals. Within the city, the Department of Health, Board of Education, and Health and Hospital Corporation are the main sources. At the state level, the Departments of Social Services and Mental Health are the two key sources, while the Department of Health and Human Services (HHS) and the Office of Health Promotion are the primary sources at the federal level. It should be noted 6 of the 11 actions could be funded from only one source, mainly the city's public sector.

Funding source	Amount	Action No.
City:Health Dept.	$ 100,000	3
City:Bd. of Educ.	100,000	4
State/Fed.:Dept. of Educ.	150,000	5
State/Fed.:NIMH	430,000	6
State/Fed.:NIMH	50,000–200,000	7
City:Dept. of Health	150,000	9
Fed.:Office of Health Promotion	60,000	14
City:Health and Hosp. Corp./Vol. Hosps.	60,000	15
City:Health and Hosp. Corp./Vol. Hosps.	100,000	16
City/State/Fed.: Medicaid/Medicare	120,000	17
City/State/Fed.: Medicaid/Medicare	300,000	18
Total	$1,620,000– 1,770,000	
City funding:	510,000	
State/federal:	$1,120,000–$1,270,000 needed	

Of the $1.6 million needed annually, almost 1 million comes from one essential source and is used to finance four actions (numbers 6, 7, 17, and 18)—Medicaid and Medicare funds. While the National Institute of Mental Health funds the initial development of its programs, their continuation depends on federal reimbursement from Medicaid and Medicare. Likewise, these sources are also needed to pay for actions 15 and 16, triage system and training the community for self-help emergencies. Obtaining funds for actions 3, 4, and 9 from the city's Department of Health may be more difficult because of the stringency of the city budget.

Funding may also be obtained from foundations and business corporations. For example, the Kellogg Foundation would be a source of funding for the nutrition education action and the Johnson Foundation for the self-help emergency training program. Corporations such as General Motors and Volkswagen might supply mobile vans for the physically handicapped, while the Council of Community Services may take responsibility for publishing the directory on cancer services. Finally, Hunter College's Institute for Health Sciences is the likely choice for recruiting Spanish-speaking physical therapy students. Thus, there are a number of alternative sources available to achieve the various actions.

Impact of Plan on District Population

Basically, most of the actions are being developed to deal with the needs of persons with particular diseases or with a high risk for developing them. Most of the emphasis is on the adult population, aged 15 to 64. Because many of the preventive, health education services are aimed at the same population, there may seem to be more persons receiving services than there are residents in the district. This appearance results from the duplication of services designed to reach high-risk populations. Since many of the same persons will be subject to different educational campaigns over the five-year life of the plan, the number being reached approximates 75,000 persons. Some 2,000 children under four years of age will be assisted with bilingual child abuse education programs. Among the senior citizens, 10,000 to 15,000 will be helped by special training programs aimed at staff in long-term care nursing facilities. Most of these programs will be established in CPD 9. At the same time, almost 50,000 blacks, most of whom reside in CPD 12, and some 60,000 whites residing in both CPDs will be beneficiaries of special hypertension education actions. The committee agreed to a general policy that, if a choice of location between CPD 9 or 12 were required for a one-of-a-kind action, CPD 19 would be given the higher priority, although the elderly in CPD 12 would be given higher priority for actions aimed at their needs.

IMPLEMENTATION

The committee and staff discussed some of the steps that would be required to implement the program. Both recognized that gaining approval from funding sources would delay the implementation of the various program components. The city's health district officer, hospital administrators, community leaders, and representatives of city and state legislators residing in the district had all taken part in the committee's deliberations. Several of the health providers had given their informal approval of individual programs they would either operate themselves or coordinate with their own services. Some had expressed concern at the duplication of effort with what their own programs were already doing or perceived a possible need to redirect them. There were differences of opinion over the development of the mental health centers by the traditional providers of such services and the more community-oriented action agencies, many of which were sponsored by antipoverty funds and were now seeking new sources of revenue.

While the committee members expressed varying degrees of support for the final plan, they all agreed that serious discussion on any aspect of it would have to await the approval of the planning agency's governing body. Once that approval is given, the staff with selected task forces will develop specific proposals for submission to HHS and the other funding sources. The agency's project review committee will have to give its approval to the individual proposals, as will the state's Department of Health and then HHS Region II office before federal or state officials will consider either the plan as a whole or specific pieces of it for funding.

Finally, the staff will develop monitoring systems to collect data on the basis of which the success of the individual programs can be evaluated as they are implemented, and their impact on the indicators the committee and staff have already developed. The committee and staff will also begin to identify possible locations in the district for the various program components and work with the health providers in order to work out the differences that exist among various proposed programs that might affect their own operations.

The committee and staff agreed that, before the next planning cycle could begin, there would have to be some beginning made in the actual implementation of the newly proposed plan. None believed the next cycle could start in less than two years. In the meantime, the committee recognized the difficult task it had ahead of itself in preparing the positive atmosphere needed to implement the action components of its plan.

NOTES

1. Boyd Palmer, *An Advanced Health Planning System* (Springfield, Va.: NTIS, 1972).

2. U.S. DHHS, *Program Policy Notice No. 79-05: Guidelines for the Development of Health Systems Plans and Annual Implementation Plans* (Hyattsville, Md.: Bureau of Health Planning, Health Resources Administration, February 23, 1979), p. 11.

3. Health Planning and Coordinating Council, *New Jersey State Health Plan: 1978–1982*, Vol. 1 (Trenton, N. J.: New Jersey State Department of Health), Section 3, pp. 10-13, 15-19.

4. *Ibid.*, p.4.

5. Andre L. Delbecq and Andrew Van de Ven, *Nominal Group Processes for Program Planning* (Middletown, Wisc.: Center for the Study of Program Administration, University of Wisconsin, 1971).

Chapter 14

Health Planning in the Context of Competition and Regulation

The inauguration of President Ronald Reagan signified a new direction in the way health services are to be provided in the United States. Three discernible principles appear to govern the new administration's dealing with health matters:

1. The rate of cost increases should be reduced through competition among medical care providers.
2. The role of the federal government in the direct provision of medical services should be reduced by transferring these responsibilities to the states.
3. The effectiveness of federally sponsored programs should be improved through block grants to the states.

These principles were stated directly or implicitly articulated in two reports that have had a pronounced influence in the thinking and actions of the Reagan administration. In a *National Agenda for the Eighties,* the President's Commission stated:

> The Commission feels, on balance, that an expansion of the role of competition, consumer choice, and market incentives rather than government control is more likely to create the much needed stimulus toward greater efficiency, cost consciousness, and responsiveness to consumer preferences so visibly lacking in our present arrangement for providing medical care.[1]

The fact that President Jimmy Carter appointed the members of the commission only tends to reenforce the thrust of the new administration's interest in competition.

The Heritage Foundation funded a study of government activity with a view to its reorganization in the event a conservative president was elected. The report, *Mandate for Leadership: Policy Management in a Conservative Administration,* has become an important document for understanding the current role and direction of the federal government in health care.[2] Two passages from the report spell out its basic thrust.

> HHS [Department of Health and Human Services] must foster legislation and an administration that fully implements a competitive approach in health care delivery. Its posture ought to be put in terms of minimizing its role as a government entity, reducing its regulation, opposing legislation that would expand its role, and instead devising statutes that would enable and at least enhance the private sector's innovative approaches.[3]

This passage focuses on the competitive aspect, the encouragement of the private sector, and the reduced role of government. In another part, the report states that "funds should be substantially redirected to block grants to the states."[4] Thus, the Heritage Foundation underlines explicitly the direction in which health care is likely to be heading. In the long run, it advocates a voucher procedure to replace Medicaid and Medicare, the use of private health care plans, and the free market for providing services to the poor and elderly.

COMPETITION

Competition has become the new buzz word in health policy circles. With the election of President Reagan and the ascendancy of those who advocate competition to positions of importance both in the new administration and in the congressional leadership, this emphasis on competition is taking stronger hold than had been previously envisioned. Disenchantment with regulation as an approach to cost containment, the burden placed on providers by these complex regulations, and the strong desire of the American public to exercise more control over decisions that affect their lives, including the costs and utilization of medical services, have all played a part in escalating the interest in competition and market forces as ways to contain medical costs. Although there are some indications that prospective rate setting and Professional Standards Review Organization (PSRO) activity may be working as intended in certain parts of the United States, the general thrust of the regulatory approach has not produced the results desired.

Factors Responsible for Rising Medical Costs

In order to understand why regulation is falling into disfavor and competition is rising in prominence, it is necessary to consider the factors involved in the rising costs of medical care.

Fee-for-Service

Physicians and hospitals have traditionally been reimbursed for services provided. The more services rendered, the more providers earn. It is assumed that physicians know what is in the best interests of their patients and that cost is not a factor to be taken into account in diagnosing and treating life-threatening conditions. In non–life-threatening situations, sometimes physicians and hospitals provide a higher level of service than required to ensure that either the physician's targeted income or a hospital's break-even occupancy rate is met. Thus, a certain percentage of service is dictated more by provider income needs than by the medical needs of patients. Emphasis on health maintenance organizations (HMOs) and their recent increase in numbers is beginning to worry providers, who foresee stiffer competition for the limited number of patients. Nonetheless, the number of prepaid health plans is too small at this time to have a major effect on the fee-for-service model, which maximizes the utilization of medical services and thus increases the aggregate cost of services.

Health Insurance Coverage

The overwhelming majority of the population is covered by one form or another of insurance for hospital and physician services. This has relieved the consumer of the burden of the high cost of medical care as illustrated by the fact that the out-of-pocket net cost to consumers of hospital care has been reduced from 50 to 12 percent between 1950 and 1975. Furthermore, by interposing a third party payer, the consumer feels a minimum of responsibility for costs and demands as much care as the physician orders. The consumer therefore tends to reinforce and accept the provider's assessment of what treatment is needed with little concern for cost. Consequently, the consumer's behavior and expectations tend to be important factors that contribute to higher medical expenditures.

Third Party Payers

Playing an essentially neutral role, third party payers simply insure the payment of medical services rendered as part of a negotiated contract. They have not generally intruded into the provider-patient relationship to assess the quality or scope of services, the place where services are offered (in or out of the hospital), or the type of provider (a generalist or a specialist). Third party payers have not served as monitors of medical services as bills are sent to them for payment, but rather as fiscal agents who passively pay medical bills as long as they are within the limits of the contract.

High Cost Medical Technology

Whether it is computerized axial tomography (CAT) scanners, kidney dialysis machines, open heart surgery, or radiation therapy, the high cost of medical technology for the treatment of patients with chronic diseases has been shown to be an important factor in the rise of medical costs. Not only are the medical devices themselves costly, but also they usually require more highly trained and expensive medical personnel to operate and maintain them. Further, even before their useful life is over, the first models of the devices are often replaced by more advanced models at higher costs; the newer models must then recapture the costs of the older devices as well as their own. Ina ddition, health economists have begun to question the efficacy and safety of many of these new devices, which have often been widely distributed even before their benefits have been fully evaluated. Their impact on the population's health status is minimal in many instances, raising further questions about their utilization and dissemination among hospitals and physicians. Although their utilization has generally posed little or no economic risks to providers, their availability may have been the attraction in the consumer's selection of a particular physician or hospital.

Increase in Medical Personnel

It has been estimated that one physician generates from $250,000 to $300,000 worth of medical expenditures annually. By 1990 the United States is expected to have more than enough physicians to meet the basic medical needs of the population. Added to this physician surplus is the newly burgeoning field of physician's assistants and nurse practitioners. When the number of physicians in a particular community is excessive so that each physician has fewer patients than expected, physicians may, within limits, maintain their income levels by charging more per patient. It has been said that physicians create their own demand. At any rate the coming surplus of medical personnel has been a factor in the increased costs of medical care.

Defensive Medicine

Physicians may ward off potential malpractice suits by practicing defensive medicine. Consumers, dissatisfied with their medical treatment, are increasingly expressing their anger by suing physicians and hospitals for medical malpractice. To reduce the chances of being charged with negligence, physicians request more tests than are ordinarily needed for a particular ailment. However, the cost of such defenses against potential malpractice suits may add an estimated three percent to the aggregate cost of medical care. Since some of these tests may result in injury to the patient, an iatrogenically induced illness adds further insult to the patient's initial injury or disease.

Aging Population

As the population grows older, chronic diseases occur more often, are more severe, and require more frequent and more costly treatment so that those who have these conditions can function with some degree of independence and comfort. Those over 65 consume a higher percentage of medical services per capita; as more people live beyond their retirement years, the costs of medical treatment can be expected to go even higher. Forecasts call for those over 65 to be the fastest growing age cohort in the United States. Their increasing numbers have already been translated into more influential political power, resulting in many new federally funded programs aimed directly at meeting their needs. Medicare has been the most costly of these programs, and its rapid growth is a cause of alarm in congressional and executive branch circles. Thus, the increasing number and the more costly and frequent treatment of the elderly combine to add significantly to the costs of medical care.

Interrelationships of Factors

It is not possible to select one or several of these factors as the most important forces exerting pressures on medical cost escalation; these factors are interrelated. For example, the elderly use high cost medical technology on a fee-for-service reimbursement pattern. Both physicians and hospitals are ready to serve them because they are assured payment under their federally sponsored medical insurance program. To protect themselves against medical malpractice suits by the elderly, physicians provide more services than those necessary to ensure an accurate diagnosis and the best available treatment. In this hypothetical example, six of the seven factors associated with increasing medical costs are clearly interrelated. To break into this pattern, Congress has passed a number of regulatory measures, each with a specific intent to reduce either the supply and/or utilization of unnecessary medical services.

Failure of the Fee-for-Service Model

Critics of fee-for-service health care have identified the perverse incentives built into the system. For example, physicians raise fees and work shorter hours if the demand for their services is reduced.[5] Another "perverse incentive" involves Medicare reimbursement policies. If the use of a prepaid health plan reduces hospital costs, providers receive no benefit from the savings. On the other hand, if the fee-for-service model results in increased utilization and higher medical costs, Medicare reimburses for the services rendered. Thus, Medicare reimburses the more expensive, but less efficient fee-for-service model by a higher percentage than the more cost conscious prepaid model.[6] In addition, because employer-paid employee health benefits are not taxable, there is no incentive for the employer or employee to accept a limited health benefit package.

Consumers have less information than they need to make rational decisions respecting their medical care. Information about the charges of hospitals and physicians is not readily available. Consumers must trust the word of a friend, go to the nearest physician, or use the telephone directory. Even local medical societies provide inquiring consumers only with the names of three physicians; they give no assessment of fees or competencies.[7] Because they lack information, consumers with regular physicians tend to rely on them to make most decisions about health problems. Arrow noted as long ago as 1963 the special relationship between patient and physician. "The patient must delegate to the physician much of his freedom of choice. He does not have the knowledge to make decisions on treatment, referral, or hospitalization." In turn, the physician feels socially bound "to give the socially prescribed 'best treatment' of the day."[8]

Union leaders likewise see no incentives to bargain for fewer health benefits than their members seek. They especially oppose cost sharing in the form of deductibles or co-insurance. Because health benefits are not taxable, union leaders and members prefer a 100 percent health benefit, since they would have to pay 30 or 40 percent in taxes if they took the benefit in the form of take-home pay. Thus, unions and their members tend to reinforce the fee-for-service system that neither puts them at risk nor offers them any incentives to purchase less expensive medical coverage.

Physicians withhold information from consumers on the ground that consumers "lack experience to make wise decisions." They benefit because it reduces not only competition but also any pressure on them to be more efficient in their use of medical services.[9] Physicians also claim that advertising would lower the quality of care. In one study of opticians who advertised and those who did not, it was found that three times as many consumers were dissatisfied with the nonadvertising opticians as were dissatisfied with those who did advertise.[10] Somers states that "I do not accept the claim, on the part of some physicians, hospitals, and other providers, that competitive pricing necessarily leads to poor quality. On the contrary, I believe that lack of concern with efficiency and price leads . . . to lack of concern with quality. . . ."[11]

Ginzberg views hospitals as quasi-utilities because they are only partially controlled by government regulation.[12] Even when hospitals are grossly inefficient, legal and regulatory practices often make it difficult to close them. Regardless of regulatory constraints, a number of constituencies will coalesce to keep a hospital open. McClure and Kligman identify these as the volunteers who support and work in the hospital, the governing body that is dedicated to the hospital's survival, the hospital administrator who construes a closing as a personal failure, the medical staff who have based their careers on the hospital, the unions that stand to lose members by the hospital's closing, the suppliers who would lose substantial business, and the political and community leaders who look upon the hospital as an important asset that makes their area attractive to industry and residents.[13] All of these constituencies rally around a hospital whenever its vital signs are beginning to weaken and it is threatened with bankruptcy.

All of these forces tend to favor maintaining fee-for-service status quo, the confidentiality and closeness of the patient-physician relationship and the consumer's dependence on the physician for medical advice, and the community hospital. Thus, any attempts to reduce medical costs must be made in the face of a formidable array of actors who are comfortable with the way medical services have been provided over the years to the consuming public.

The Regulatory Approach

In a competitive market, there are many buyers and many sellers. In a monopolistic market, there is one seller and many buyers. Since there are few hospitals in any but the largest urban communities, since physicians generally send most of their patients to the hospital where they have admitting privileges, and since consumers tend to rely on their personal physician for their course of medical treatment, the health care industry more closely resembles a monopolistic market than a competitive one. All the factors mentioned are likely to limit consumer choice in the use of hospitals and physicians.[14]

To deal with this problem, economic regulation is often used to "repair the structural failures in competitive markets."[15] In other words, in an effort to restructure the market, regulatory controls are introduced to simulate a competitive market. However, there are two levels of economic regulation: the comprehensive and the conduct forms. Comprehensive economic regulation is concerned with the total management of the enterprise, i.e., determining the rate of profit, deciding the services consumers really want, and setting the prices to be charged. Except in a few instances, such as the Tennessee Valley Authority or municipal utilities, total regulation of an industry is usually avoided. Conduct regulation, on the other hand, "establishes a general set of rules within which detailed resource decisions can still be made on the basis of market-determined prices."[16] Regulation of hospitals began this way.

The regulatory strategies used by Congress and the executive branch are designed to curb costs mainly by limiting the supply of services. The certificate-of-need requirement limits the expansion of new medical services. Appropriateness review is aimed at identifying currently inefficient medical services and encouraging their elimination or improvement. Prospective rate review governs the amount a hospital may spend by setting a "cap" on expenditure before that institution's fiscal year begins; the institution must live within that cap figure. One of the major goals of a PSRO is to limit utilization of hospital, ambulatory care, and nursing home services or to use less costly, more appropriate services where feasible.

All of these supply strategies were initiated as conduct type regulations, i.e., providers had considerable flexibility in their implementation. However, as providers used these flexible guidelines to continue business as usual, later congressional amendments made them mandatory and more detailed, moving them strongly in the direction of comprehensive regulations. It is this movement toward greater control over the everyday management of medical institutions and physician activities that has drawn criticism and resistance from providers.

Of all the regulatory mechanisms currently in place, only prospective rate review has shown any indication of achieving its objectives. It is not clear why, after a clearly weak start, this strategy has begun to produce a significant improvement. It has been suggested that its success is due to the mandatory aspects of the program and especially in those states with a strong certificate-of-need program, to its use in conjunction with rate review. However, Bauer's study of rate review is clearly skeptical of its achieving its objectives in the future.[17]

An ICF report, summarizing a landmark work by Alfred Kahn, points to five basic characteristics that inhibit the effectiveness of the regulatory approach.

1. The regulator does not own the regulated firm, or manage it day-to-day; both functions typically reside entirely in private hands.

2. The regulator has minimal power to compel private action in a positive direction; initiative rests with the regulated firm.

3. The regulator does not have the same amount of quality of management or technical resources as the regulated firm (measured in terms of information, funds, or calibre of personnel).

4. The regulator has no clearly defined objective to guide his decisions, but rather a vaguely defined, difficult to measure, and often contradictory regulatory mandate to protect the "public interest." This mandate can become even more confused because the "public interest" is typically reflected in a constituency with conflicting views, including investors, employees and consumers.

5. Finally, the regulator must make his interrelated decisions in a piecemeal fashion in whatever order the regulated firm elects to bring them forth. Moreover, he must do so leaving a trail of documents capable of withstanding tests of due process.[18]

Thus, regulation in the United States starts with some strong constraints that prevent regulators from achieving their objectives. Regulation is based primarily on the regulating agency's interpretation of legislative intent. If the agency is too liberal in its interpretation, it will be criticized for overstepping its bounds; if the agency does less than the legislature intended, it will be criticized for failure to achieve its objective(s). Consequently, the regulatory agency will adhere closely to the explicit meaning of the legislation, whether or not that interpretation works in the public interest. This approach of regulators leads to several outcomes:

1. Regulatory agencies tend to focus on written rules and procedures rather than on the substance of the issues. In this way, they take on a judicial type function.

2. They make decisions by consensus. By avoiding controversial issues, they tend to deal with mundane, routinized issues.

3. They tend to create adversary relationships with the regulated institutions mainly on narrow, procedural issues. This prevents their taking a larger, more comprehensive approach to regulating the market and leads to repeated confrontations on the same narrow issues.[19]

Under these circumstances, it is not surprising that regulating agencies are soon captured by the regulated. In order to avoid controversy and maintain favor with the legislative bodies, they look on the regulated institutions as their allies in making necessary changes in the legislation. This, of course, has the unfortunate effect of protecting the status quo instead of serving the public interest and achieving regulatory goals of economic efficiency. Thus, not only are the structural deficiencies not corrected, but also, under the guise of regulation, they are reinforced and given public sanction through legislative actions. The public is lulled into thinking the regulations are protecting its interests when, in fact, it is the providers' interests that are protected.

With appropriate resources, with legislative commitment to the goals, and with a staff dedicated to achieving its objectives, regulation can work effectively. It has been shown clearly that, in those states or localities with these characteristics, such as the New York City PSRO, the Rhode Island or Massachusetts certificate-of-need agency, or Maryland's Rate Review Commission, there have been successes. In all of these cases, however, special circumstances have given impetus to their achievements. Where these characteristics are not present or the environment is inimical to them, regulation cannot succeed. This is particularly true in those areas, such as the Sun Belt and the mountain states, where services are still increasing to meet demand. Since the political power in the United States is shifting from the Northeast and Midwest to these regions, the regulatory approach, no matter how conducive to correcting the structural defects in the fee-for-service model through supply strategies, is no longer feasible as the primary means of setting limits on rising medical costs. The advocates of competition are demanding their day in court.

Inducing Competition

If there is to be competition, then there must be enough suppliers of services in the community to provide consumers with alternatives. The chief exponents of the competition movement have been Havighurst, Enthoven, and Ellwood. Havighurst has long decried the monopolistic practices and powers of physicians and their organizations. He has articulated the need for genuine competition and has advocated bringing legal action where antitrust activities are blatantly manifested. He has urged the creation of other types of organizations to compete with the existing fee-for-service, solo, and group medical practices.[20] Ellwood was the first in recent years to press for prepaid medical services modeled after the Kaiser-Permanente program in California (and later the prototype espoused in the HMO Act of 1973).[21] Most recently, Enthoven refined the HMO concept into an alternative national health plan to foster competition in the medical field as public policy.[22] Ellwood et al. coined a new term to express all the various combinations of competitive organizational arrangements that the ingenious mind of man has been innovating—the Competitive Medical Plan. This refers to "all combined arrangements of physician and hospital services that are purchased on a price-competitive basis, ranging from preferred provider organizations to closed-panel HMOs."[23] Included in this concept are fee-for-service organized health plans as well as prepaid HMOs.

The central focus of the movement is not on the mode of payment, but on a climate of true competition among medical providers, including physicians and hospitals. Proponents of this concept believe competing health plans can survive best in an atmosphere that rewards efficient organizations. It is not the presence or absence of a prepaid HMO, for example, that is considered essential, but whether the physicians and hospitals in a community or region are forced to compete for consumer favor.

There are a number of propitious forces at work that appear to be creating an environment in which competition may, in fact, have a real chance to operate. Public policy is now being set by an administration that strongly favors a competitive approach in the provision of medical services. In several test grounds, e.g., Minneapolis-St. Paul, Denver, and Hawaii, competing health plans have succeeded in restraining the costs of medical care, largely by decreasing the utilization of hospital care. The surplus of physicians expected by 1990 will not permit physicians to continue charging more for doing less. Not only will they have to lower their fees, but some will have to migrate to communities lacking physicians in order to practice. Likewise, shifting populations, are resulting in a glut of hospital beds in certain parts of the United States, forcing the financially weaker, smaller, and more inefficient institutions to close, go bankrupt, or merge. In New York City alone, more than 3,000 beds have been retired in the 1970s. Finally, there is a growing recognition that, although medical care is continuing to take a slightly increased percentage of the gross national product, there is a limit to how much these expenditures can be increased. A growth limitation philosophy is slowly replacing the open-ended economic policy followed since the end of World War II.

The combination of these forces is requiring decision makers to reexamine the way in which medical services have been financed in the past and to consider a structural reorganization of those services in the future. Furthermore, large-scale profit-making corporations are slowly emerging as a force that cannot be ignored. This is evidenced by the spectacular growth of health care corporations such as Humana and Hospital Corporation of America, which had a gross revenue of $1 billion each in 1979, and national corporations such as Connecticut General Insurance Company, Prudential Insurance, and American Medical International. All are producing high profits and attracting the favorable attention of Wall Street stock analysts. A nonprofit hospital can no longer rest on its public interest laurels; it also must be efficient. It is in this atmosphere of dynamic change that one must understand Enthoven's Consumer Choice Health Plan (CCHP).

Enthoven identifies four principles needed to produce fair economic competition:

1. Consumers must have at least annually a choice of multiple health plans.
2. Each consumer must be guaranteed a fixed dollar subsidy to cover basic acute care and ambulatory care services. This should be guaranteed by union contracts, employers, and tax levy funds.
3. The same rules should apply to all health plans; rules should cover such topics as enrollment procedures, setting of premiums, and information disclosure.
4. Physicians should be organized in competing plans. This would provide a way of measuring their effectiveness in controlling costs.

Following these principles would help to ensure that medical care services are accessible to all people, that the factor of risk falls on the provider, and that consumers have a choice among several health plans. Most important, consumers would be given sufficient information to make a choice among competing health plans as well as among the optional levels of coverage they might desire. Consumers would pay extra for the service components in the package above the basic plan benefits. These benefits might include contact lenses, prescription payments, or mental health care.

Based on these principles, CCHP would be under consumer control rather than employer-union control; i.e., instead of having unions negotiate medical benefits as part of labor contracts, consumers would select from among existing community health plans the one that best suits their needs. Second, the distribution of public funds would be improved. Only that portion of the benefits covered in the basic, fixed price health plan would be tax-free. Any benefits above that amount would be paid by the consumer and be taken as a normal tax deduction on the consumer's tax return. Third, the aim of CCHP is to encourage the medical care system to reform itself. This is done, not by forcing any change upon providers, but by requiring the development of competing organized health plans. Those physicians opting to practice on a fee-for-service basis would then be competing with the organized groups and would be under pressure to show their patients that they can offer services at least as efficiently as the organized plans. Incentives are thus given to physicians to become more cost conscious and efficient, to consumers to make their own choices, and to government to provide sufficient funds for basic medical services for the needy. Finally, government has the major role of setting the ground rules and providing sufficient information to make the system work. As such, government plays a monitoring, oversight role, but it does not interfere in the actual operation of the competing plans. The free market choices of consumers determine which plans survive and grow, which remain stagnant, and which go bankrupt.

Enthoven specifies eight criteria that all health plans would have to meet:

1. open enrollment without discrimination of any kind.
2. community rating in order to ensure the plan does not discriminate against high-risk consumers.
3. availability of a minimal level of basic health services to all consumers. He suggests the use of the list contained in the HMO Act of 1973.
4. premium rating by market area so that those in low-level areas are not subsidizing those in high-level areas.
5. two or more options for all consumers, with the low option containing the basic health services. Consumers would be required to pay for services in a higher option plan.
6. catastrophic expense protection to ensure that no consumer has to pay out-of-pocket expenses beyond a basic figure. He suggests $1,500 with a 20 or 25 percent coinsurance. This means that the consumer would pay $20 to $25 for every $100 of medical benefits of covered expenses, up to a family limit of $1,500. All expenses beyond that would be the responsibility of the health plan.
7. federal government approval of all promotional materials publicizing a health plan before they are used to recruit new plan members.
8. health plan identification cards for all members so they would be assured of basic health services regardless of where they became sick. The burden of collection would be on the health plan, not the consumer.

Enthoven is realistic enough to know that the passage of a federal law will not change things overnight. He believes it will take at least ten years for 50 percent of the population to be covered by these competing organized health plans. He also knows the behavior of consumers, physicians, union leaders, hospitals, and employers does not change rapidly. Ellwood predicts the forces at work in the economy will result in 40 percent of the population being covered by health plans by 1990, yet he states quite candidly that "it is impossible to escape the conclusion that, on a national scale, full-scale competition will be a long time in coming."[24]

Ellwood and others have noted that consumers are for the most part capable of making the best choice for their circumstances. This has been shown by studies of consumer satisfaction with current health plans. A 1980 Harris poll showed, for example, that a higher percentage of consumers enrolled in HMOs reported they were "very satisfied" with their health care compared to the percentage of those satisfied in the general public. Further, only three percent of the HMO members sampled stated they were not reenrolling, mostly for eligibility reasons.[25] Likewise, previously noted, a study by Benham showed that more than three times as many consumers stated they would not return to a nonadvertising optometrist or optician than to one who advertised. Although not all consumers would make choices in their best interest or make them based on full information, many more would have the opportunity to make such decisions under CCHP than under the fee-for-service system.

CCHP, Enthoven admits, would not ensure basic health services for those residing in rural areas. There simply are too few people scattered over a large geographical area to make such a plan economically feasible. However, through telecommunication, use of physician's assistants, and emergency transport of the acutely ill, services would be improved, because all residents would be guaranteed a basic set of services.

Potential Benefits of Competition

An analysis of CCHP reveals that it deals with most of the major forces pushing the costs of medical care upward. In a prepaid practice, for example, physicians themselves would be at risk, because using more services will cost them personally. Consumers would no longer be immune in their demands for medical services under CCHP. By paying directly for high-option plans, they would forego extra take-home pay. They also would pay either a deductible or a copayment for services used. In both instances, they would be made conscious of the cost of medical care and their responsibility in paying for it. Third party health insurance companies could not take a neutral role in CCHP. Hospitals and prepaid plans would use carriers that gave them the best rates. Therefore, the insurance companies would have to be more active in monitoring the costs of the health plans and hospitals to ensure that both the utilization and quality of medical services rendered are reasonable. Likewise, because CCHP patients would use fewer high medical technology procedures, the cost of both hospitalization and clinic care would be reduced. Internal audits would be used to ensure that services would be used only when their benefits and safety have been clearly established and they are considered medically necessary. The numbers of medical personnel would reach a point of equilibrium in urban and suburban communities so that new entrants would be able to practice only as others retired, moved, or died. Physicians would no longer be able to charge higher fees for fewer patients to maintain their levels of income. Peer control and consumer choice would keep fees in line with prevailing rates. Physicians and hospitals would not be able to practice defensive medicine; cost conscious consumers and plan managers would question the use of any unnecessary services.

CCHP may be responsible for more persons living longer; however, by emphasizing preventive medicine during the population's younger years, it might alleviate some of the more expensive and debilitating chronic diseases in the later years. Over several decades, the aging population should become healthier, which should retard the rise in the cost of services to the elderly and possibly keep costs constant even as the number of the elderly increases.

Constraints on CCHP Competition

If prepaid medicine has all these benefits, why has it not proliferated over the years? After all, the prepaid concept has been around for a number of decades. There is a wide range of reasons why prepaid plans have been limited in their expansion. Enthoven himself identifies the most important:

> People value their established relationships with their physicians, and they will change them only slowly and usually not for a small difference in price. Doctors and patients are understandably wary of new organizational schemes. They will want to see how each innovation works before they can be confident that it is a change for the better. . . . Many people will change their health plans only reluctantly and slowly.[26]

In an assessment of bills before the 97th Congress, the Health Insurance Association of America concluded, "Sponsors of some of the pro-competition bills have candidly stated that they are not now looking for immediate enactment of their entire bills. Rather, they are trying to lay out a road map of where they believe the medical care system should be several years hence. In other words, their proposal is a statement of philosophy. . . ."[27]

Technical and political forces also serve as constraints. Politically, Enthoven identifies a great many groups who stand to lose power, status, income, or livelihood by the implementation of CCHP. Hospitals will lose patients; physicians will lose some of their freedom and income; union leaders will lose some influence and control over their union members; employers will lose a bargaining chip in negotiating with unions; employees will lose some of their tax-free health insurance benefits; hospitals, group practices, clinics, and health plans that are inefficient will cease to exist; and health insurers will lose their passive role. It can be expected that none of these actors and their political representatives will accept changes of this magnitude without a struggle.

Technically, there are many other issues that must be confronted. CCHP requires the federal government to involve itself initially with the development of conduct type regulations rather than comprehensive type regulations. Enthoven recognizes that the federal government must serve in the important role of "gatekeeper." In this role, it would

- determine the basic package of medical services
- set the upper limit or range of out-of-pocket costs to the consumer
- review all health plans to ensure they meet minimum standards
- approve all literature to inform consumers about the various plans, and
- ensure continuity of coverage for all those who might lose benefits due to death, loss of employment, or divorce.

While initially the federal government would be required to set guidelines within which suitable alternatives could be offered by various health plans, it is the nature of American society that innumerable questions and nuances not covered directly by the guidelines would arise. As these issues are resolved, conduct regulation would become incrementally converted into comprehensive regulation. Further, regulations dealing with Medicaid, Medicare, Veterans Administration, and dependents of those in the armed forces would have to be rewritten for consistency with CCHP legislation. Finally, since two systems, a fee-for-service model and CCHP, would coexist for several decades, the behavior and actions permitted under both systems would have to be regulated. Thus, for a long while, it appears that more rather than less regulation would be needed.

A second set of technical implications deals with the handling of special cases. Enthoven accepts the fact that CCHPs would have to be differentiated by actuarial categories such as age, sex, location, and size of family. The need to figure each of these characteristics into the charges of a health plan would tend to complicate the administration of the plan. Further, over a ten-year period, Enthoven advocates reducing the difference between the costs of the basic plans in high and low cost medical areas to zero. Regions failing to reduce their high cost services would be penalized, while those that started out as low cost areas would benefit. However, McMahon and Drake have shown that hospitals have little control over many factors that affect their costs, e.g., inflation and higher costs of supplies and utilities.[28] Also, communities such as Manhattan, Boston, and Chicago would have to be excluded from the national standards because of their high concentration of tertiary level medical schools and hospitals. The costs associated with medical schools/hospitals, teaching hospitals, and community hospitals differ according to their roles and function and the high cost medical technology used by each type.

The Health Insurance Association of America has identified a number of technical issues that must be addressed.[29] It notes that consumers would not necessarily reject a high option plan just because they must pay a tax beyond the exempted cost of the basic plan. With respect to the rebate for those who choose a low option plan, the report noted that healthy, younger consumers would be more likely to opt for a low option plan and a rebate, while the unhealthy consumers (mostly older) would opt for a high option plan. The association therefore suggests that an age factor would be needed in computing the refund. This, of course, adds to the administrative complexity of the regulations and the CCHPs. In addition, two-paycheck families would tend to choose low cost plans because the benefits of each could be coordinated so that the result resembled a high cost plan. This would produce two rebates, increasing the cost to the employer, particularly if one or both required heavy medical expenses.

CCHP attempts to substitute competition among insurance plans for competition among providers. This has the effect of specifying which hospitals and providers are eligible under the plans. However, it is not feasible for insurance companies to remove free choice of providers from all plans. "Limiting coverage to services provided by only selected, licensed providers would run afoul of current state insurance legislation and regulation, create dissatisfaction among insureds whose physicians were excluded, and subject insurers to charges of restraint of trade."[30]

Physicians who favor the continuation of the fee-for-service model have already been experimenting with HMOs that permit this. The eligibility of this type of HMO under CCHP is one issue that must be resolved. Another is the possibility that such HMOs violate antitrust laws. Where the full membership of a local medical society participates in an HMO, they might be violating such antitrust laws. Further, as Egdahl et al. note, they may set up common physician fee schedules that may also be a violation of antitrust laws.[31]

Hospitals will be the most immediate victims of CCHP. Most studies have clearly indicated that, as prepaid health plans proliferate in a hospital service area, the number of hospital days per 1,000 plan members will drop by 30 to 50 percent. This forces hospitals to raise their per diem rates to make up for the loss of patient days. It also puts pressure on the hospital either to close low use services, even if they are considered necessary in the community, or to add new services to compensate for their losses. A number of hospital watchers are already fully aware of this potential problem and have suggested ways the hospitals could respond, e.g., forming their own HMOs or serving as the community health center by vertically integrating inpatient, outpatient, and community services.[32] Hospitals will be able to adjust to the decrease in hospital utilization if it is gradual; should it become rapid, however, they will need compensation while they make the necessary adjustments to fewer patients. Means for this compensation should be built into federal regulations.

Finally, in a utopia where the whole nation is covered by one or another CCHP, will a new, though lower, plateau be reached from which costs will escalate once more? At this point, CCHPs would no longer be competing with less efficient fee-for-service physicians or hospitals, but mainly with each other. The price range among CCHPs would be fairly narrow for similar services. The inefficient and poorly managed CCHPs would have already disappeared. It has been noted that an HMO generally requires 30,000 enrolled persons to break even; since most cities in the United States have less than 100,000 population, most communities can support two health plans at the most. What is to prevent the same sort of informal professional practices that have resulted in the high costs of medical care under the present system from developing in the new system? After all, the price range of automobile producers or toothpaste manufacturers for similar quality products is quite comparable; when one company increases prices, the others follow suit. In short, a new form of collusion becomes possible and the "free choice" system may then become a facade.

CCHP may well be a system whose time has come. If it is not accepted by the American public under current conditions, which are most auspicious to its acceptance, then it will never become an important alternative system for providing medical services. This writer is personally in favor of prepaid medical services, but many pitfalls and technical, legal, and political problems must be overcome before prepaid services can become a reality for a substantial portion of the American public.

THE STATES AND BLOCK GRANTS

In the late 1960s and early 1970s, a major congressional battle was fought over general revenue sharing. It culminated in 1972 when a bill was passed that authorized the distribution of allotted federal funds to cities (2/3) and states (1/3). This was the major federal initiative for block grants. Along with the general revenue sharing, efforts were made to pass special revenue sharing block grants, one of which would have dealt with health. The first health plan block grant had been passed as part of the Comprehensive Health Planning Act of 1965. Section 314(d) gave funds to the states, and 15 percent of these funds were to be disseminated for mental health services. However, at this later date, only personnel requirements and community development block grants were passed. In essence, the Reagan administration is gearing itself up to complete the task first considered by President Lyndon Johnson, championed by the liberal economist Walter Heller, and later enacted under President Richard Nixon with special assistance from Representative Wilbur Mills. For varying reasons, the concept has thus been embraced by political leaders with both liberal and conservative philosophies.

A block grant is the transfer of an allotment of funds from one level of government to another based on an accepted formula. The accountability of the giving level of government as to how these funds are spent is limited.* For this reason, block grants have a number of advantages:

- They require a relatively minimal form of administration on the part of the receiving government.
- They can be used in a highly flexible manner by the receiving government because there are no conditions attached to them as there are with categorical grants.
- They transfer decision-making and therefore responsibility and authority from the giving to the receiving government.
- Because the use of the funds at the lower level of government is not restricted, block grants generate greater community participation in their allocation. Likewise, the focus of attention shifts from the federal to the state or local government.
- They facilitate the coordination of funds because the usually restrictive eligibility requirements of individual grant programs no longer exist.
- The receiving government has complete control, determining its priorities and naming the agency to allocate the use of funds in meeting priority goals.

---

*The nature of block grants is to severely limit the giving government's accountability of how the receiving government spends those funds. This is supposed to give the receiving government maximum flexibility in spending them within some broad parameters set by the giving government level. The main accountability will be occasionally from the public and the interest groups that represent them. To the extent they get their share of the block grants, the interest groups are happy and no one really asks how the funds are spent, who they help, or how effective the programs are.

Local and state governments have long supported the concept of block grants for these very reasons. Specialized block grants for health and social services would tend to make it easier for governments to meet their state and local health needs. As with all new concepts, however, there are costs as well as benefits. A review of some of the negative criticisms of block grants will uncover some of these costs:

- Block grants in the Reagan administration would be accompanied by a 25 percent reduction in the current levels of the categorical programs included. There would thus be a decrease in funds allocated at the state and local levels.
- The federal government will not be in a position to monitor the spending priorities of states or local municipalities. It must accept the negative as well as the positive results of those allocations.
- Congressional leaders who formerly championed one or more of the categorical health grant programs would lose this source of influence and thus could not score points with local constituents in their election battles.
- Special interest groups would be forced to transfer their battles for funding for their special programs from a few committees at the federal level to the 50 states; the battle ground is thus transferred from the giving to the receiving government.
- The most influential groups would tend to get a larger share of the funds. Funds might be distributed on the basis of political influence rather than priority health goals. There would thus be discrimination against the weak in favor of the strong state/local lobbies.*
- Since the federal government would have only limited power to determine how funds are allocated, the federal quality control studies made in the past for grant programs would no longer be undertaken to determine the effectiveness and the beneficiaries of programs.
- Block grant funds might be merged with the regular funds of the receiving governments. Well over half the states merged their general revenue sharing funds with their state revenues. This may result in a substitution of federal for state funds.
- Funds might be allocated to existing programs with little or no effort at innovation. This would be consistent with one of the findings in a study of how general revenue funds were spent.[33]

---

*Weak interest groups are able to focus their energies with considerable impact at one or two target groups, such as a Congressional committee. Where they must deal with 50 different targets, their weak resources are so meager that they are unable to compete with stronger interest groups at the local or state level.

Proponents of block grants view them as a positive administrative concept that will make it possible to carry out programs in a more coordinated, goal-directed way than would be possible with a number of separate grant programs. Critics of block grants view them as a political strategy to break up the gains made under the programs of Presidents Kennedy and Johnson. Furthermore, the reduced level of funding will harm primarily the poor, traditionally the main constituency served by programs included in block grants.

The one level of government that gains power from block grants is the state. While states have more funds to allocate, their allocation is not an easy task. The block grants for health cover two major areas:

1. *basic health services*
       community health centers
       primary health care research and development
       black lung services
       migrant health
       home health services
       maternal and child health
       sudden infant death syndrome
       hemophilia
       emergency medical services
       mental health services
       alcohol abuse services
       drug abuse services
2. *preventive health services*
       high blood pressure
       adolescent health services
       genetic diseases
       family planning
       health incentive grants
       health education
       lead-based paint
       venereal disease
       rat control
       fluoridation
       immunizations

Funding for these programs would be reduced by 25 percent on the premise that the administrative costs would be substantially lowered and states with a special interest in any particular program could add to the funding level as they consider necessary. Some of the older and better financed programs, such as mental health, community health centers, and family planning, would obviously be considered more important than those programs that are funded at a lower level and affect fewer consumers, such as hemophilia and sudden infant death.

Unless the state government has a plan that sets goals and priorities and identifies the resources needed to implement them, the constituents who normally support each program will be waging political battles to obtain their fair share of the block grants. Since the responsibility for all health programs is likely to be concentrated in one agency, usually the health department, that commissioner and the bureau chiefs would be the object of these political power strategies by the various interest groups. Local political and government officials, local nonprofit health agencies with specialized interests, universities, consulting firms, and unions can all be expected to exert their special brands of influence. Whether better decisions can be made in this process than would have been made at the federal level is open to question. Because states no longer have to account for the expenditure of these funds to the federal government, they have less need to collect and analyze data, to determine the effectiveness of their programs, or to be overly concerned about their administrative efficiency.

In the best of all possible worlds, planning would precede the distribution of block grant funds; but, in a world where existing programs have built-in constituencies and persons are suffering from various diseases and conditions, it is impossible to plan rationally and deliberately how these funds should be allocated. Rather, planning tends to be the result of political influence and various mixed motives bound up in political and legislative decision making. Sometimes such a process meets the health care needs of local communities; sometimes it does not. Until the allocation process has had an opportunity to work itself out, there is no way to predict what the end results will be.

THE ROLE OF HEALTH PLANNING

The current role of health planning can be understood only in the context of the new thrusts toward competition and state control of federally funded block grants. For competition to work well in a relatively free market, consumers must be knowledgeable and there must be alternative sellers of services. In the medical field, these conditions are found mainly with regard to the sophisticated, upper income populations, who can afford more expensive levels of service (a specialist instead of a generalist, a teaching or medical school hospital facility instead of a clinic or community hospital) and can either pay for the best medical advice or educate themselves about the risks and benefits of various types of treatments. However, consumers in rural areas, small urban areas, and poor communities generally have limited medical care services available to them and/or lack the information to make the best decision. In most instances, the typical American defers to the decisions of his or her physician for most medical care. Thus, under present conditions, the market is competitive for only a part of the population, not for the greater portion.

For normal goods and services, consumers make purchase decisions based on price. Wealthier persons purchase the higher priced theater tickets and automobiles; lower income persons sit in the balcony and buy lower priced new or used automobiles. Where goods and services are not essential to the well-being of a family or community, price is an excellent gauge of what the market will bear. Where goods and services are essential, such as utilities and medical services, price cannot be the sole arbiter of who gets what services. Access to medical services when illness and disease are life-threatening or debilitating to physical and mental well-being cannot depend on price alone. Yet, in the United States, the cost of medical care is a major concern. It is rapidly rising to the point where certain consumers, especially those dependent on public expenditures and those with limited health plans, cannot afford certain types of medical interventions, such as renal dialysis or open heart surgery.

Thus, rising costs, consumers' dependence on their physicians for information and medical decisions, uneven distribution of medical resources, and dependence of a large segment of the population on public funds are factors that severely retard the efficient operation of a competitive market in the medical care field.

The response to this set of circumstances has been the development of regulations to ensure that basic quality medical services are accessible and affordable to all persons, whether through work-based health plans or through public taxation mechanisms. This body of regulation has grown incrementally in reaction to specific problems that the medical marketplace failed to resolve on its own, e.g., duplication of high cost medical technology in hospitals, overutilization of hospital facilities, uneven geographical distribution of physicians and hospitals, and a gross disparity in levels of quality care provided by individual practitioners and hospitals. Yet, it should be underscored that regulation is a poor substitute for a relatively free competitive market.

Our industrial democracy fosters certain behavior by individuals that is consistent with our economic philosophy of competition. Independence of action, self-reliance, ability to make decisions that maximize one's own best interests, initiative, and aggressiveness are characteristics valued in the United States. In a quasi-monopolistic industry such as medical care, these behavior characteristics can be seen in the competition among physicians and medical institutions for patients to maximize their own incomes, profits or prestige. Since the providers, not the consumers, make decisions that are in their own best interests, the perverse incentives that abound in health care come to the surface. If an extra, unneeded medical encounter adds to the income of the provider and does no real harm to the consumer, then the medical marketplace has lost its competitive strength. It is indeed difficult for the provider, who benefits from this unnecessary service, who operates primarily in his or her own self-interest, to take those self-imposed actions that permit the market to correct itself. When to this economic self-interest is added the incentive to achieve prestige and status among peers, the market is further distorted. Although there may be a surplus of open heart surgery units in a community, a hospital without one goes to great expense to develop this service, even at the risk of doing economic harm to itself. Although family practitioners are in great demand, few physicians opt for this field of practice because it lacks the glamour, prestige, and status of a specialty; the result is a surplus of surgeons and a deficit of family physicians.

The promulgation of regulations seeks to change, constrain, or reverse these perverse incentives in an economic environment calling forth behavior that is exactly the opposite of the behavior required by regulation. Regulations require cooperation, coordination, integration, and restraint, characteristics that are alien to an industrial democracy. Regulations are often perceived by providers as one more challenge to be overcome in pursuit of their own interests. Provider ingenuity knows no bounds when it comes to finding ways of subverting the intent of regulations. An all-inclusive service fee to a self-paying patient may become a series of separate charges to a Medicaid patient, resulting in an equivalent if not higher charge for a similar service. Hospitals reimbursed on a per diem basis may simply add more days to the patient's length of stay. If the PSRO limits the length of stay, then more intensive and more expensive medical procedures are used. If neither are permitted, costs are shifted to self-paying or nonregulated patients. In the medical field, competition and regulation can be viewed as a yin-yang situation; the excesses of one breeds the conditions for the entrance of the other. Competition, has been succeeded by regulation. Regulation, having become too onerous is succeeded by a return to competition.

In response to the perceived overregulation of the medical care field, Congress is giving careful attention to CCHP as advocated by Enthoven. Since competition has not worked satisfactorily and the behavior of providers prevents regulation from working at all, it is felt that CCHP may be the answer. The real irony of the CCHP model is that it, too, requires a regulatory mechanism to work. Without the federal monitoring role, without a federal definition of what constitutes a basic package of medical services, without federal intervention to mandate a minimum number of health plans to guarantee a competition and consumer choice, without federal changes in tax laws regarding the treatment of medical benefits, and without a host of other federal policies and decisions, the medical marketplace could not even begin to function as envisioned by Enthoven. Furthermore, CCHP requires a major shift in the economic behavior of medical providers. While this author is personally in favor of CCHP, he shares with others a pessimism concerning the probability that any real changes will occur in our medical structure. Mechanic states it this way, "In sum, it is difficult to be very optimistic about the possibilities of constructive change in a context so complicated, so fettered with entrenched traditions and deeply felt interests, and so perverse in its incentives."[34] He also questions the validity of CCHP assumptions, as do others, that consumers would cease to rely on physicians for medical decisions, that hospitals would put constraints on the many adverse economic decisions made by physicians, or that physicians would be willing to give up their current mode of practice and their freedom of action to a more structured prepaid model.

Both economic models thus have their built-in limitations. The innate conflict between the competition and regulatory models in terms of goals, economic behavior required, and impact on use of resources creates an insoluble dilemma. There must be a third force that calls attention to the problems that arise under either model. This is the basic role of health planning.

Health planning is essential when resources are scarce and there is a basic conflict between market and regulatory forces. The planning process is a way to identify the gaps in service, the overutilization of service, the inappropriate use of services, and the inaccessibility of services. When the most recent round of regional health plans was developed, for example, many inadequacies in the medical care system were revealed. Because resources were limited, health planning agencies were forced to select priorities from among alternative choices. These choices, in a sense, represented the community's statement of its highest priority goals and the changes it desired in the medical care system. Such health plans transcend the individual self-interests of providers by focusing on community interests. Unlike regulation, health plans are blueprints, guidelines to what is desired. They are not demands, nor do they have any form of legal authority. They do, however, carry a strong community sanction of what ought to be.

Health planners and their decision-making community boards have been placed in the role of mediators in determining what actions individual institutions ought to take to reduce waste, improve the quality of care, and develop new services for populations with unmet needs. It is, thus, the deliberate actions taken in the health planning process that indicate what medical services are desirable for the community. Although health plans themselves lack the power and authority to mandate change, regulations dealing with certificates of need, appropriateness review, quality review, and rate review do have such power and authority. Regulatory decision makers are increasingly using health plans' priority goal statements as bench marks against which to justify their decisions. Because of the limited resources, medical providers are, in a sense, forced to compete with each other for approval of their plans on the basis of cost, quality, access, and other such factors—the criteria regulatory agencies use in making their decisions. In the absence of health plans and their priority goal statements, regulatory agencies would render decisions without considering the impact of the decisions on the community's health needs. Thus, planning fosters competition within the context of a community's medical needs by setting the parameters within which regulatory decisions are made. Furthermore, unlike regulations, health plans are dynamic, living documents subject to change as new discoveries, new needs, and new patterns of service delivery emerge.

Implementation of a health plan requires cooperation from all the actors involved; however, as noted earlier, this cooperative spirit is difficult to obtain from providers traditionally concerned mainly with their own best interests. Thus, in spite of the moral sanction their priorities carry, the goals of community health plans are not automatically realized. Authority such as that found in regulatory mechanisms is necessary to compel a forced cooperation. It is this threat to use the authority of regulations that promotes cooperation.

With the temporary demise of community health planning, it can be expected that institutional planning will flourish. In a competitive environment, each institution must use its resources in the most economical manner and must meet the needs of targeted populations or the geographical areas it serves. The planning process and concepts will be the same, but the scope will be limited to smaller service areas than has been the case with regional health planning. Data will be collected and analyzed, alternatives noted and selected, priority goals stated, and resources needed to implement them identified. Institutional planning will emphasize implementation rather than the diagnostic aspect of planning. It will also be concerned as much, if not more, with the internal operations of the institution as with an analysis of its service population and their needs. Therefore, implementation methods and techniques noted in earlier chapters will take on greater importance than other methods. (See Chapters 5, 7, and 8.) Many states will find it useful to maintain some type of regulation, most probably certificate-of-need and rate review, to prevent the competing institutions from concentrating only on their own best interests.

In time, especially during the next 10 to 15 years while the CCHP system is developing, there will be periodic efforts to reinstitute communitywide planning. Community decision makers will survey the system to determine where it is weak and where it is strong. The impetus for these surveys will come from two sources. First, potential confrontations between local communities and state jurisdictions over the distribution of block grants will necessitate some type of community and/or statewide planning effort to determine the allocation of these funds. Planning will therefore be used as a means of reducing tension between the two levels of government. Second, the state will require guidelines for making regulatory decisions. Hill-Burton and state medical facility plans have traditionally been used as the standards for rendering such decisions, and the state will most likely take the lead in calling for the periodic development and updating of such plans.

As now, two types of plans, institutional and community health plans, will be needed. Each will address a different set of needs. Compromises will consequently have to be negotiated to ensure that both types of plans are at least partially implemented.

While competition will help to make the utilization of resources more efficient, health plans and state regulations will be used to identify unmet needs and to reinforce the efficiency produced by competition. As resources become more and more scarce, planning and regulation will become more, rather than less, important. Competition serves mainly to underscore the need for efficient use of resources; planning spotlights to whom and how these resources might be directed. Thus, in the coming decade, this author foresees the continued coexistence of planning, regulation, and competition in an uneasy but necessary dynamic relationship.

NOTES

1. President's Commission, *National Agenda for the Eighties* (Washington, D.C.: U.S. Government Printing Office, 1980), p. 78.

2. Charles L. Heatherly, ed., *Mandate for Leadership: Policy Management in a Conservative Administration* (Washington, D.C.: The Heritage Foundation, 1980).

3. *Ibid.*, p. 248.

4. *Ibid.*, p. 255.

5. Alain C. Enthoven, "Competition of Alternative Delivery Systems," in *Competition in the Health Care Sector*, ed. Warren Greenberg (Rockville, Md.: Aspen Systems Corporation, 1978), pp. 267–269.

6. *Ibid.*, pp. 267–269.

7. Clark C. Havighurst, "The Role of Competition in Cost Containment," in Greenberg, *Health Care Sector,* p. 330.

8. Stuart H. Altman, "Regulation as a Second Best," in Greenberg, *Health Care Sector,* p. 344, quoting Arrow.

9. Lee Benham, "Guilds and the Form of Competition in the Health Care Sector," in Greenberg, *Health Care Sector,* pp. 368–369.

10. Benham, "Guilds and Competition," p. 372.

11. Anne R. Somers, "Comment," in Greenberg, *Health Care Sector,* pp. 376–377.

12. Eli Ginzberg, "Health Reform: The Outlook for the 1980s," *Inquiry* 15 (1978): 311–326.

13. Walter McClure and Lenore Kligman, *Conversion and Other Policy to Reduce Excess Hospital Capacity,* Health Planning Information Series No. 16 (Hyattsville, Md.: Health Resources Administration, U.S. Department of Health and Human Services, September, 1979).

14. David S. Salkever, "Competition among Hospitals," in Greenberg, *Health Care Sector,* pp. 149–154.

15. ICF, Inc., *Selected Use of Competition by Health Systems Agencies.* (Hyattsville, Md.: Bureau of Health Planning, Health Resources Administration, DHHS, December, 1976), p. A–17.

16. *Ibid.,* p. A–4.

17. Katharine G. Bauer, "Hospital Rate Setting—This Way to Salvation?" in *Hospital Cost Containment,* ed. Michael Zubkoff (New York: Prodist, 1978), pp. 324–369. See also Brian Biles et al.: "Hospital Cost Inflation under State Rate-Setting Programs," *The New England Journal of Medicine,* 303, no. 12 (September 1980): 664–668; Mark R. Chassin, "The Containment of Hospital Costs: A Strategic Assessment," *Medical Care Supplement* 16, no. 10 (October 1978): 1–55.

18. ICF, *Selected Use of Competition,* p. A–35.

19. *Ibid.,* p. A–43.

20. Clark C. Havighurst, "Speculations on the Market's Future in Health Care," *Regulating Health Facilities Construction,* ed. Clark C. Havighurst (Washington, D.C.: American Enterprise Institute, 1974).

21. Although there is no specific reference for this statement, it is generally known that President Richard Nixon used Paul Ellwood as a consultant in the legislative development and conceptualization of the HMO Act of 1973. This is inferred in his recent statement. Paul M. Ellwood, Jan K. Malcolm, and JoElyn McDonald, *Competition: Medicine's Creeping Revolution,* mimeographed (Excelsior, Minn.: InterStudy, March 23, 1981), p. 1.

22. Alain C. Enthoven, *Health Plan* (Reading, Mass.: Addison-Wesley Publishing Co., 1980).

23. Paul M. Ellwood, Jan K. Malcolm, and JoElyn McDonald, *Competition: Medicine's Creeping Revolution,* mimeographed (Excelsior, Minn.: InterStudy, 1981), p. 2.

24. *Ibid.,* p. 41.

25. *Ibid.,* p. 27, quoting Harris Poll.

26. Enthoven, *Health Plan,* p. 91.

27. Technical Advisory Committee, *Competition in the Health Care System* (Washington, D.C.: Health Insurance Association of America, March, 1981), p. 15.

28. John A. McMahon and David F. Drake, "The American Hospital Association Perspective," in Zubkoff, *Hospital Cost Containment,* pp. 76–102.

29. Technical Advisory Committee, *Competition in the Health Care System.*

30. *Ibid.,* p. 7.

31. Richard H. Egdahl et al., "Fee-for-Service: Health Maintenance Organizations," *Journal of the American Medical Association* 241, no. 6 (1979): 588–591.

32. Linda A. Burns, "Lessons Learned through Hospital Involvement in HMO," *Hospitals,* August 16, 1979, pp. 73–74; Gail Warden and Edwin Tuller, "HMOs and Hospitals: What Are the Options?" *Hospitals,* August 16, 1979, pp. 63–65; Jan Malcolm and Paul M. Ellwood, "Competitive Approach May Ease Problems in Delivery System," *Hospitals,* August 16, 1979, pp. 66–69; Paul Ellwood and Linda Krane Ellwein, "Physician Glut Will Force Hospitals to Look Outward," *Hospitals,* January 16, 1981, pp. 81–85.

33. "Block Grant Approach to Services, Reagan Budget Cuts Will Hurt Poor," *NASW News* 26, no. 3 (March 1981), p. 1. See also "Reagan Budget: A Real Shift," *The Nation's Health* April, 1981. p. 5.

34. David Mechanic, "Some Dilemmas in Health Care Policy," *Milbank Memorial Fund Quarterly: Health and Society* 59, no. 1 (1981), p. 13.

Index

About the Author

Herbert Harvey Hyman, Ph.D., is a Professor in the Graduate Program on Urban Affairs, Hunter College, City University of New York. He has served as a consultant to HEW for the implementation of PL 93-641, and has been active for a number of years as an executive, project director, and consultant in health planning and community health programs. He is co-author of *Basic Health Planning Methods,* published in 1978; the editor of *Health Regulation: Certificate of Need and 1122,* published in 1977; and the author of *Health Planning: A Systematic Approach,* published in 1975, and *The Politics of Health Planning,* published in 1973. Dr. Hyman received his Ph.D. from Brandeis University. He holds a B.A. degree from Ohio University and a Master's Degree in Social Work from the University of Connecticut.